Enjoy Good HEALTH

Caring for your body and personal wellness

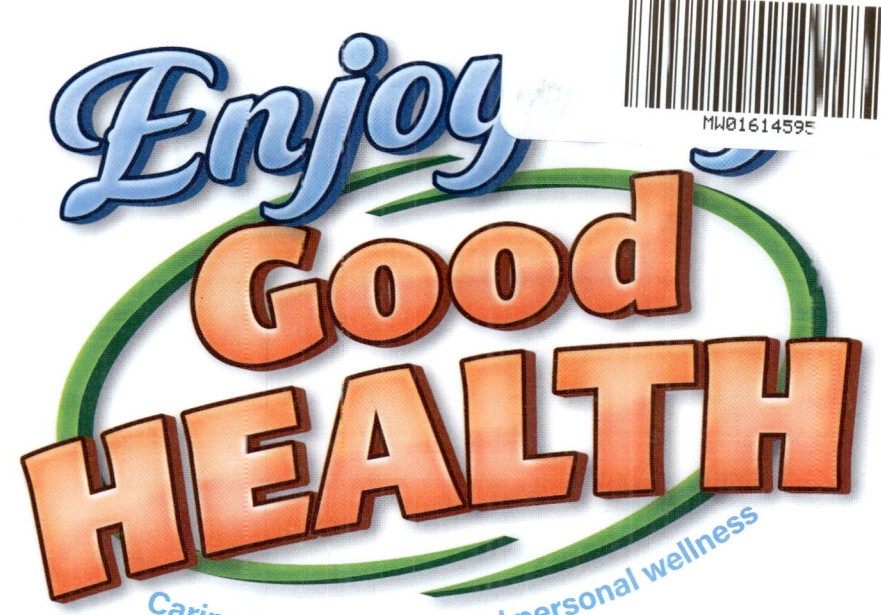

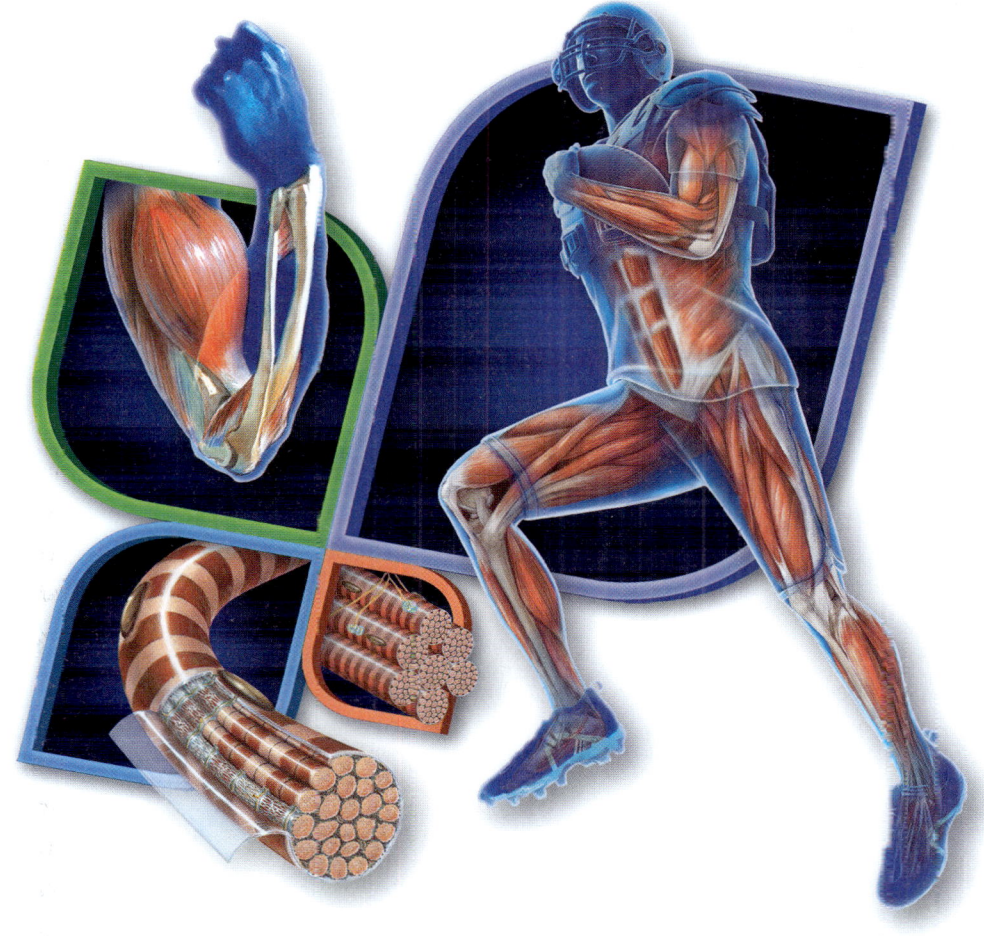

abeka.
Pensacola, FL 32523-9100
an affiliate of PENSACOLA CHRISTIAN COLLEGE®

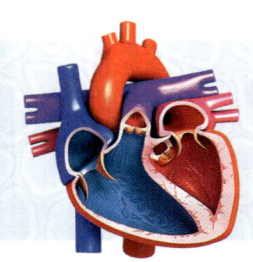

Explore God's design of the human body and discover how its *systems work together* using a *balanced diet* to fuel and energize itself for *Enjoying* **Good Health**.

To Teachers and Parents

The human body is a product of God's intentional and masterful design, but it requires care to maintain proper function. In *Enjoying Good Health*, students will increase their ability to apply health concepts in their own lives. They will gain a deeper knowledge of the proper anatomy and function of the body systems. Then, they will apply this knowledge to understand the influence of healthy habits on physical, mental, and spiritual health. Mental Workouts are designed to encourage higher-level thinking, while Build on Truth, Live It Out, and Hands-On Health activities demonstrate practical applications of the lessons. Diagrams, Comprehension Checks, Terms boxes, and Chapter Concepts Review sections are designed to prepare students for written evaluation.

Enjoying Good Health
Fourth Edition

Staff Credits
Authors: Tiffany Middlebrooke, Jeremy Foster, Delores Shimmin
Managing Editor: Amy Yohe
Product Manager: Barbie Tupua
Edition Editors: Elizabeth Betonio, Edwin Oksanen
Contributor: Hilary Hasty
Designer: Tammy McLaughlin
Production Artists: Karen Kisner, Thomas McKeen
Illustrators: Brian Jekel, Jeremy Gorman, Peter Kothe, Abigail Beaty, Caleb Tyndall,
    Joshua Burylo, Lydia Broc, Bobby Dalrymple, Ashlyn Deaton, and
    Abeka Staff

Credits appear on pp. 221–222 which is considered an extension of copyright page.

Cataloging Data
    Enjoying Good Health/Tiffany Middlebrooke, et. al. -- 4th edition
    iv, 232 p. : col. ill. ; 25 cm. (Abeka science and health series)
    ISBN 978-1-63223-358-5
    1. Health education (Elementary) 2. Middlebrooke, Tiffany. III. Abeka Book, Inc.
Library of Congress: RA440 .M52 E9 2025
Dewey System: 372.3

Contents

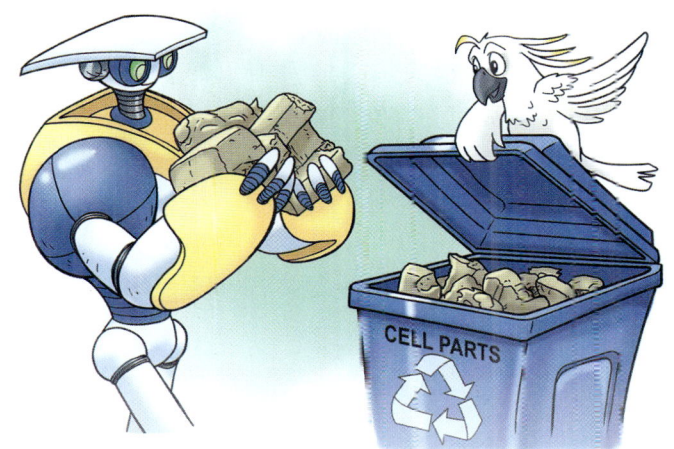

Health Activities Key

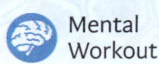 Mental Workout

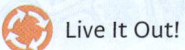 Live It Out!

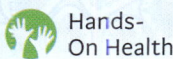 Hands-On Health

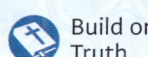 Build on Truth

 Recipes

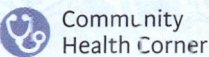 Community Health Corner

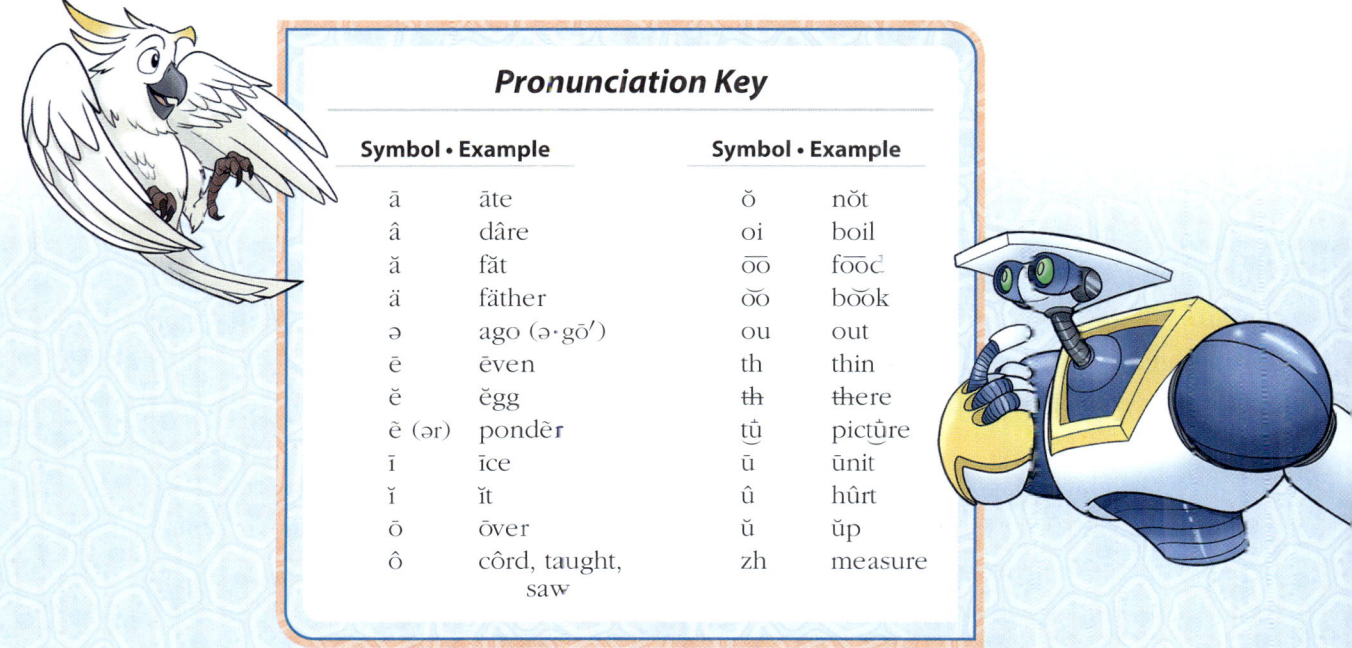

Pronunciation Key

Symbol · Example		Symbol · Example	
ā	āte	ŏ	nŏt
â	dâre	oi	boil
ă	făt	o͞o	fo͞od
ä	fäther	o͝o	bo͝ok
ə	ago (ə·gō′)	ou	out
ē	ēven	th	thin
ĕ	ĕgg	t͟h	t͟here
ê (ər)	pondêr	tū̆	pictū̆re
ī	īce	ū	ūnit
ĭ	ĭt	û	hûrt
ō	ōver	ŭ	ŭp
ô	côrd, taught, saw	zh	measure

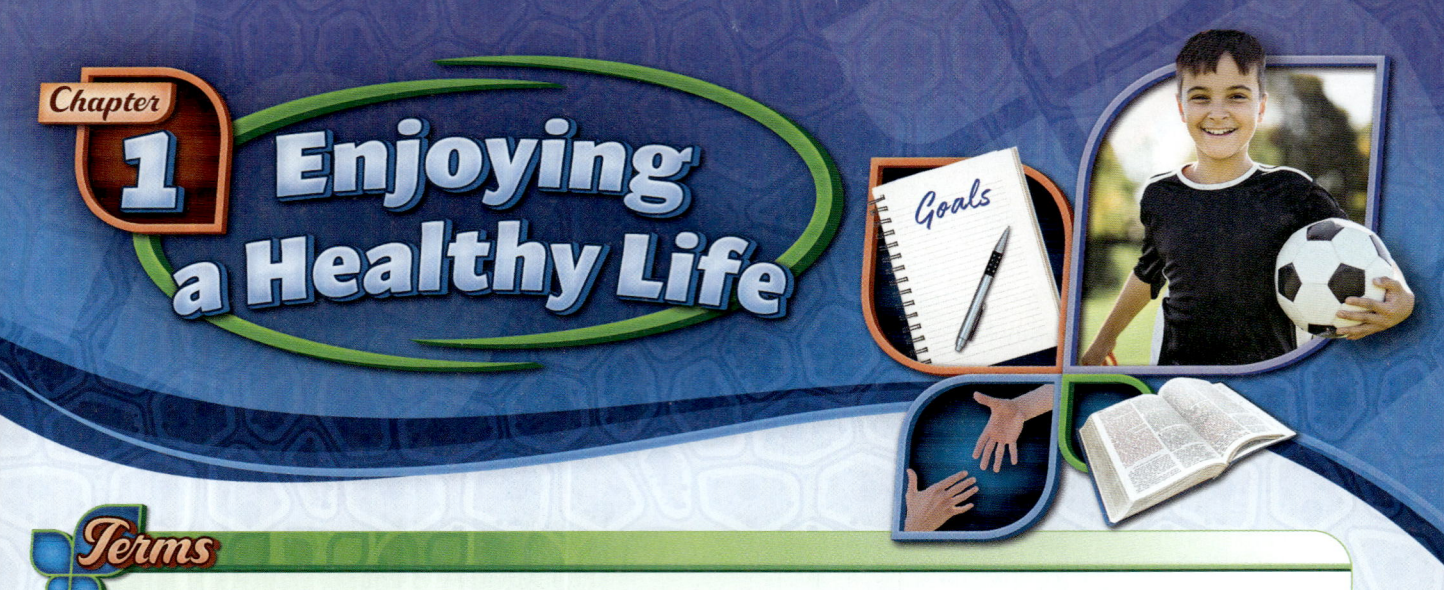

Terms

anatomy: study of the structure and parts of the body

health: complete well-being of a person; includes the material body and immaterial spirit

stewardship: managing what belongs to someone else as a caretaker

Fearfully and Wonderfully Made

> I will praise Thee; for I am fearfully and wonderfully made: marvelous are Thy works; and that my soul knoweth right well. **Psalm 139:14**

On the sixth day of Creation, God formed the bodies of the first man and woman and gave them life (Gen. 1:26–31). The human body—*your* body—is a wonderfully designed creation of God. Human engineers develop complex devices, but God, the Master Designer, made the human body more complex than any manmade device.

We can glorify God through science, the study of His creation. One branch of science is **anatomy**, *the study of the structure and parts of the body*. Learning about

the complex and marvelous design of your body should lead you to praise and worship the God Who made it.

Your body is made out of matter. It has outside parts, such as your skin and eyes, and inside parts that you do not normally see, such as your bones and muscles. All the parts that make up your body are *material, or made of matter*. But God made you more than just a material body. He made you in His image, with parts that are invisible and *immaterial, or not made of matter*. The Bible uses words such as *spirit*, *soul*, *mind*, and *heart* to describe the immaterial parts of you. Your immaterial parts give you thoughts and feelings. They let you learn Who God is and how to love and trust Him. God's image is a unique gift given only to humans.

> *And God said, Let Us make man in Our image, after Our likeness: and let them have dominion over the fish of the sea, and over the fowl of the air, and over the cattle, and over all the earth, and over every creeping thing that creepeth upon the earth. So God created man in His own image, in the image of God created He him; male and female created He them.* **Genesis 1:26–27**

Health Stewardship

Health is *the complete well-being of a person. Your health includes both your material body and immaterial spirit.* Both are gifts from God through His creation of you. Christians are also purchased by Jesus' blood and should glorify God through their bodies and spirits. **Stewardship** is *managing what belongs to someone else as a caretaker.* Your body and spirit belong to God; you should practice stewardship by taking care of them. Health stewardship is one way to glorify God.

> *What? know ye not that your body is the temple of the Holy Ghost Which is in you, Which ye have of God, and ye are not your own? For ye are bought with a price: therefore glorify God in your body, and in your spirit, which are God's.* **1 Corinthians 6:19–20**

What Affects Your Health?

Many factors can affect your health. One important factor that you cannot control is *heredity, the passing of characteristics from parents to offspring.* Some diseases run in families; heredity affects the likelihood of developing the disease. Your age, where you live, and your environment are other factors that you have little, if any, control over.

Important factors that you can control are your health behaviors, your actions that either help or harm your overall health. Your health behaviors can be influenced by those around you. You and your family members probably have some of the same health behaviors. Your neighbors and community encourage you to practice some health behaviors and avoid others. Messages from media, including the internet, books, and magazines, can also influence your health behaviors. Influences can be helpful by encouraging healthy behaviors or can be harmful by making unhealthy behaviors look normal, fun, or popular. Although these factors can influence you, *health stewardship means that you are ultimately responsible for your health behaviors.*

What Health Stewardship Skills Can You Develop?

Health stewardship requires understanding how your body works. Your study of health will include the structure of your body and its parts. Once you know how each part is supposed to work, you can learn what factors affect how it works and what health behaviors help it work correctly.

Much of health stewardship is about developing good habits. You should use your knowledge of how your body works to practice healthy behaviors. Changing how you behave can be difficult, but with effort and practice, healthy behaviors will become habits. These good habits will make managing your health easier. Of course, practice can also develop bad health habits. You should begin developing healthy habits now, because unhealthy behaviors are harder to change once they become habits.

Developing good habits requires making decisions to set health goals. Every person has different strengths and challenges that affect his health behaviors. You must decide how to apply general health principles in your own life. Consider how different options affect both you and others around you. Once you make a decision, use it to set specific goals. Some goals will be long term; these are health habits that you want to develop or skills that you want to learn. Other goals will be short term; these goals are small steps to meeting long-term goals. A long-term goal can be to run a mile without stopping. A short-term goal can be to daily go a mile, alternating running and walking; this builds the endurance needed to meet the goal of running the entire distance.

To meet health goals, you must make a plan. If your goal is to be more physically active, plan when you will be active and what activities you will do. Consider potential challenges, like weather that prevents outdoor activities; plan indoor activities for when the weather is poor. A plan may be complex, with several short-term goals. Or a plan may be simple, like planning to refuse alcoholic beverages.

You cannot develop healthy habits alone. *An important part of health stewardship is seeking help, or support, to make decisions and reach health goals.* Ask a parent or trusted adult for guidance and support. Other friends and family members can also provide support. If your goal is to eat more fruit, your parents may be able to include fruit in family meals. If your goal is to run regularly, you can ask someone to join you in your running.

Health stewardship also includes helping others maintain good health. You can encourage those around you to practice healthy behaviors. If someone needs support to meet a health goal, you may be able to provide that support. You can also work with others to increase the health of your community. Environmental factors that affect health are often too large for one person to change. But the community can work together to improve these factors so that everyone benefits.

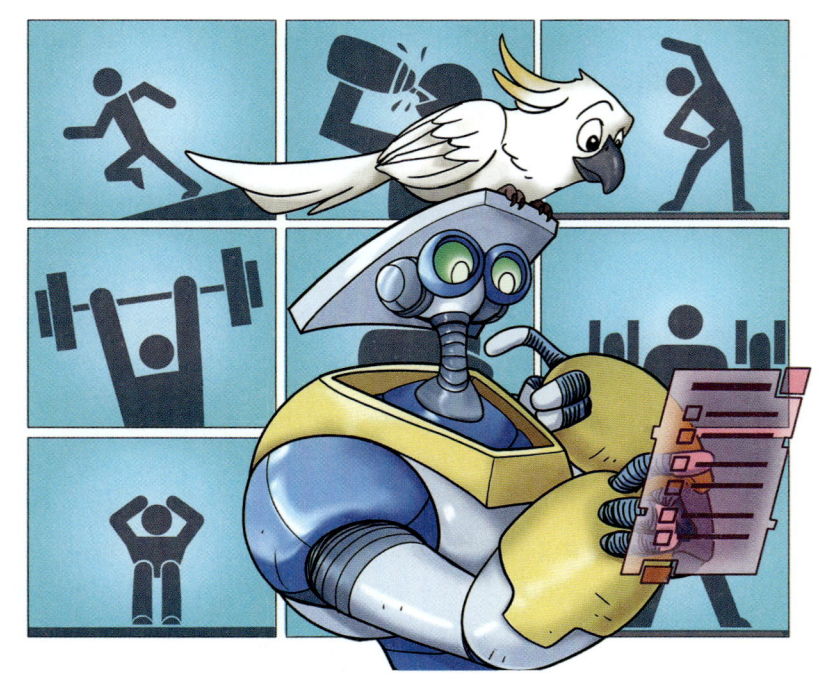

Where Can You Find Health Information and Services?

Being a wise steward of your health requires obtaining accurate health information. This begins with your parents or others caring for you. Their wisdom and experience can help you find accurate answers to your questions. When you tell your parents about your physical, emotional, or spiritual concerns, you are working together to find the best solutions for your overall health.

Your doctor can answer many health questions or concerns you may have, offering trustworthy advice based on your current health. Your doctor can also give you medication and direct you to other health services. Your community health department is also a reliable source for health information and services. Beware of any health service or product that promises a quick but often expensive solution to a health problem. Such services and products often give little health benefit or may even be harmful.

Media, such as the internet, books, and magazines, can provide both accurate and inaccurate information. Ask your parents or a trusted adult to help you research the most reliable sources. Trustworthy and accurate health information has the following characteristics:

- **It comes from a reliable source.**
  Is the writer or publisher an expert? An expert has degrees or extensive professional experience in his specific area of knowledge. The things he says or writes are accepted by other experts. Public-health organizations, like your community health department, are also reliable sources of health information. In contrast, a social-media post by an individual who is not an expert is *not* a reliable source of health information.

- **It is current.**
  Was the information published recently or a long time ago? In science and health, information is updated as new discoveries are made. Current information is usually most accurate, but the very latest discoveries may not have been verified by other experts yet.

- **It is unbiased.**
  Sometimes, people base decisions or information on opinions rather than on facts; this is called bias. Many sources of health information are biased. Bias is especially common when someone is trying to sell a health product or service. The seller may try to make the product or service seem better than it is. This bias appears in advertisements, on product packaging, or in reviews by individuals paid to promote the product or service.

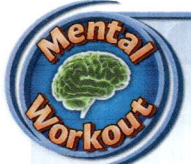

Study these statements and decide which one is likely the more accurate information. Explain your choice. _____

_____

_____

_____

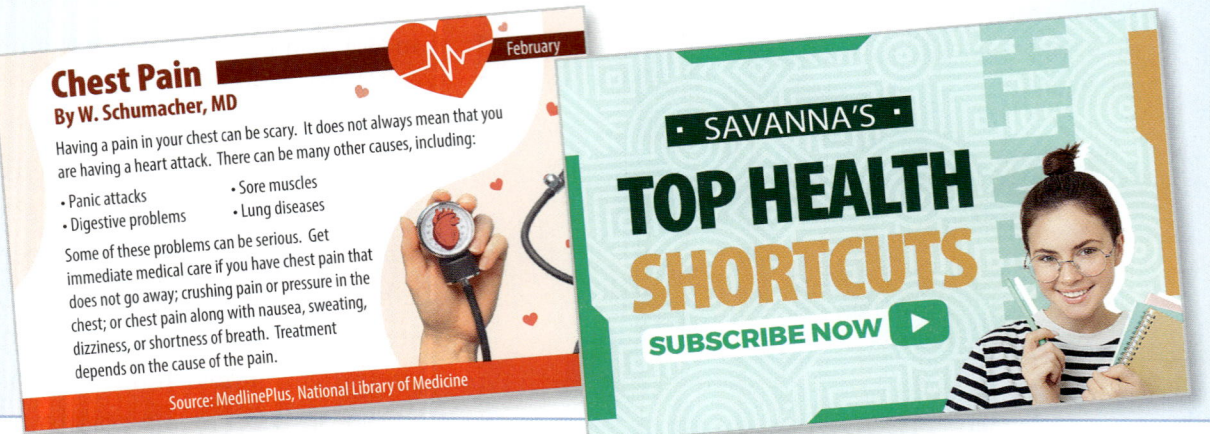

Chest Pain
By W. Schumacher, MD

Having a pain in your chest can be scary. It does not always mean that you are having a heart attack. There can be many other causes, including:

- Panic attacks
- Digestive problems
- Sore muscles
- Lung diseases

Some of these problems can be serious. Get immediate medical care if you have chest pain that does not go away; crushing pain or pressure in the chest; or chest pain along with nausea, sweating, dizziness, or shortness of breath. Treatment depends on the cause of the pain.

Source: MedlinePlus, National Library of Medicine

February

SAVANNA'S TOP HEALTH SHORTCUTS
SUBSCRIBE NOW

Community HEALTH CORNER

Physician

A physician, or medical doctor, is an expert who is trained in diagnosing (identifying) and treating diseases. All physicians receive detailed education about the body, how it works, and what can go wrong with it. Each physician also chooses to receive additional training in a specialty, or particular field of medicine. A person's main source for non-emergency health care should be a primary care physician. A primary care physician chooses a specialty that covers treating many of the most common diseases and conditions that affect the body.

When you visit your primary care physician, you will be cared for by a medical team that includes not only the physician but also nurses and possibly other medical professionals. Your exam will include making body measurements such as your height and weight, questions about your personal and family medical history, and any areas of pain or other symptoms. Your physician will examine you for common indications of disease and may also order tests, like x-rays or blood tests, that can help identify a disease.

Your physician may recommend changes to your health behaviors. If needed, he will also prescribe medicine for you to take. For some conditions, your primary care physician will send you to a specialized physician or to another medical professional for additional care and treatment. By treating common diseases and helping to identify serious diseases early, a primary care physician plays an important part in the health of individuals and of the whole community.

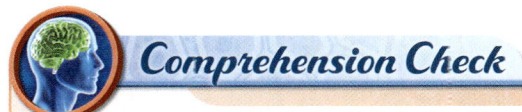

Comprehension Check

True/False: *If the statement is true, write* true *in the blank. If the statement is false, replace the underlined word with a word that will make the statement true. Do not write* false *in any blank.*

_____ 1. The study of the structure and parts of the body is called <u>ecology</u>.

_____ 2. Managing what belongs to someone else as a caretaker is <u>stewardship</u>.

Short Answer: *Write the correct answer in the blank.*

3. What is health? _____

4. What are health behaviors? Who is ultimately responsible for your health

behaviors? _____

_____

5. What are three health stewardship skills that you should develop?

_____

_____

_____

_____

_____

_____

_____

_____

Classify: *If the source of health information is trustworthy, write* T; *if it is not trustworthy, write* N.

_____ 6. An advertisement encourages those with certain symptoms to take a particular medicine.

_____ 7. A community health department distributes pamphlets about preventing the spread of whooping cough.

_____ 8. Someone who posts funny videos online encourages people to buy a new brand of running shoes.

_____ 9. A book published in 1950 says that you are likely to drown if you swim within an hour after eating.

Enjoying a Healthy Life **7**

Cells, Tissues, Organs, and Systems

cell: smallest unit of any living thing

tissue: group of cells working together to perform a single function for the body

organ: structure made of several types of tissue to perform a definite function for a system

system: group of organs working together to do a specific job for the body

2.1 Human Anatomy

Cells

Genesis 2 tells us that God created Adam and Eve, the first man and woman, and placed them in the Garden of Eden to live. An artist can paint a picture showing what he thinks it may have looked like in the Garden of Eden. To paint an animal such as a tiger, the artist has to make several parts, such as the head, the body, the legs, and the tail. Each of these parts is made of many individual brushstrokes. If you saw just one of these brushstrokes by itself, it may look like a black line or an

orange blob, but when all the brushstrokes come together, they form a painting of a tiger. Each of the other things in the painting is

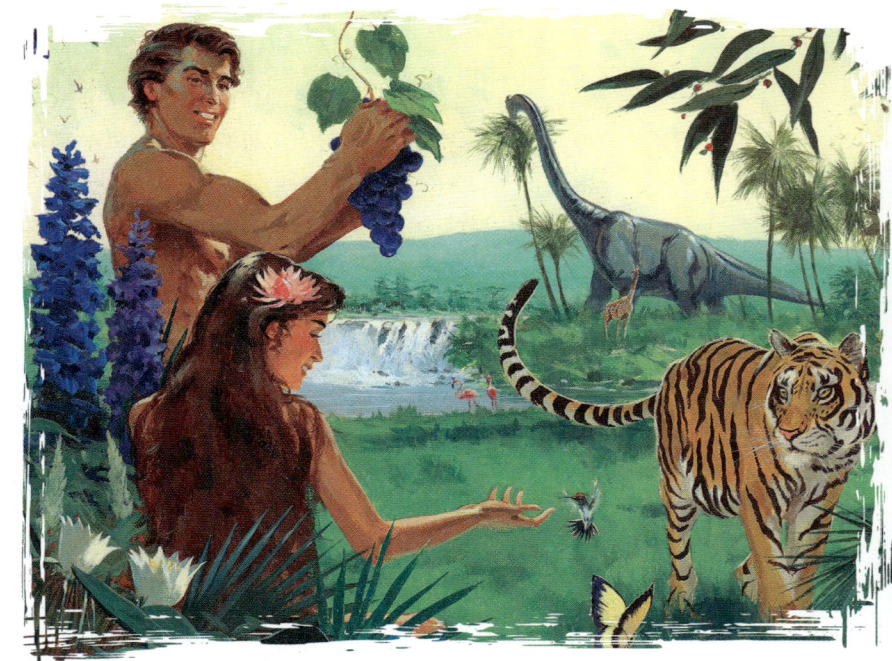

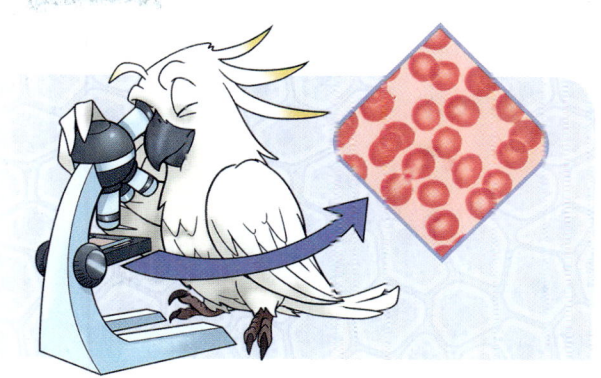

also made of many brushstrokes. All the parts put together form a beautiful picture!

Much as an artist paints a painting, God, as the Master Artist, designed His creation as a work of art. Just as a painting is made of many smaller parts and individual brush-strokes, God created the human body to be made of many smaller parts. Just as a brushstroke is one of the smallest parts of a painting, a **cell** is *the smallest unit of any living thing*. Cells are found not only in your body but also in all other living things. Each tiny bacterium or protozoan is a single living cell. Your body contains trillions of cells, all working together to keep you alive. Most cells are so tiny that they can be seen only through a microscope.

Each cell of your body has a certain task that it must perform. Long, thin nerve cells act as living wires to carry messages throughout your body. The skin cells that cover your body are flat and relatively hard so that they can form a strong and water-proof covering. Red blood cells are round disks that can bend to travel through even the tiniest blood vessels. *God designed each type of cell with a size and shape suited to its task.*

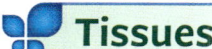

Tissues

No single cell can do all the tasks that your body needs to do; instead, cells must work together. *A group of cells working together to perform a single function for the body* is a **tissue**. Just as there are many types of cells, there are many types of tissues. Each tissue performs a particular function.

A tissue contains not only cells but also nonliving material made by cells. Blood is a tissue formed of blood cells surrounded by a nonliving liquid called plasma. Living bone cells produce a nonliving solid called bone matrix; the bone matrix gives bone tissue its strength and hardness. Cartilage is a tissue found in the tip of your nose and in your outer ear. The nonliving material in carti-lage makes it rubbery and flexible. *Different types of tissue have different types of cells and different types of nonliving material around the cells.*

Organs

If you could look inside your body, you would see large structures like your heart, lungs, and stomach. Each of these is an **organ**, *a structure made of several types of tissue to perform a definite function for a system*. Your heart's function is to pump blood throughout the body. The heart is mostly muscle tissue, but other tissues cover the muscle tissue and give the heart its shape. The lungs transfer gases between the air and your blood. They need stiff tis-sue to form air tubes and stretchy tissue to change size as you breathe in and out. The stomach contains muscle tissue to mix and churn food and other tissue to make chemi-cals that break down the food. By combin-ing types of tissue, each organ can do its own special job.

Systems

The organs are combined into eleven body systems. A **system** *is a group of organs working together to do a specific job for the body.* The circulatory system consists of the heart, blood vessels, and blood. Its job is to deliver needed materials to cells and remove the cells' wastes. The nervous system senses your environment and controls your body. It consists of the brain, spinal cord, nerves, and sense organs like the eyes and ears. The skeletal system gives your body its overall structure. Each bone of the skeletal system is its own organ. In your study of health, you will learn about how the body systems work and how you can keep them healthy.

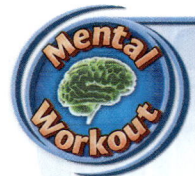

Why is it important that the organs in each system work together?

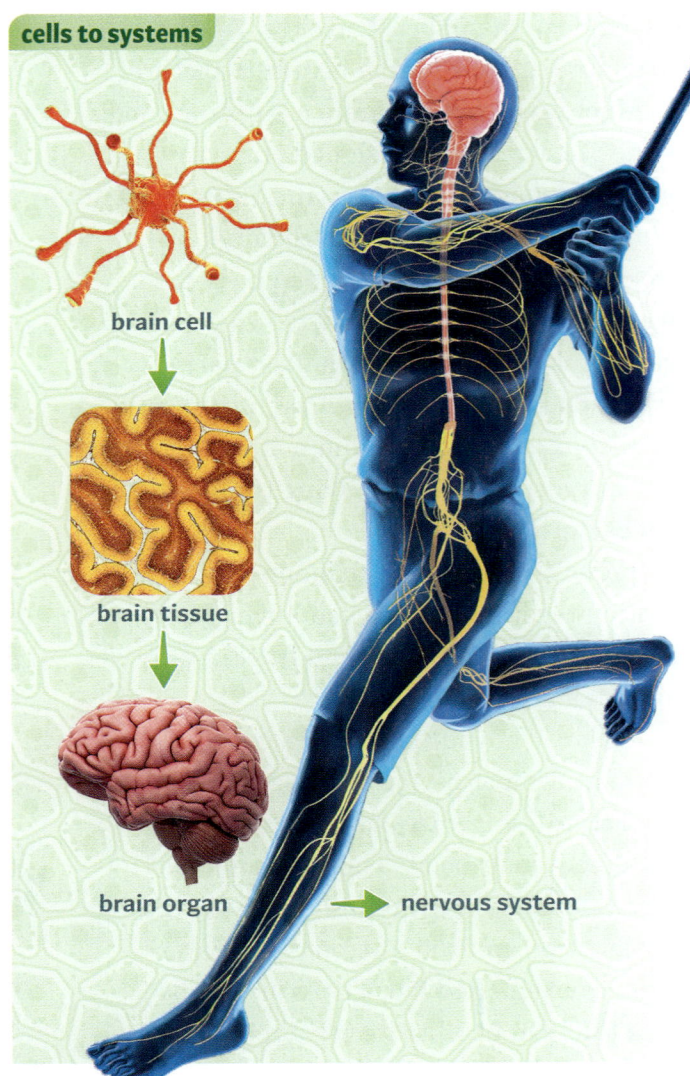

cells to systems

brain cell

brain tissue

brain organ

nervous system

Although you have many organs, they all work together to form one body. The body needs all organs to do their jobs; none of them are unimportant. The apostle Paul compares the church to the parts (members) of the human body. All Christians are baptized into the body of Christ. The members of the church have different abilities and different jobs within the church. All these jobs are important. Even the jobs that are not attention getting will glorify God when they are done for Christ through the power of the Holy Spirit.

For as the body is one, and hath many members, and all the members of that one body, being many, are one body: so also is Christ. For by one Spirit are we all baptized into one body, whether we be Jews or Gentiles, whether we be bond or free; and have been all made to drink into one Spirit. For the body is not one member, but many. **1 Corinthians 12:12–14**

Organ Donation

Do you know someone in your community who needs an organ donation? A person may need an organ donation if an important organ, such as the heart, liver, kidneys, or lungs, stops working properly. A sick person's life can be saved when he receives an organ from a healthy person who chooses to become an organ donor. Doctors will match the sick person with an organ donor using a computer system that compares factors including blood type, body size, and available organs. Organ donations can come from any family member, friend, or stranger that matches well with the sick person. The doctors can remove the sick organ and quickly replace it with a healthy organ from the donor. Damaged bone, skin, or nerve tissues can also be replaced with healthy tissue from another person.

In the United States, over 100,000 people need organ transplants. Since only 40,000 transplants take place each year, about

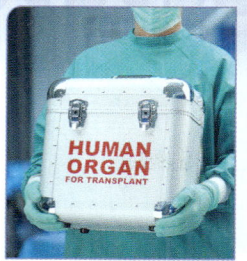
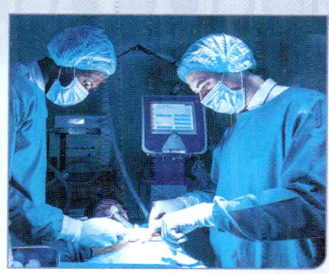

seventeen people waiting for transplants die each day. There is a huge need for more healthy organs that can be donated. A person who wants to become an organ donor can sign up on a donor registry. This will allow doctors to match his healthy organs with someone on the transplant list.

Although you are not yet old enough to register as an organ donor, you can still learn more about organ donation. Learning more will let you make an informed choice about whether to become a donor when you are older. You can also suggest that adults in your family and community consider the impact of registering as an organ donor.

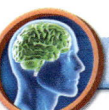

Comprehension Check 2.1

Short Answer: *Write the correct answer in the blank.*

1. What is the smallest unit of any living thing? _____

2. What is a group of cells working together to perform a single function for the body? _____

3. What are the two things that make up a tissue? _____

   _____

4. What is an organ? _____

   _____

5. What is a system? _____

   _____

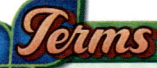

circulatory system: body system that circulates blood throughout the body; main parts are blood, heart, and blood vessels

blood: liquid tissue that carries substances throughout the body; main parts are plasma, red blood cells, white blood cells, and platelets

plasma: straw-colored liquid part of blood; makes up over 50% of blood

red blood cells: blood cells that absorb oxygen in the lungs and carry it throughout the body

hemoglobin: special protein that red blood cells use to carry oxygen; contains the mineral iron

white blood cells: blood cells that defend the body by fighting disease and infection

platelets: part of blood that covers open wounds and enables blood to clot

circulation: the continuous flow of blood within the body

heart: main organ of the circulatory system; powerful muscle that circulates blood throughout the body

blood vessels: tubes that carry blood throughout the body; arteries, capillaries, and veins

artery: blood vessel that takes blood away from the heart

capillary: the smallest type of blood vessel; links arteries and veins

vein: blood vessel that returns blood to the heart

2.2 The Circulatory System

Think of the way that a transportation system works. For example, a bus carries passengers to the bus station. Some passengers get off as new passengers get on the bus. The bus then travels on roads to various destinations, where some passengers depart and additional passengers get on the bus. The bus then returns to the station for another round trip. Your body has a transportation system called the **circulatory system**. *The circulatory system transports blood throughout your entire body.* Like a bus, the blood carries passengers that it drops off and picks up at different parts of the body. The blood travels through blood vessels in the same way that a bus drives on roads. Each part of your circulatory system has an important role in keeping your body healthy. *The three main parts of your circulatory system are the blood, heart, and blood vessels.*

What Is Blood?

Blood is a *liquid tissue that carries substances throughout the body.* God has designed your blood to sustain life. *Every cell in your body needs a continual supply of oxygen and food.* Your blood transports these life-giving substances throughout the body. It also removes carbon dioxide and waste products that the cells no longer need. Some parts of your blood help fight diseases and heal wounds. Your body has about three quarts of blood traveling through it; an adult has about five quarts of blood. *The main parts of the blood are plasma, red blood cells, white blood cells, and platelets.*

Plasma is the *straw-colored liquid part of blood. Over 50% of your blood is plasma.* Digested nutrients are added to the plasma by the small intestine and taken to every part of the body. Waste materials are collected in the plasma. These wastes are removed from the body by the kidneys, lungs, liver, and sweat glands. Plasma also helps fight infection and helps the blood to clot, or thicken. The plasma contains substances called *antibodies*, which help protect the body from disease and infection.

The **red blood cells** *absorb oxygen in your lungs and carry it throughout your body.* Your blood appears to be red because every drop contains millions of red blood cells. *Red blood cells use a special protein called* **hemoglobin** [hē′mə•glō′bĭn] *to carry the oxygen.* When red blood cells carry oxygen, they are bright red. After they give up the oxygen to other cells, they turn a dull, bluish-red color.

Remember that every part of your body needs oxygen to do its work. If there are not enough red blood cells to supply oxygen to the body, the whole body is weakened and slowed down. Red blood cells wear out after about 120 days, so the body must constantly replace them. About 2 million red blood cells are replaced per second. To replace the worn-out red blood cells, your body requires iron. *Iron is a mineral that is an important part of hemoglobin molecules.* The iron in hemoglobin gives red blood cells their color. Most of the iron needed to make new red blood cells comes from old red blood cells. Your liver breaks down the old cells

and recycles their parts; this natural recycling shows God's wise design of your body. *Additional iron can be obtained from iron-rich foods such as red meat, yogurt, and green leafy vegetables.*

The primary purpose of the **white blood cells** is to *defend your body by fighting disease and infection.* The blood contains fewer white cells than red cells. White cells are usually larger than the red cells and are not swept along by the bloodstream as red cells are. Instead, they can move around by themselves. When your skin is cut or punctured, disease-causing germs enter the bloodstream. Your body's army of white blood cells are instantly called into action. Millions of white blood cells quickly surround and begin to destroy the germs. This action keeps the germs from spreading through your body. You must take proper care of your body by eating a variety of good foods and getting enough rest and exercise. These healthy choices help the white blood cells prevent infections and diseases.

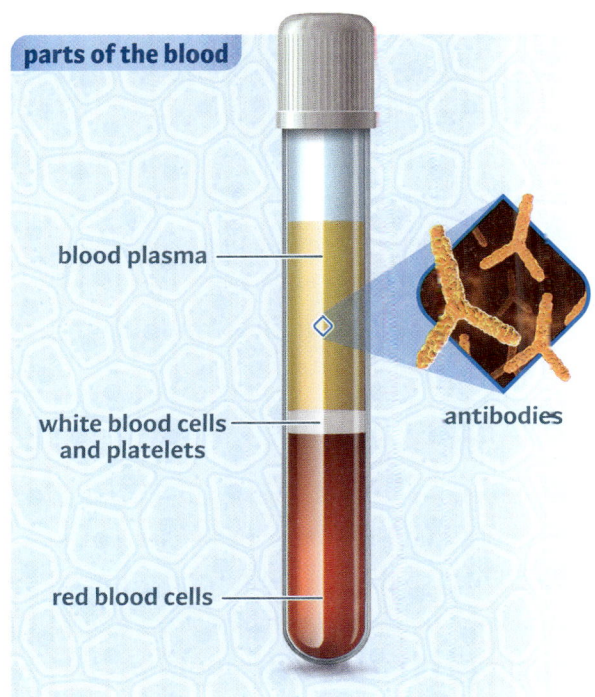

parts of the blood

blood plasma

white blood cells and platelets

antibodies

red blood cells

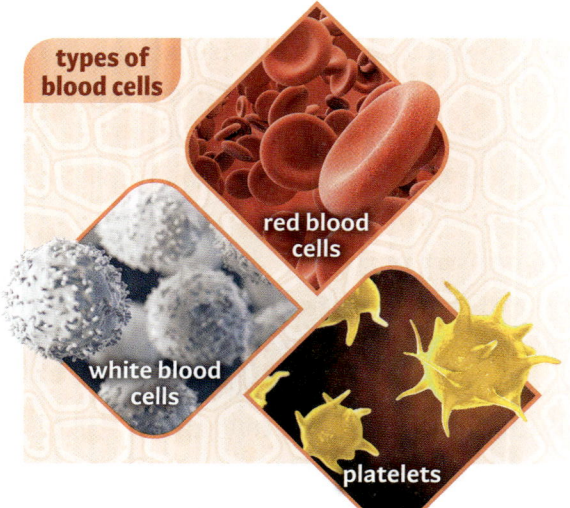

types of
blood cells

red blood
cells

white blood
cells

platelets

main organ of your circulatory system is your
heart, the *powerful muscle that circulates
blood throughout your body*. This muscle
pumps blood through 60,000 miles of blood
vessels. Though only about the size of your
fist, your heart is able to pump about five
quarts of blood every minute.
It contracts and relaxes for

Platelets are the
*part of blood that covers open wounds
and enables blood to clot* when a blood
vessel gets cut. Platelets in the blood
stick to the rough edges of the wound
and to each other. They pile up to form
a temporary covering over the injury.
The platelets also work with plasma
proteins to help the blood clot. A blood
clot on your skin, called a scab, prevents the wound from bleeding and
helps keep the wound clean. If the
body does not have enough vitamin K, the blood will not clot properly. A person without enough vitamin K can lose too much blood from
even a small cut or scratch. Most vitamin K is produced by bacteria in the colon.
*Green leafy vegetables, soybeans, and carrots
help provide your body with vitamin K.*

Pumping Blood

Just as a bus travels from the bus station,
along roads, and then back to the station,
the blood also makes a round trip throughout the body. *The continuous flow of blood
within the body* is called **circulation**. *The*

types of
blood vessels

vein

artery

capillary

veins (carry blood to
the heart)

arteries (carry blood
away from the heart)

your whole life, without stopping. Your heart automatically adjusts to the needs of your body—sleep slows it down; excitement and exercise speed it up.

Blood vessels are *the tubes that carry blood throughout the body. There are three types of blood vessels: arteries, capillaries, and veins. The blood vessels that take blood away from the heart* are called **arteries**. Arteries have thick elastic, or stretchy, walls that can expand to make room for the blood as it is pumped by the heart. Arteries branch into tiny **capillaries**, *the smallest blood vessels. Capillaries link arteries and veins.* Capillaries have the thinnest walls. These very thin walls allow food, oxygen, carbon dioxide, and waste products to move back and forth between the bloodstream and the body's cells. **Veins** collect the blood from the capillaries and *return blood to the heart*.

Community HEALTH CORNER

Cardiologist

Your heart works hard pumping blood through your body all the time. God designed our hearts to work perfectly so that we can live forever, but the effects of sin introduced sickness and death to our bodies. Therefore, it is essential that you make wise choices to keep your heart healthy. Sometimes a person's heart stops working properly, causing chest pain, shortness of breath, or heart flutters. If you begin to experience heart problems, you may need to see a cardiologist. A cardiologist is a doctor who specializes in caring for the heart by treating diseases and disorders of the circulatory system. A pediatric cardiologist treats children who were born with or develop heart problems.

Some people are born with heart problems or inherit heart conditions, while other people develop heart disease as they get older. Many heart conditions develop because of improper care of the body. A cardiologist will first diagnose the condition by performing tests. Some tests use electricity to study the heart's activity. Other tests take a picture of the heart or observe how the heart functions during exercise. These tests allow the cardiologist to diagnose the condition. They can then treat the condition by prescribing medicine or performing surgery.

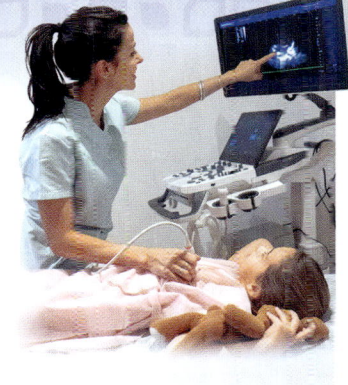

One of the simplest ways to take care of your heart is by living a healthy lifestyle. Exercising, eating a nutritious diet, and avoiding cigarette smoke can all help to make your heart healthier. You can influence others to care for their hearts by participating in community activities that promote heart health. One activity that occurs every year in the United States is Heart Health Month in February, with the first Friday of the month celebrated as National Wear Red Day. Your family can also be part of a run or walk that promotes heart health at any time of year. By participating in community activities, you can influence others to join you in promoting heart health. What are some other specific ways that you can promote heart health in your family and community?

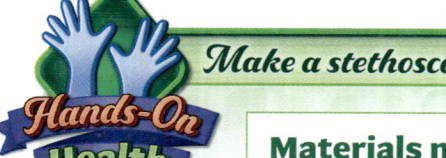

Hands-On Health

Make a stethoscope.

Materials needed:

- plastic funnel
- cardboard tube
- data sheet (from *Activity Book*)
- duct tape
- plastic wrap
- scissors
- stopwatch

BEEP!... BEEP!...

When you have a doctor's appointment, the doctor may use a *stethoscope*. A stethoscope has a sound-detecting device on one end and an earpiece on the other end. It is used to listen to the sounds inside your body. Some sounds that the doctor may listen to are your heartbeat, air going in and out of your lungs, and the movements in your stomach.

You can make your own stethoscope by following these steps:

1. Place the narrow end of the funnel inside the cardboard tube. Tape them together with a strip of duct tape.

2. Cover the wide end of the funnel with plastic wrap. Pull the plastic wrap smooth and tight and then tape it down.

3. Place the funnel flat against your friend's chest. Put your ear against the hole at the end of the cardboard tube. Count how many times your friend's heart beats in 30 seconds.

4. Have your friend do some jumping jacks until he starts to breathe heavily. Place the funnel on his chest again and count the number of heartbeats in 30 seconds. How did your friend's heart rate change after exercising?

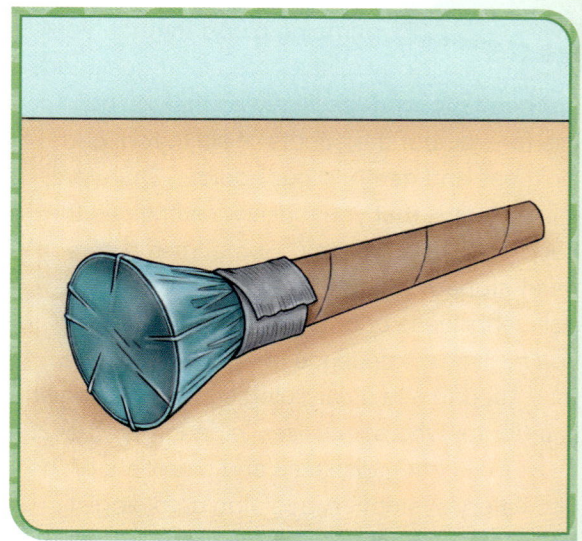

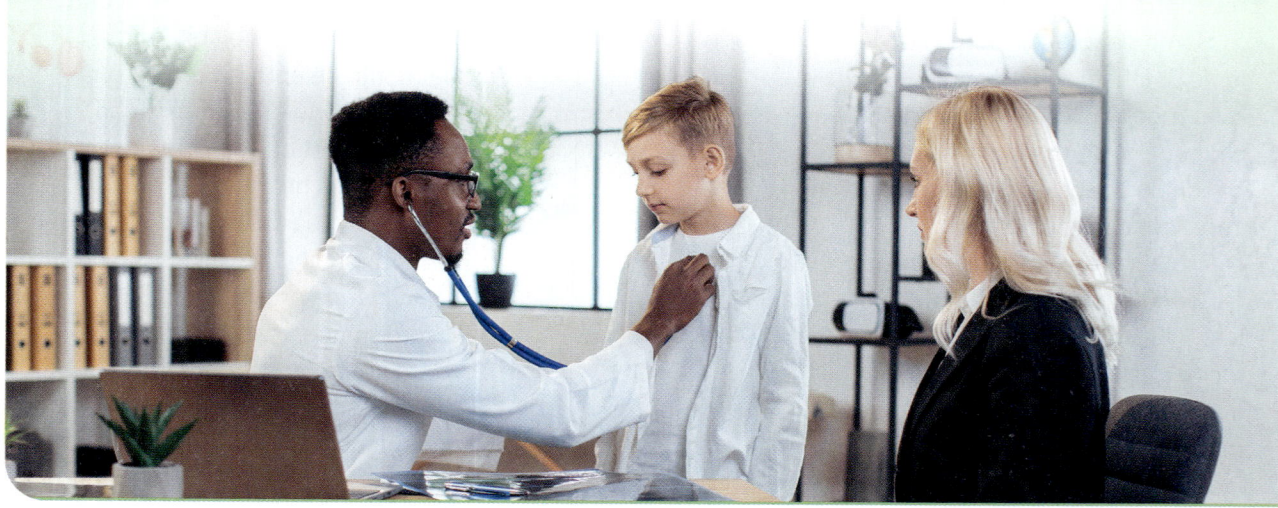

Matching: *Write the letter of the correct answer in the blank.*

_____ 1. blood part that makes up over 50% of blood

_____ 2. cell that carries oxygen throughout the body

_____ 3. blood part that defends against disease

_____ 4. blood part that helps the blood to clot

_____ 5. tube that carries blood throughout the body

A. blood vessel
B. heart
C. plasma
D. platelet
E. red blood cell
F. white blood cell

True/False: *If the statement is true, write* true *in the blank. If the statement is false, replace the underlined word with a word that will make the statement true. Do not write* false *in any blank.*

_____ 6. The protein that helps red blood cells carry oxygen is <u>calcium</u>.

_____ 7. The blood vessels with the thickest walls are <u>arteries</u>.

_____ 8. The smallest blood vessels are <u>veins</u>.

_____ 9. The blood vessels that return blood to the heart are <u>arteries</u>.

Short Answer: *Write the correct answer in the blank.*

10. What system moves nutrients and oxygen throughout the body? _____

_____

11. What mineral is an important part of hemoglobin molecules? _____

12. How can foods like green leafy vegetables help your circulatory system?

_____

_____

_____

_____

_____

_____

_____

Terms

respiratory system: body system that brings oxygen into the body and exchanges it with carbon dioxide

pharynx: throat

trachea: windpipe

larynx: voice box

bronchi: the air tubes that allow air to enter the lungs (bronchus, *sing.*)

lungs: main organs of the respiratory system; absorb oxygen from the air into the blood and release carbon dioxide from the blood into the air

bronchioles: the smallest air tubes in the lungs

alveoli: the tiny air sacs in the lungs; thin walls allow the exchange of gases between the air and blood (alveolus, *sing.*)

respiration: the process of inhaling (breathing in) and exhaling (breathing out) air

diaphragm: main muscle of breathing; moves down to inhale and up to exhale

2.3　The Respiratory System

You have learned that one job of the circulatory system is to deliver oxygen to every cell of the body. How does the blood get this oxygen? *Oxygen is brought into the body and exchanged with carbon dioxide* by the **respiratory system**. Your respiratory organs work together to make a powerful breathing machine.

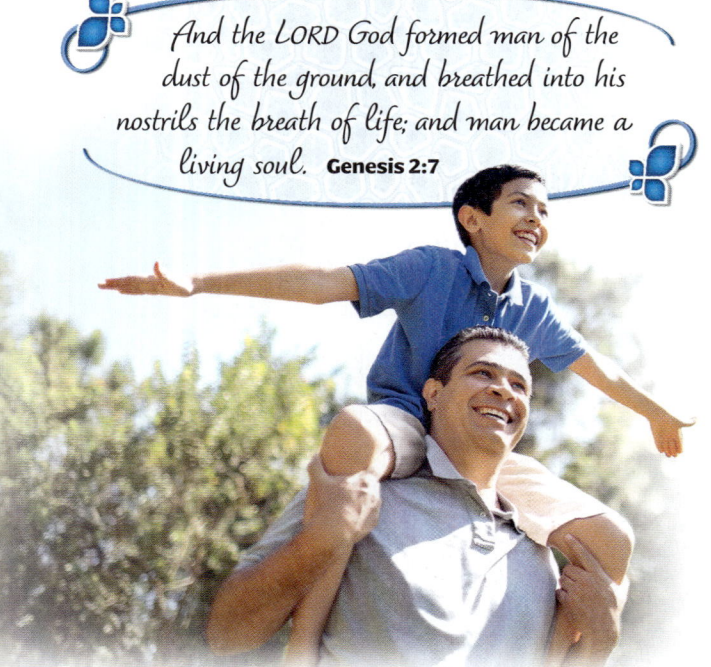

And the LORD God formed man of the dust of the ground, and breathed into his nostrils the breath of life; and man became a living soul. **Genesis 2:7**

The Respiratory Organs

The respiratory system is designed to bring air deep into your lungs. Air enters your body through your nose and mouth. Here, dust particles and other solids are trapped by sticky mucus. Hairs in the nose also trap solid particles. The air passes into your **pharynx** [făr′ĭngks], or *throat*. Next, the air travels down the **trachea** [trā′kē·ə], or *windpipe*. The **larynx** [lăr′ĭngks], or *voice box*, is at the top of your trachea. The larynx contains the *vocal cords*, two folds of tissue that produce sounds for speech when air flows over them. The trachea splits into *two air tubes* called **bronchi** [brŏng′kī′]. *Each bronchus* [brŏng′kəs] *goes into one of your lungs.*

The main organs of the respiratory system are the **lungs**. Your two lungs are large, spongy organs located on either side of your heart. To make room for your heart, your left lung is slightly smaller than your right lung. Your lungs are protected by your rib cage. *The lungs are the organs that absorb oxygen from the air into the blood and release carbon dioxide from the blood into the air.*

Once a bronchus enters a lung, the bronchus splits into many smaller air tubes, or *bronchial tubes*. *The smallest air tubes*, called **bronchioles** [brŏng′kē·ōlz′], end in *tiny air sacs* called **alveoli** [ăl·vē′ə·lī′]. There are millions of alveoli in the lungs. Each alveolus [ăl·vē′ə·ləs] has very thin walls and is surrounded by tiny capillaries. *The thin walls of the alveoli allow the exchange of gases between the blood and air.* Oxygen from the air passes into the blood. The oxygen molecules attach to hemoglobin in the red blood cells to be carried throughout the body. The blood also contains dissolved carbon dioxide produced by body cells. In the alveoli, this carbon dioxide passes out of the blood into the air.

🍃 The Breathing Process

The process of breathing in and out is called **respiration**. When you *inhale*, or breathe in, the air brings oxygen deep inside your lungs. The oxygen crosses the thin walls of the alveoli and capillaries and enters the bloodstream. At the same time, carbon dioxide in the bloodstream flows from the capillaries into the alveoli. You then *exhale*, or breathe out. Exhaling releases the carbon dioxide into the atmosphere. God designed plants to use this carbon dioxide in the process of photosynthesis, which makes food for the plants and releases oxygen.

Your body is designed to inhale and exhale without your thinking about it. Your brain controls the **diaphragm** [dī′ə·frăm′], *the main muscle of breathing. When you inhale, the diaphragm moves down*, and muscles in your chest also lift the rib cage up. These motions increase the space in your

chest and allow air to flow into your lungs. *When you exhale, the diaphragm moves back up*, and the chest muscles let the rib cage drop down. These motions decrease the space in your chest, and the air rushes out of your lungs.

You can control your breathing by holding your breath or breathing faster or slower. *But if your body does not have enough oxygen, your brain will automatically tell your diaphragm to move.* This is why you can hold your breath for only a short time. When the oxygen levels in your blood get low, your brain forces you to breathe. Your body needs extra oxygen during physical activity. If you run or play hard, your diaphragm will move faster to help bring in more air. Your heart will also beat more powerfully to get the extra oxygen to the cells quickly.

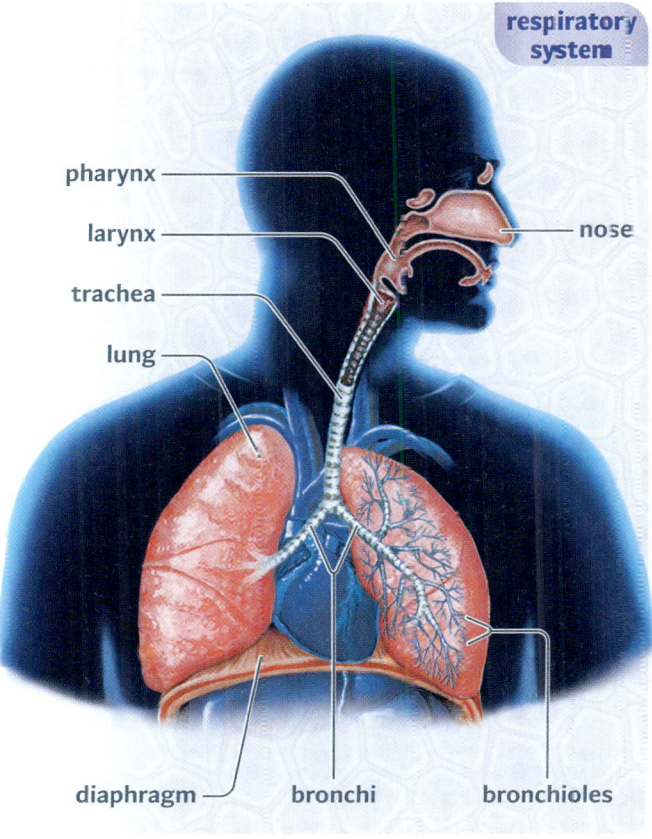

respiratory system

pharynx
larynx
trachea
lung
nose
diaphragm
bronchi
bronchioles

Community HEALTH CORNER

Air Pollution

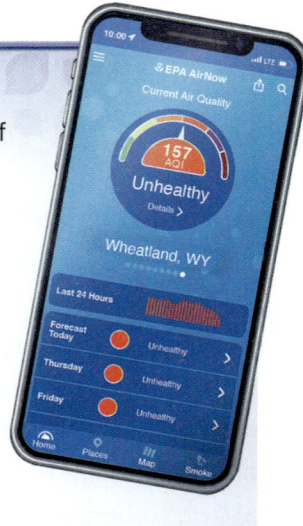

If you have ever lived in or visited a large city, you may have noticed that the air looked smoky or cloudy. It also may have had a bad smell or yellowish-brown color. This poor air quality, or air pollution, is caused by aerosols [âr′ə·sôlz′], small solid or liquid particles floating in the air. Aerosols can be found in both cities and rural areas, although they are usually more abundant in cities. Aerosols can come from both manmade and natural sources. Volcanic eruptions, forest fires, and methane gas are natural sources of pollution. Manmade sources of aerosols include factories, motor vehicles, and fuels. Fuels like coal and natural gas are used to heat homes and run power plants. In addition to aerosols, air pollution can be caused by poisonous gases in the atmosphere. These gases include ozone and carbon monoxide. Smog is a smoky fog that forms when chemical pollutants react with sunlight.

Air pollution can cause serious damage to your respiratory system. It can increase asthma attacks as well as cause many respiratory diseases and cancer. People living near busy roads or in areas with high ozone levels can be severely affected. Some cities issue air advisory warnings. These warnings recommend that people stay inside because of how poor the air quality is.

Air pollution from natural sources cannot be eliminated or reduced, only avoided. A single individual has little direct control of manmade air pollution, but many individuals making small decisions to reduce air pollution can have a large effect. Governments can enact laws and policies to help reduce manmade pollution. Businesses like factories and power plants can also work to limit their release of pollution. Sometimes, a factory can switch to a process that produces less aerosols or harmful gases. Other times, it can use techniques that remove polluting substances from gases released to the environment. You can work with your community to encourage individuals to reduce their air pollution. You can also promote laws, government policies, and business policies that seek to limit manmade air pollution.

Stewardship: Air Pollution

Motor vehicles such as cars and trucks are a major source of air pollution. Although you are not old enough to drive, you can still think about how you will make wise transportation decisions in the future. Think about how you would respond in each of these situations:

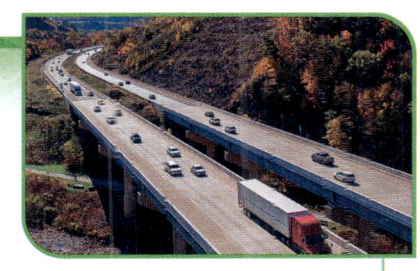

1. Your friend wants to play with you at a park down the street. What are some ways that you could get to the park without causing air pollution? _____

   _____

   _____

   _____

2. Your sports team is scheduled to play a game in a different town. Which of the following do you think would cause the least air pollution: every family driving individually, each family taking several team members, or the whole team going by bus? Explain your choice. _____

   _____

   _____

   _____

   _____

Pulmonologist

Have you ever had a persistent cough or cold that wouldn't go away? If you suffer from respiratory problems like shortness of breath or a cough that lasts more than three weeks, you may need to see a pulmonologist [pŏŏl/mə·nŏl/ə·jĭst]. A pulmonologist is a doctor who specializes in disorders of the respiratory system. Pulmonologists can also be thought of as lung doctors or chest doctors. A pulmonologist must complete over fourteen years of training and pass a board certification exam. Pulmonologists can specialize in various respiratory conditions.

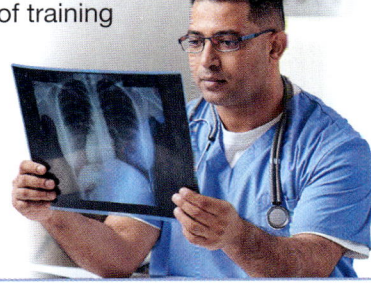

A visit to a pulmonologist will begin with conducting several tests to diagnose the respiratory disease. Chest x-rays and CT scans take pictures of the lungs. Other tests measure how well the lungs work. The pulmonologist may also schedule a sleep test, in which breathing is observed during sleep. These tests can help diagnose diseases such as cystic fibrosis [sĭs/tĭk fī·brō/sĭs], emphysema [ĕm/fĭ·sē/mə], asthma, or pneumonia [nŏŏ·mōn/yə]. The pulmonologist may treat the condition by prescribing medicine or recommending lifestyle changes. Medical devices can help the lungs do their job. A CPAP machine helps keep the bronchial tubes open while a person sleeps. An oxygen concentrator or oxygen tank provides extra oxygen for the lungs to absorb. A pulmonologist helps the community by helping people breathe better.

Identify: Label the parts of the respiratory system.

1. _____

2. _____

3. _____

4. _____

5. _____

6. _____

7. _____

Matching: Write the letter of the correct answer in the blank.

_____ 8. windpipe

_____ 9. voice box

_____ 10. air tube that allows air to enter the lungs

_____ 11. smallest type of air tube in the lungs

A. bronchiole
B. bronchus
C. larynx
D. pharynx
E. trachea

Short Answer: Write the correct answer in the blank.

12. What are the air sacs in the lungs called? _____

13. What is the process of breathing in and out? _____

14. What is the main muscle of breathing? _____

15. What will your body do if you try to hold your breath for too long? _____

_____

_____

Think about It.

16. Explain one aspect of the respiratory system that reflects the intentional and
    loving design of our Creator. _____

_____

_____

_____

septum: wall of muscle that separates the right side of the heart from the left side

atrium: upper chamber of the heart (atria, *plural*)

ventricle: lower chamber of the heart

vena cava: large vein that brings blood from the body to the right atrium of the heart (venae cavae, *plural*)

aorta: the body's largest artery; receives blood from the left ventricle of the heart; branches into arteries that carry blood to the rest of the body

blood pressure: the pressure of blood against the artery walls

pulse: the expanding of the arteries after each heartbeat; used to measure heart rate

aerobic endurance: ability of the body to do strenuous work over long periods of time

lung capacity: the amount of air that the lungs can hold

atherosclerosis: buildup of fatty deposits in an artery

2.4 Two Systems in Coordination

God has designed your circulatory and respiratory systems to work together closely. Your respiratory system brings oxygen into your body and removes carbon dioxide. Your circulatory system brings blood to every cell of your body to deliver oxygen and food and to remove carbon dioxide and waste. *The continuous flow of blood around the body is called circulation.* It takes less than one minute for the blood to flow from your heart, through your entire body, and back to your heart.

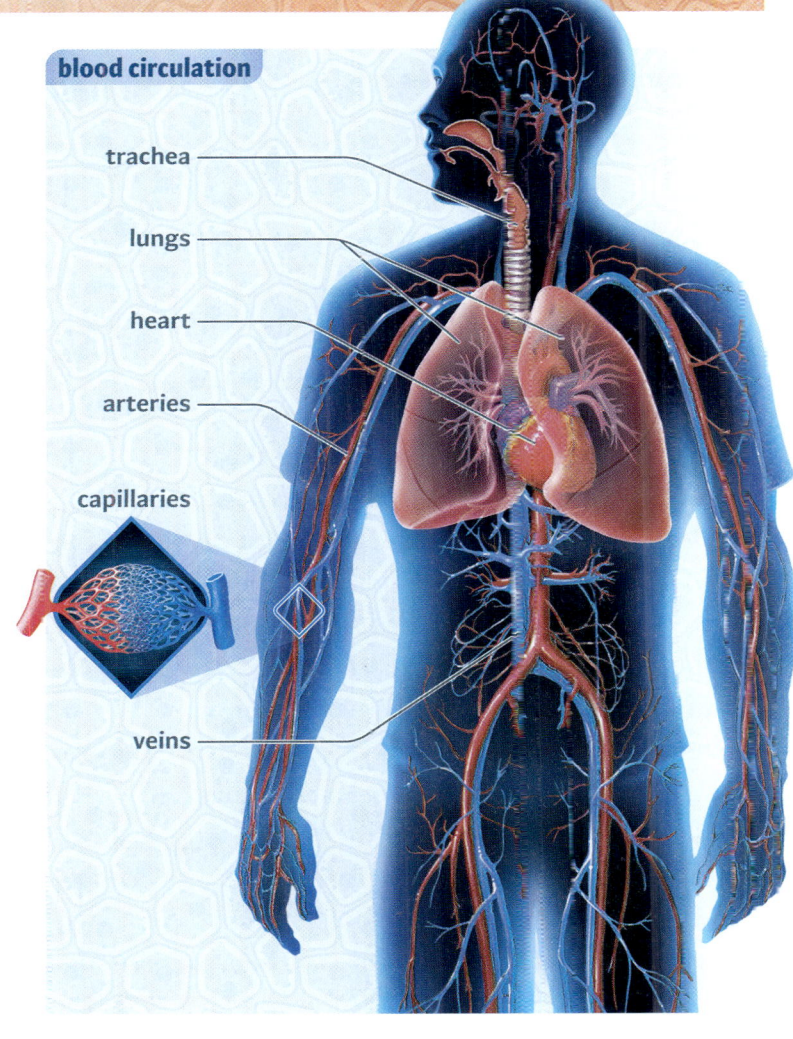

blood circulation

- trachea
- lungs
- heart
- arteries
- capillaries
- veins

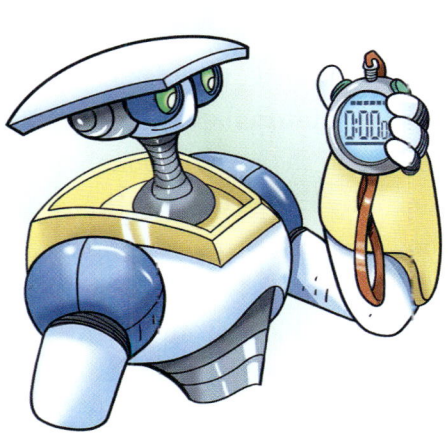

The Pumping Heart

Remember that your heart is the muscle that pumps blood throughout your body. *Your heart is really two pumps, placed side by side, that work at the same time.* A *wall of muscle called the* **septum** [sĕp′təm] *is between the two pumps. The septum separates the right side of the heart from the left side.* Each side of the heart has two hollow spaces called *chambers*. The *upper chambers* on each side are the **atria** [ā′trē·ə]. The two *lower chambers* are the **ventricles** [vĕn′trĭ·kəlz].

The two sides of your heart pump blood to different places. The right side of the heart receives oxygen-poor, or deoxygenated [dē·ŏk′sə·jə·nāt′əd], blood from the body and sends it to the lungs. The left side of the heart receives oxygen-rich, or oxygenated [ŏk′sĭ·jə·nāt′əd], blood from the lungs and pumps it to the rest of the body.

Deoxygenated blood from the rest of the body enters the right atrium [ā′trē·əm] *through two large veins called the* **venae cavae** [vē′nē kā′vē]. The *superior (upper) vena cava* [vē′nə kā′və] brings blood from the head, shoulders, arms, chest, and upper back. The *inferior (lower) vena cava* brings blood from the lower parts of the body.

From the right atrium, deoxygenated blood enters the right ventricle. The right ventricle then contracts to pump the blood through arteries to the lungs. After the lungs exchange oxygen and carbon dioxide,

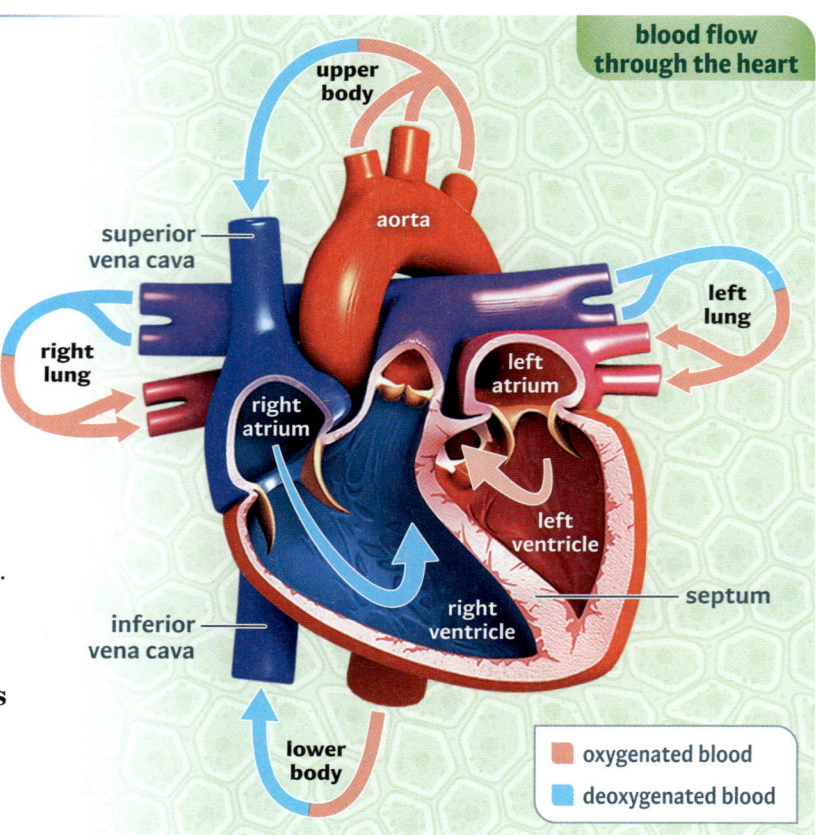

blood flow through the heart

oxygenated blood
deoxygenated blood

veins carry the newly oxygenated blood back to the heart. This round trip from the heart to the lungs and back again is called *pulmonary circulation*. (*Pulmonary* means "having to do with the lungs.")

The left atrium receives oxygenated blood from the lungs. The left ventricle pumps this blood into the **aorta** [ā·ôr′tə], the *body's largest artery. The aorta branches into arteries that carry blood to the rest of the body.* In the capillaries, the blood exchanges gases and other materials with body cells. It then returns to the heart through veins, which eventually merge to form the venae cavae. The venae cavae deposit the blood in the right atrium so that the cycle can begin again. The flow of blood from the heart to the rest of the body and then back to the heart is called *systemic circulation*.

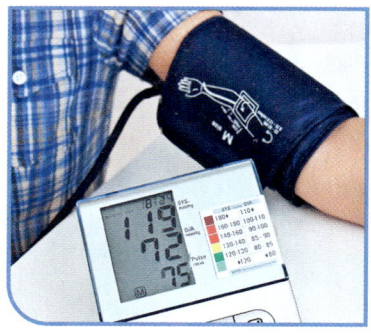
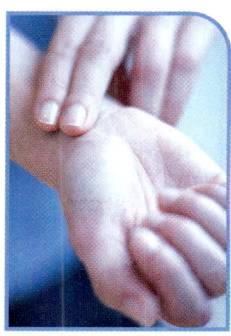

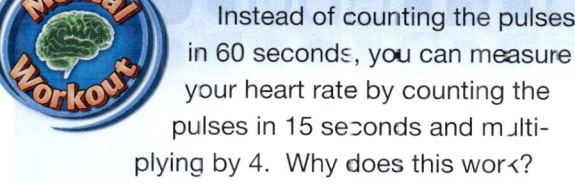

Instead of counting the pulses in 60 seconds, you can measure your heart rate by counting the pulses in 15 seconds and multiplying by 4. Why does this work?

Blood Pressure and Pulse

As blood flows through your arteries, it pushes against the artery walls. *The pressure of the blood against the artery walls* is called **blood pressure**. At a checkup, your doctor will usually measure your blood pressure. It is measured as two numbers. The larger number, which is written first, is the pressure when the ventricles are contracting. The smaller number is the pressure while the heart is resting, between beats. Blood pressure that is either too high or too low can indicate a problem with the circulatory system. You can help yourself avoid many of these problems by having a healthy diet and getting regular physical activity.

When your heart rests between contractions, the arteries spring back to their original size, forcing the blood along. *The expanding of the arteries after each heartbeat* is called a **pulse**. You can feel the pulse in your body wherever an artery is close to your skin, such as in your neck, wrist, or side of your face. *You can measure your heart rate by measuring the rate of your pulse*; the number of pulses in 60 seconds is your heart rate in beats per minute. Because your body needs more oxygen during physical activity, your pulse is lowest when you are at rest and increases during activity.

Aerobic Endurance

Part of developing good health is taking care of both your circulatory and respiratory systems. **Aerobic** [â·rō′bĭk] **endurance** is the *ability of your body to do strenuous work over long periods of time.* *Periods of strenuous physical activity help build your endurance by strengthening your heart and lungs.* Physical activity can also increase your **lung capacity**, or *the amount of air that your lungs can hold.* The U.S. Department of Health Physical Activity Guidelines for Americans recommends that young people get at least 60 minutes of physical activity every day.

Another way that you can take care of your heart is by eating a healthy diet. High levels of *cholesterol* [kə·lĕs′tə·rôl′], a fatty substance in the blood, can harm the heart. Solid fats, found in animal fat and fried food, can raise the level of cholesterol in the blood. Liquid fats, found in vegetable oils and fish oils, do not increase cholesterol. *Layers of cholesterol can build up in the arteries*, creating a condition called **atherosclerosis** [ăth′ə·rō·sklə·rō′sĭs].

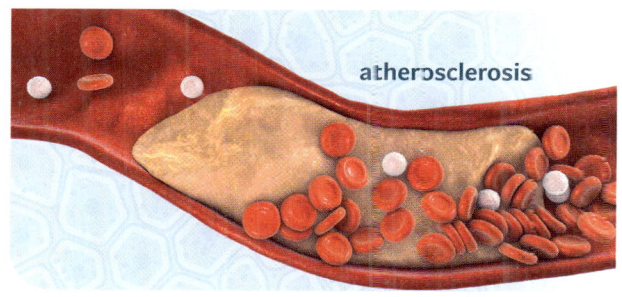

atherosclerosis

Atherosclerosis can be dangerous because it narrows the blood vessels and restricts blood flow. A proper diet and regular aerobic exercise will help prevent atherosclerosis.

When your body is in good condition, it is easier for it to recover from any illness. Medical research shows that people with well-conditioned bodies have fewer heart attacks. If they do have heart attacks, they recover faster. Although many people die of heart and lung disease every year, these diseases can often be prevented. Physical activity and good nutrition help to keep your heart and lungs healthy.

LIVE IT OUT!

Planning for Aerobic Endurance

The following questions will help you prepare to set goals for developing or maintaining aerobic endurance.

1. List one strength you have that can help you develop or maintain aerobic endurance.

   _____

   _____

   _____

   _____

   _____

2. Describe how you can use this strength to help you meet an endurance goal. _____

   _____

   _____

   _____

   _____

   _____

3. List one challenge you face that can make it harder to develop or maintain aerobic endurance. _____

   _____

   _____

   _____

   _____

4. Describe a way that you can overcome this challenge. _____

   _____

   _____

   _____

   _____

   _____

   _____

5. Who can you go to for support in meeting a goal for aerobic endurance? _____

   _____

   _____

   _____

   _____

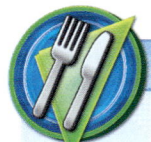

Heart-Healthy Snack Platter

You can make a heart-healthy snack platter to share with your family.
Be aware of allergies or sensitivities before you handle or eat food.

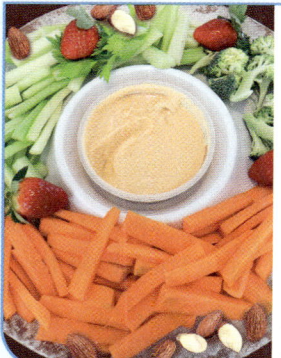

Ingredients:

- fresh-cut vegetables, such as broccoli, cauliflower, carrots, peppers, and celery
- fresh fruit, such as apple slices, berries, and bananas
- hummus dip or guacamole
- nuts, such as almonds and walnuts

Directions:

1. Place the dip in the center of the platter; then arrange fruits and veggies around it.
2. Add nuts where you can fit them.
3. Share with your family and enjoy!

Community HEALTH CORNER

Managing Asthma

Your lungs and airways are designed to bring in the air that your body needs, but sometimes they do not function properly. One common disease that affects the lungs and airways is asthma. During an asthma attack, the muscles in the airways tighten, causing the airways to become too narrow for air to flow freely. The lining of the airways also becomes swollen and produces sticky mucus, making it even harder for air to flow. Someone with asthma may experience shortness of breath, wheezing, coughing, or trouble sleeping. According to the Centers for Disease Control, asthma affects more than 22 million people in the United States, including 4.5 million children.

Asthma can be life threatening, and there is currently no cure. But asthma can be managed by reducing triggers. Common triggers include cigarette smoke, seasonal allergies, and air pollution. Mold, pests,

and dust mites are common indoor triggers. Strenuous exercise can also trigger an asthma attack. Heat during the late spring and summer months can make asthma symptoms worse. Hot, humid air can trap air pollution and other triggers. Improving air quality in both the home and community can help reduce triggers. Doctors can prescribe inhalers or other medications to stop or prevent an asthma attack. An active lifestyle also helps keep your lungs healthy.

Health organizations promote Asthma Awareness Month during May, when many individuals' asthma symptoms are worst. What can you do to raise awareness about asthma in your community? Encourage your friends and family to work together to maintain good respiratory health.

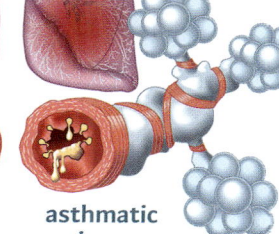

normal airway   asthmatic airway

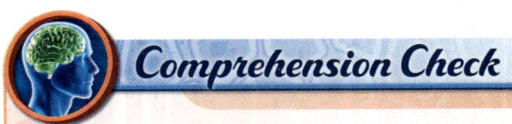

Fill in the Blank: *Write the correct word in the blank.*

Blood from the body flows into the _____, one of the upper chambers of the heart. It then flows into the _____. From there, blood is pumped to the _____, where it releases carbon dioxide and picks up oxygen. The oxygenated blood flows to the _____ of the heart. It then flows into the _____. The _____ is the large artery that takes the blood from the heart to the rest of the body. After passing through the organs, the blood returns to the heart through large veins called the _____.

Short Answer: *Write the correct answer in the blank.*

1. What is the wall of muscle that separates the right side of the heart from the left side of the heart called? _____

2. What is the expanding of the arteries after each heartbeat? _____

3. What is the ability of the body to do strenuous work over long periods of time?

   _____

4. What is lung capacity? _____

   _____

5. What is the buildup of fatty deposits in an artery? _____

Think about It.

6. The left side of the heart has to be able to pump more strongly than the right side does. Why is this?

   _____

   _____

   _____

   _____

   _____

   _____

   _____

1 Human Anatomy (2.1)

Matching: Write the letter of the correct answer in the blank.

_____ 1. the smallest living units of your body

_____ 2. includes blood, bone, and cartilage

_____ 3. includes heart, lungs, and stomach

_____ 4. your body has eleven of them

A. cells

B. organs

C. systems

D. tissues

2 The Circulatory System (2.2)

A. Classify: *Read the statement. Write A for artery,*
V for vein, and C for capillary.

_____ 1. returns blood to the heart

_____ 2. smallest blood vessel

_____ 3. has thick elastic walls

_____ 4. has the thinnest walls

_____ 5. carries blood away from the heart

artery

vein

capillary

B. Multiple Choice: *Write the letter of the correct answer in the blank.*

_____ 1. What part of the blood carries oxygen to every part of the body?
    a. plasma   c. red blood cells
    b. platelets   d. white blood cells

_____ 2. What part of the blood helps you heal when you scrape your knee?
    a. plasma   c. red blood cells
    b. platelets   d. white blood cells

C. Short Answer: *Write the correct answer in the blank.*

1. What is the straw-colored liquid part of the blood? _____

2. What protein do red blood cells use to carry oxygen? _____

3. Which two parts of the blood defend against infection and disease? _____

_____

4. What vitamin is important for platelets to do their job? _____

5. What is the continuous flow of blood within the body? _____

3 The Respiratory System (2.3)

A. Crossword: *Fill in the answers to complete the crossword puzzle.*

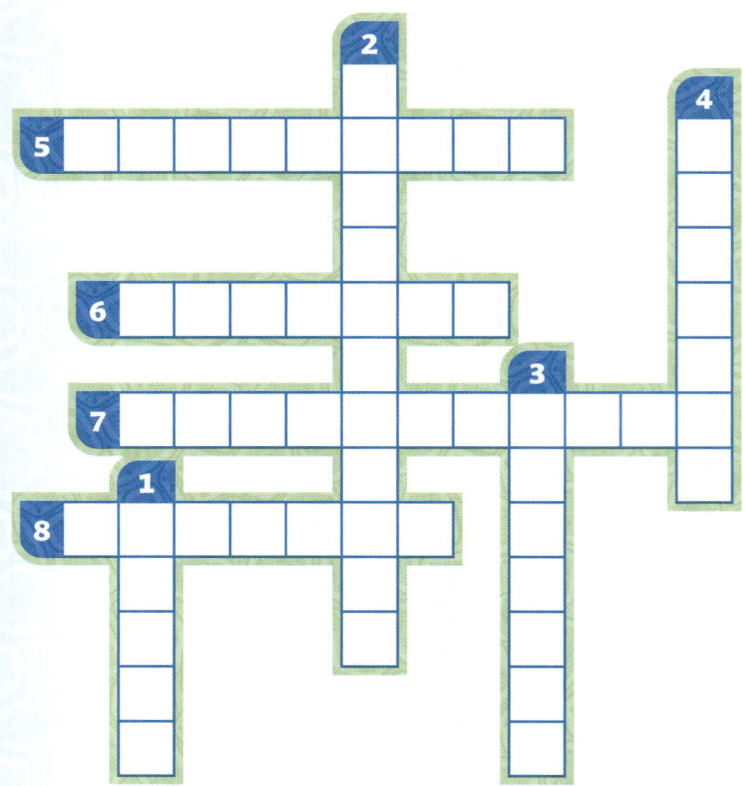

Down

1. main organs of the respiratory system
2. the smallest air tubes inside the lungs
3. the windpipe
4. the throat

Across

5. main muscle of breathing
6. two large air tubes that enter the lungs
7. process of breathing in and out
8. air sacs in the lungs

B. Short Answer: *Write the correct answer in the blank.*

1. How does the respiratory system help the body? _____

   _____

   _____

2. What is the scientific name of the voice box? _____

3. Describe what happens inside your chest when you inhale. _____

   _____

   _____

   _____

   _____

   _____

   _____

   _____

   _____

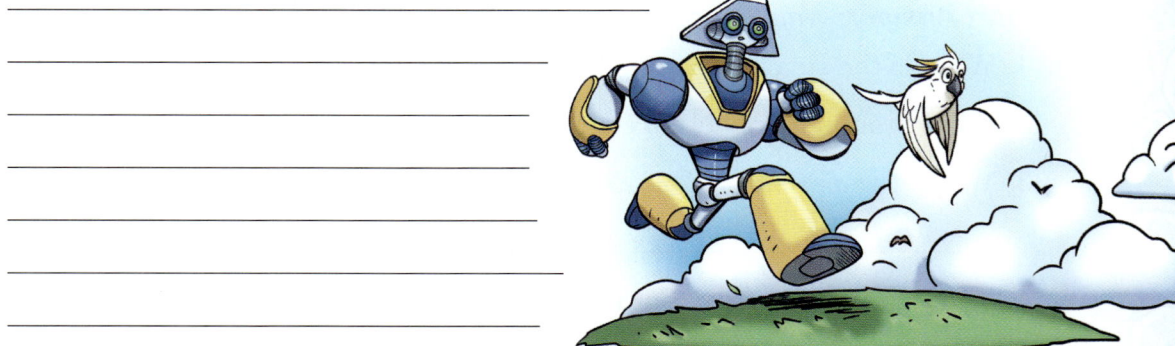

4 Two Systems in Coordination (2.4)

A. Identify: *Label the parts of the heart.*

1. _____

2. _____

3. _____

4. _____

5. _____

B. True/False: *If the statement is true, write* true *in the blank. If the statement is false, replace the underlined word(s) with a word that will make the statement true. Do not write* false *in any blank.*

_____ 1. The upper chambers of the heart are the <u>ventricles</u>.

_____ 2. The largest artery in the body is the <u>vena cava</u>.

_____ 3. The expanding of the arteries after each heartbeat, which is used to measure heart rate, is the <u>blood pressure</u>.

_____ 4. The body's ability to do strenuous work over long periods of time is aerobic <u>endurance</u>.

_____ 5. The buildup of fatty deposits in an artery is <u>atherosclerosis</u>.

C. Short Answer: *Write the correct answer in the blank.*

1. What is the pressure of blood against the arteries? _____

2. What is the amount of air that your lungs can hold called? _____

3. What are two ways that you can take care of your heart? _____

_____

D. Think!

1. What is the difference between the right side of the heart and the left side of the heart? _____

_____

_____

_____

2. Why are liquid fats healthier than solid fats? _____

_____

_____

Terms

nervous system: body system that coordinates and controls all activities of the body; brain, spinal cord, and nerves

neurology: medical study of the nervous system

central nervous system (CNS): major part of the nervous system consisting of the brain and spinal cord

peripheral nervous system (PNS): major part of the nervous system consisting of nerves and of sense organs

neuron: nerve cell; cell that transmits messages within the body

cell body: central part of a neuron containing the nucleus and organelles

dendrite: short, branching part of a neuron that extends from the cell body

axon: long, straight part of a neuron that extends from the cell body

3.1 Neurology

Think of a group that you are a part of, such as a sports team, orchestra, band, or choir. Each of these groups has many people working together for a common goal. The members of a sports team work together for the goal of winning a game. The members of a music group work together for the goal of performing their music. For the group to meet its goal, each member has a specific task to do. Each group has a leader, such as a coach or director. An important part of the leader's job is to coordinate the group's activity. Doing this requires clear communication between the leader and the group members.

Your body is a group of many organs and systems. All the organs and systems work toward the common goal of keeping you alive and healthy. Like a sports team or choir, your body needs good coordination and clear communication. God designed the **nervous system** to *coordinate and control all activities of the body*. These activities include movement, respiration, and heart rate. The nervous system sends messages to all parts of the body and receives messages from all parts of the body. *The main organs of the nervous system are the brain, spinal cord, and nerves.*

The nervous system is so important that the *medical study of the nervous system* is its own field of medicine, called **neurology**. Neurology includes learning how the nervous system works and how to identify and treat diseases of the nervous system.

Parts of the Nervous System

The nervous system has two major parts. *One major part is the* **central nervous system**, *or* **CNS**, *which consists of the brain and spinal cord.* These organs receive messages from senses like touch, taste, and sight. They make the decisions that control the body. And they send messages to the rest of the body.

The other major part is the **peripheral** [pə·rĭf′ər·əl] **nervous system**, or **PNS**. *The peripheral nervous system consists of nerves* that branch out from the brain and spinal cord. *Sense organs* like the ears and eyes are also part of the peripheral nervous system. Each nerve is a bundle of nerve cells. The nerves transmit messages from the sense organs and from sense receptors in other organs to the central nervous system. The nerves also transmit messages from the central nervous system to other organs.

When you pick up your pen and write a word, your brain decides to write and determines exactly what body movements are needed. It then sends out messages that travel through the spinal cord and through nerves. These messages tell every part of the body what to do. They tell your arm to reach for your pen, your fingers to grasp the pen, and so on. Your sense of touch feels your fingers pressing on your pen. This sense also feels the slight change in pressure when your pen touches the paper. This information travels back to your brain through your nerves and spinal cord. Your brain then knows to send the messages for your arm to move and form the letters.

While you are writing, the nervous system is also busy coordinating other parts of the body. Your heartbeat and breathing must continue. The brain receives messages about your blood pressure and the oxygen in the blood. It uses this information to send messages that control your heart and diaphragm. Your body has many other automatic functions. Your nervous system controls and coordinates these automatic functions all the time, whether you are awake or asleep, without you having to think about it.

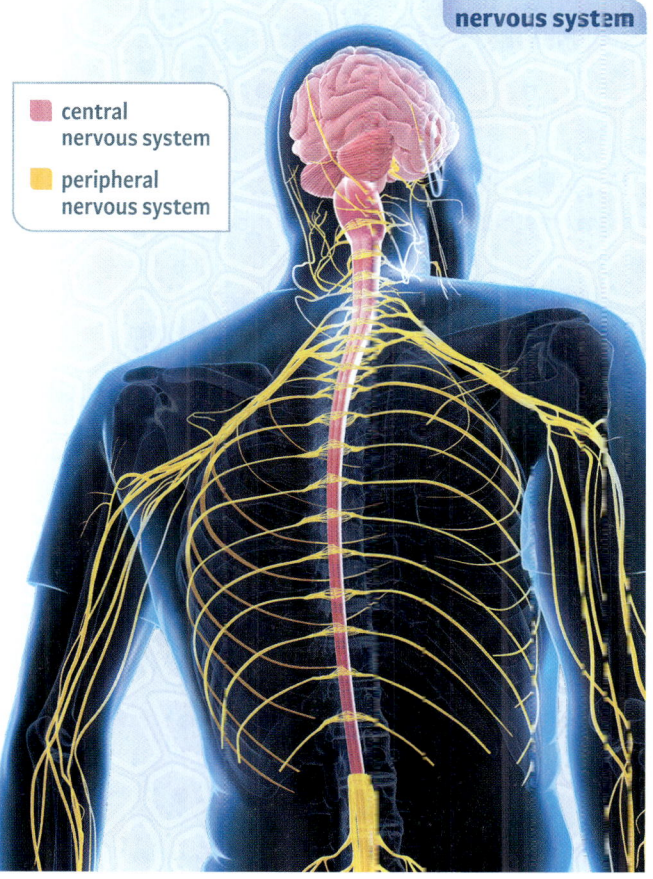

nervous system

central nervous system

peripheral nervous system

Neurologist

Your local community offers resources to keep your nervous system healthy. If you have a problem with your brain or nerves, your physician may send you to see a neurologist, a physician who specializes in treating disorders of the brain and nervous system. A neurologist must complete many years of special training to gain the knowledge necessary to work on the nervous system.

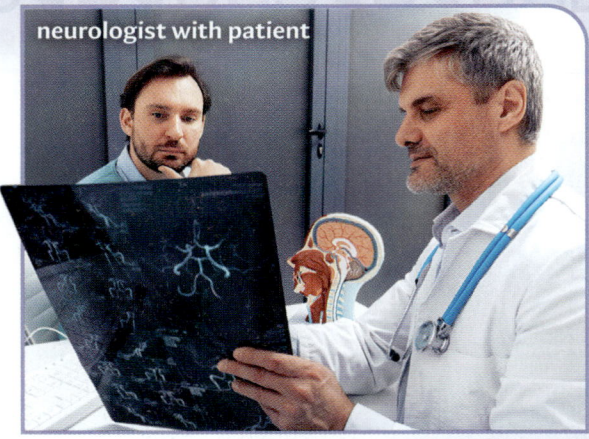
neurologist with patient

There are many neurological disorders that are treated by a neurologist. A stroke may occur when there is not enough blood flow to the brain. A seizure—a sudden lack of muscle control that causes convulsions (spasms) or loss of consciousness—occurs when there is a sudden change in how the brain works. Some diseases result from infections that attack the brain and spinal cord. Other disorders develop as the person grows older. Sometimes, injuries to the brain and spinal cord can cause severe problems.

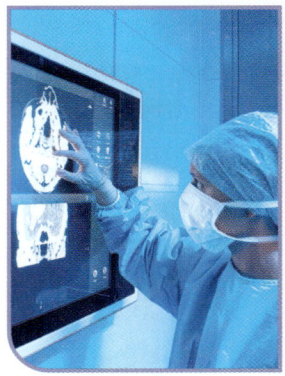
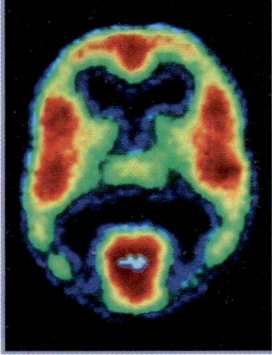
neurosurgeon looking at brain scans   brain scan

A neurologist may perform several tests to diagnose disorders of the brain or nervous system. He can use specialized machinery and tests to take pictures of the brain or to observe brain and nerve function. He may also do a spinal tap, in which he takes fluid from the spine to look for infection. Once the neurologist has diagnosed the condition, he will prescribe medicine. He may also recommend surgery. The surgery will be performed by a neurosurgeon, a doctor who specializes in performing surgery on the nervous system. Whatever the condition is, a neurologist knows how to work with you and your family to keep your nervous system healthy.

Your community can work together to promote healthy nervous systems. A nutritious diet and physical activity improve your brain's health. Another way to improve health is to limit the amount of time you spend looking at the screens of televisions, computers, and cellphones. Although screens are often needed for education and work, too much exposure can harm your nervous system. You can encourage others in your family and community to make time for hobbies, relationships, and fun activities.

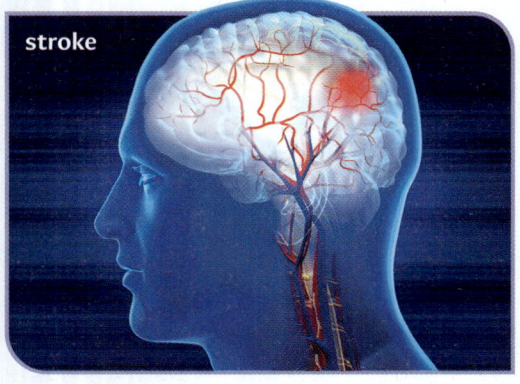
stroke

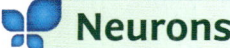

Neurons

The main cells of the nervous system are nerve cells, or **neurons**. *Neurons are the cells that actually transmit messages within the body.* There are different types of neurons for carrying different kinds of messages, but they all have the same basic structure. The three main parts of every neuron are the cell body, the dendrites, and the axon.

Every cell of your body has a *nucleus* that controls the cell and *organelles* [ôr′gə·nĕlz′] that do various jobs for the cell. *A neuron's nucleus and organelles are in the central part of the cell*, called the **cell body**. *The cell body is where the cell performs the functions that all cells need to live.* These functions include releasing energy from sugar, making and recycling cell parts, and disposing of waste products. Materials needed by the dendrites and axon are made in the cell body. These materials are then delivered by special "machines" within the cell.

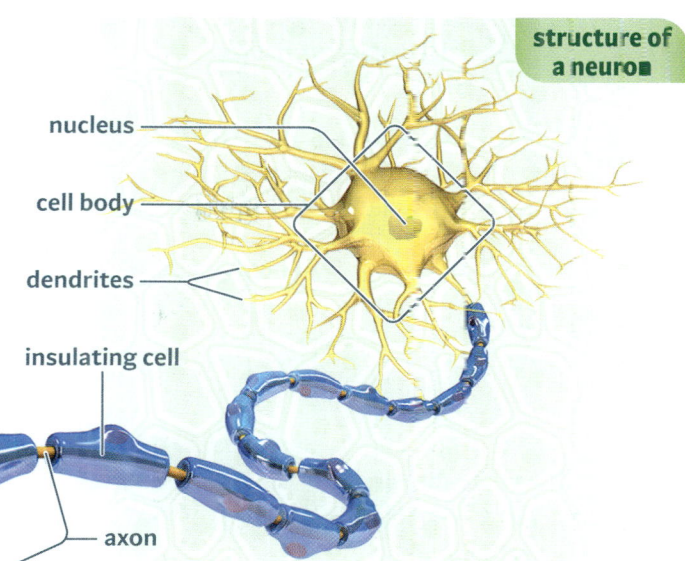

structure of a neuron

nucleus

cell body

dendrites

insulating cell

axon

Each **dendrite** is a short, branching part of a neuron that extends from the cell body. A single neuron may have hundreds or thousands of dendrites. *The job of the dendrites is to receive messages from other neurons and transmit those messages to the cell body.*

The third part of the neuron is the **axon**, *the long, straight part of a neuron that extends from the cell body. The job of the axon is to transmit messages from the cell body to other neurons.* Although a neuron usually has many dendrites, a neuron always has only one axon. *An axon is also called a nerve fiber.*

An axon is like a long wire that transmits a message as a pulse of electric current. A metal wire is insulated by a plastic coating. Similarly, an axon is insulated by special insulating cells that wrap around it. Most of the axon is long and straight, with no branches, but it may split into several small branches at the end. Each branch delivers the same message to one of several nearby cells.

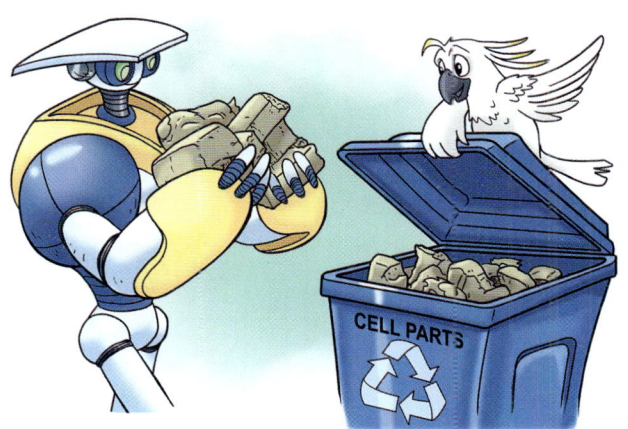

CELL PARTS

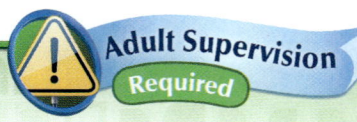

Hands-On Health

Make a neuron model.

Materials needed:

- large drinking cup or glass with a 3 in. to 4 in. opening
- piece of white construction paper or white cardboard
- pencil
- scissors
- utility knife
- piece of regular brown cardboard (optional)
- glue (optional)
- colored pencils or crayons
- 15–20 in. yarn
- glue gun
- small craft beads

1. Set the drinking cup or glass upside down on the white construction paper or white cardboard. Trace around the rim of the glass with the pencil.

2. Cut out the circle of paper or cardboard. If the cardboard is too thick to cut with scissors, have an adult cut it with the utility knife.

3. If you are using construction paper, trace a second circle on a piece of regular brown cardboard. Either cut it out with scissors or have an adult cut it out with the utility knife. Glue the construction paper to the cardboard.

4. Color the white circle to represent a neuron's cell body. Be sure to include the nucleus.

5. Cut a piece of yarn 3–4 in. long and set it aside. Have an adult use the glue gun to attach one end of the remaining yarn to the underside of the "cell body" circle. About ½ in. should be on the circle, with the rest hanging off. This piece of yarn is the axon.

6. Slide a craft bead onto the axon. Tie a knot after the bead to hold the bead in place. This bead is an insulating cell.

7. Continue adding beads and knots until you are near the end of the axon. Leave about 2 in. after the last knot.

8. Untwist the end of the axon (after the knot) into separate strands. These strands represent the axon branching.

9. Cut the short piece of yarn that you set aside in step 5 in half, so that you have two 1½–2 in. long pieces. Completely untwist both of these short pieces into separate strands.

10. Have an adult attach the short strands around the back of the "cell body" circle with the glue gun. About ½ in. of each strand should be on the circle, with the rest hanging off. These short strands are the dendrites.

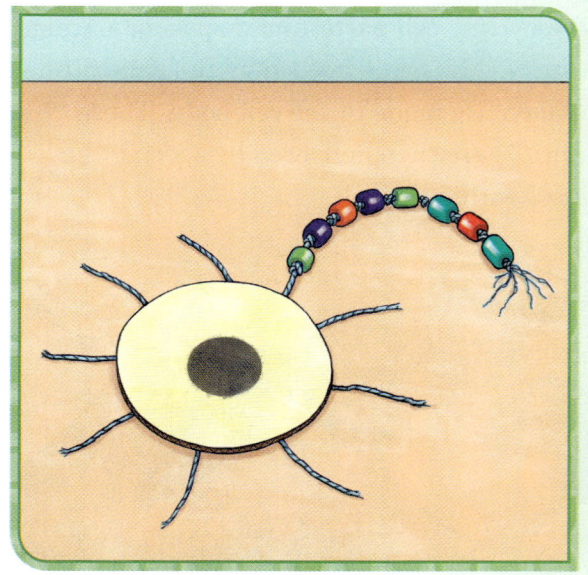

Short Answer: *Write the correct answer in the blank.*

1. What are the nervous system's two main jobs? _____

   _____

2. What is the medical study of the nervous system called? _____

3. What are the two major parts of the nervous system? _____

   _____

4. What is a nerve cell called? _____

5. What part of a neuron contains the nucleus and organelles? _____

Identify: *Label the parts of a neuron.*

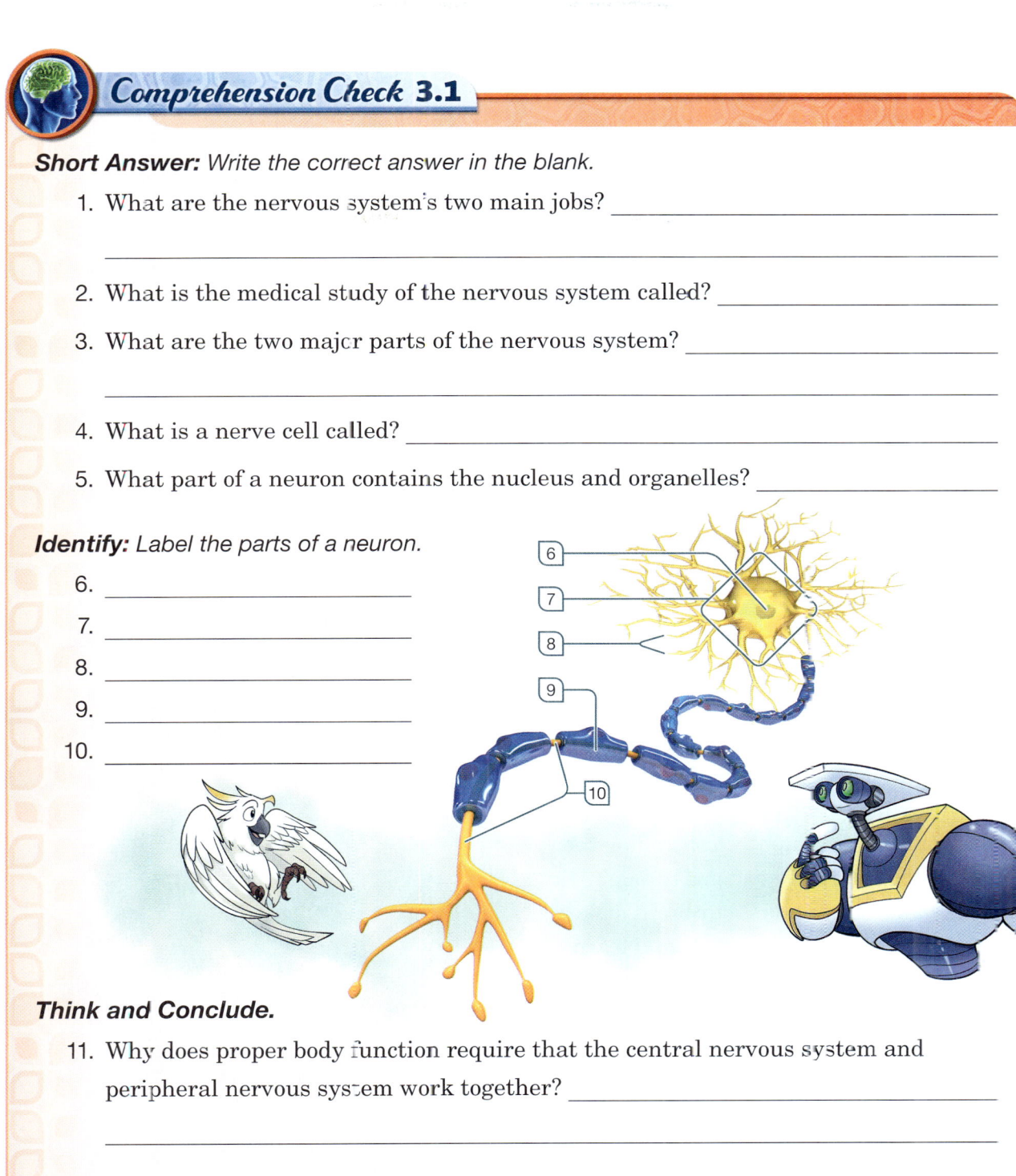

6. _____

7. _____

8. _____

9. _____

10. _____

Think and Conclude.

11. Why does proper body function require that the central nervous system and peripheral nervous system work together? _____

   _____

   _____

   _____

   _____

   _____

   _____

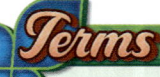

brain: main organ of the nervous system; controls the body

cerebrum: largest part of the brain; controls the process of thinking and reasoning; receives and interprets information from sense organs

cerebellum: part of the brain that controls balance and coordination of voluntary muscles

brain stem: controls involuntary functions of the body; "turns off" and "turns on" cerebrum for sleeping and waking

limbic system: part of the brain that helps you coordinate emotions, alerts you of physical needs, and is important for forming memories; includes an emotional reward system

spinal cord: bundle of nerve cells attached to the base of the brain stem; carries messages between the brain and the rest of the body

reflex: quick, automatic action that the body does in response to something else

3.2 The Central Nervous System

The Brain

As you have learned, the central nervous system consists of the brain and the spinal cord. The **brain** is the *main organ of the nervous system; its job is to control the whole body.* It is a soft, spongy organ weighing between two and three pounds. Your brain acts as your body's computer, controlling the functions of all the body systems through messages and commands. Your brain makes it possible for you to move, think, and learn. Your brain controls automatic functions, including your heartbeat, your breathing, and your digestion of food.

God gave you a brain to help you experience life. What are some things you enjoy doing? Without your brain, you could not enjoy a game of soccer, taste delicious food, or hear beautiful music. Your brain also helps you feel emotions, such as happiness and sadness. Because your brain is such an important organ, God enclosed it in the bones of your skull for protection.

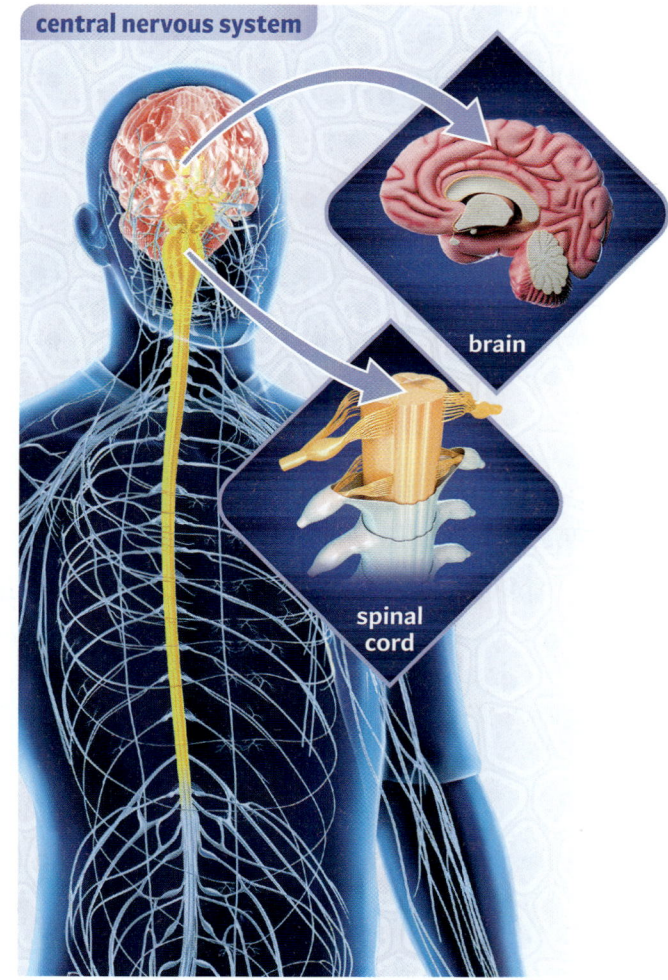

central nervous system

brain

spinal cord

Cerebrum

Your brain has three main parts: the cerebrum, the cerebellum, and the brain stem. The **cerebrum** is *the largest part of the brain; it controls the process of thinking and reasoning.* It lets you remember, solve problems, speak, and write. *The cerebrum receives and interprets information from your sense organs.* Sense organs like your eyes, ears, tongue, nose, and skin detect things in your environment and send messages to your brain. Your cerebrum interprets the messages to identify what you are seeing, hearing, tasting, smelling, or feeling.

The cerebrum has two halves, or *hemispheres. The right hemisphere controls the left side of your body, and the left hemisphere controls the right side of your body.* Each hemisphere specializes in certain types of thinking. The left hemisphere specializes in language, mathematics, and logic, or reasoning to a conclusion. The right hemisphere specializes in creativity, imagination, and intuition, or making a conclusion without having to stop and think.

Cerebellum

At the back of your brain, below the cerebrum, is the **cerebellum**. The cerebellum is only about the size of your fist. *It controls balance and the coordination of your voluntary muscles.* When you first learned to ride a bike, you had to think about each movement. You used your cerebrum to coordinate your muscles for pedaling, steering, and balancing. As you practiced, your cerebellum learned how to make your muscles move in coordination. Once your cerebellum learned what to do, it took over. Now, you do not have to think about how to ride a bike; you just get on your bike and go. Your cerebellum has helped you develop other skills like walking, brushing your teeth, and tying your shoes. Anytime you need coordination and balance, you can depend on your cerebellum.

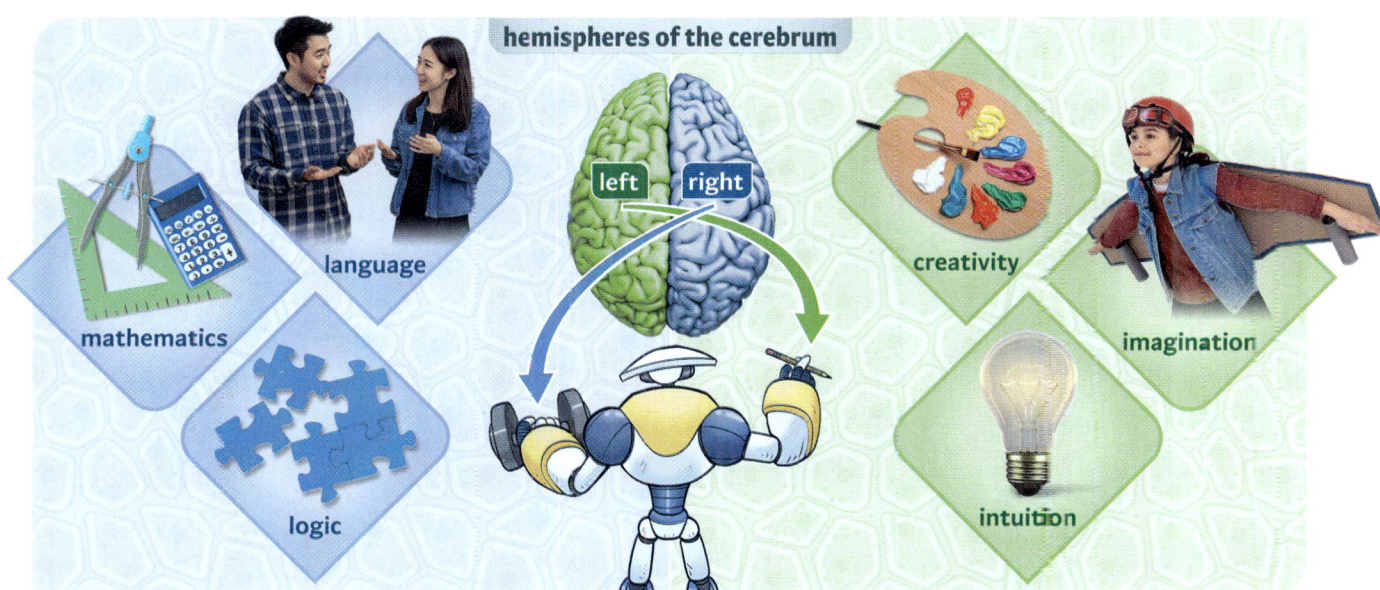

hemispheres of the cerebrum

left right

language

mathematics

logic

creativity

imagination

intuition

Brain Stem

Between the cerebellum and the spinal cord is the brain stem. *The **brain stem** controls the automatic, or involuntary, functions of the body* that keep you alive. Do you remember what some of these functions are? The circulatory, respiratory, and digestive systems are all controlled by the brain stem. *The brain stem also "turns off" and "turns on" the cerebrum when you go to sleep and wake up.* All nerve fibers (axons) that connect the brain and the spinal cord pass through the brain stem.

Limbic System

In the middle of your brain, just above the brain stem, is a group of structures called the **limbic system**. Your limbic system has several functions. *It helps you coordinate emotions, such as love and anger. It alerts you to physical needs, like the need for sleep or food. It plays an important role in forming long-term memories.*

Your limbic system also includes an emotional reward system. When you think about an action, the reward system predicts the emotions the action will produce. If the reward system predicts positive emotions, it releases chemical messengers that trigger a desire to do the action. If the reward system predicts negative emotions, it releases chemical messengers that trigger a desire to avoid the action. The system also learns from your experiences. If an action or situation causes negative emotions like pain or fear, the system changes its circuits to produce a desire to avoid that action or situation in the future.

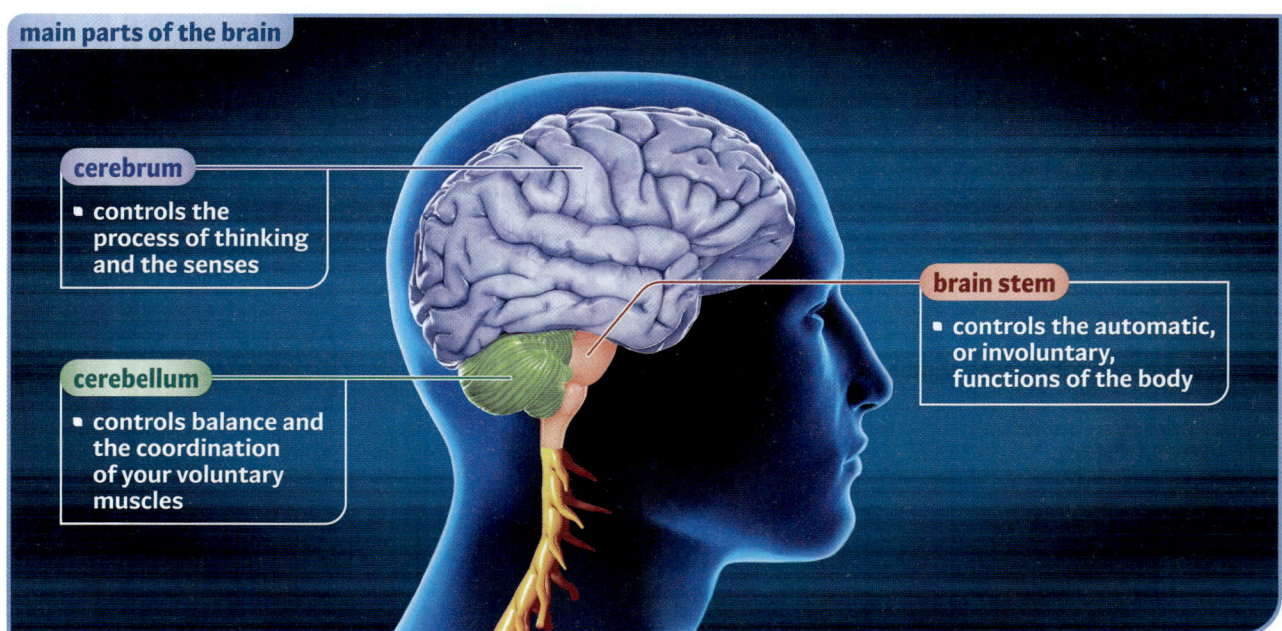

main parts of the brain

cerebrum
- controls the process of thinking and the senses

cerebellum
- controls balance and the coordination of your voluntary muscles

brain stem
- controls the automatic, or involuntary, functions of the body

God designed the limbic system to make us desire His good physical gifts, like rest (Ps. 127:2; Prov. 3:24) and food (Ps. 104:14–15; 136:25). Because of our sinfulness, we often misuse these gifts by being lazy or overeating. We also have other desires that are themselves sinful and can lead us to sinful actions. We might deal with sinful desires to do things that are wrong or to avoid doing things that we should do. As Christians, we are not to give into any of these wrong desires. Instead, we are to surrender ourselves and our desires to God, so that we serve Him and do right.

> *Let not sin therefore reign in your mortal body, that ye should obey it in the lusts* [strong desires] *thereof. Neither yield ye your members as instruments of unrighteousness unto sin: but yield yourselves unto God, as those that are alive from the dead, and your members as instruments of righteousness unto God. For sin shall not have dominion over you: for ye are not under the law, but under grace.* **Romans 6:12–14**

Brain Development

During your first few years of life, your brain grew rapidly. When you were six or seven, it was already nine-tenths of its adult size. By your early teens, it will have reached its adult size. Although your brain will not grow any larger, it will still develop and mature. It will not be fully mature until your early to mid-twenties.

During your preteen and early teenage years, your limbic system and emotional reward system develop. This development means that you will probably feel stronger emotions than you did when you were younger. Your emotional reward system will also give you stronger desires to do things that you think will be fun or will make you happy. Some of these desires will be to do things that are safe and good. But others will be to do things that are dangerous or wrong.

At this age, you need to learn to manage your emotions and desires. Before acting on a desire, stop and think. Is it a desire to do something wrong? Is acting on the desire likely to harm yourself or others? If the action is wrong or harmful, you should reject the desire. You need to make the right choice no matter how much fun an action seems or how strong the desire is.

Managing your desires is not easy, but it will become easier as you practice and as other parts of your brain mature. Make a plan to resist wrong or harmful desires. Also seek help from those in your community, especially parents and other trusted adults who can guide you through these years. Most importantly *pray and give your desires to God*. Through the Holy Spirit, He will give you strength to overcome wrong desires and do His will.

> *This I say then, Walk in the Spirit, and ye shall not fulfill the lust* [strong desire] *of the flesh. For the flesh lusteth against the Spirit, and the Spirit against the flesh: and these are contrary the one to the other: so that ye cannot do the things that ye would.* **Galatians 5:16–17**

The Spinal Cord

The brain communicates with the body through the **spinal cord**. Your spinal cord is *a bundle of nerve cells that is attached to the base of your brain stem. It carries messages back and forth between the brain and the rest of the body.* Like the brain, the spinal cord is protected by a covering of bone. Instead of being inside a rigid shell like your skull, your spinal cord runs through a flexible channel inside your backbone.

The spinal cord also controls your simple reflexes. A **reflex** is *a quick, automatic action that your body does in response to something else.* One simple reflex is pulling your hand back from a hot or sharp object. When your spinal cord receives the pain message, it sends your muscles emergency commands to jerk your hand back. The reflex begins

moving your hand away from danger even before your cerebrum has time to interpret the pain signal. During regular checkups, your physician will test your reflexes to check the health of your nervous system. He or she may tap your knee, causing your leg to kick out without your thinking about it.

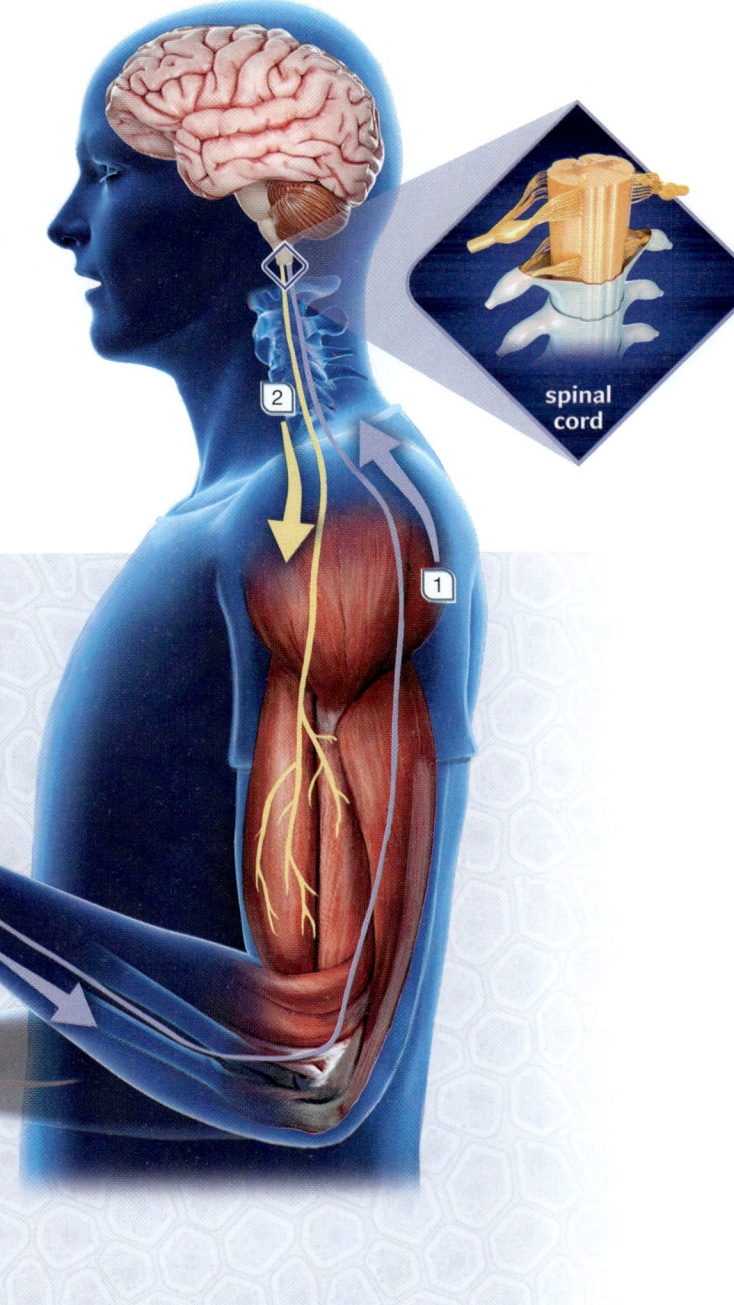

spinal cord

sense of touch: reflex process

1. Pain message travels to spinal cord.
2. Spinal cord sends message to arm muscles.
3. Hand jerks back.

True/False: *If the statement is true, write* true *in the blank. If the statement is false, replace the underlined word(s) with a word or phrase that will make the statement true. Do not write* false *in any blank.*

_____ 1. The main organ of the nervous system is the <u>spinal cord</u>.

_____ 2. The right hemisphere of the cerebrum controls the <u>left</u> half of the body.

_____ 3. The cerebrum is "turned on" and "turned off" by the <u>limbic system</u>.

_____ 4. A quick, automatic action that the body does in response to something else is a <u>reflex</u>.

Matching: *Write the letter of the correct answer in the blank. Answers may be used more than once.*

_____ 5. largest part of the brain

_____ 6. controls thinking and reasoning

_____ 7. controls balance and coordinating of voluntary muscles

_____ 8. controls involuntary functions of the body

_____ 9. helps coordinate emotions and alerts you to physical needs

_____ 10. carries messages between the brain and the rest of the body

_____ 11. controls simple reflexes

A. brain stem
B. cerebellum
C. cerebrum
D. limbic system
E. spinal cord

Think about It.

12. Suppose you are copying your spelling words. How are the cerebrum, cerebellum, and brain stem involved in this activity? _____

_____
_____
_____
_____
_____
_____

3.3 The Peripheral Nervous System

The job of the CNS is to make decisions and to coordinate body activities. Communication between your CNS and the rest of your body occurs through the peripheral nervous system, consisting of nerves that branch out from the brain and spinal cord.

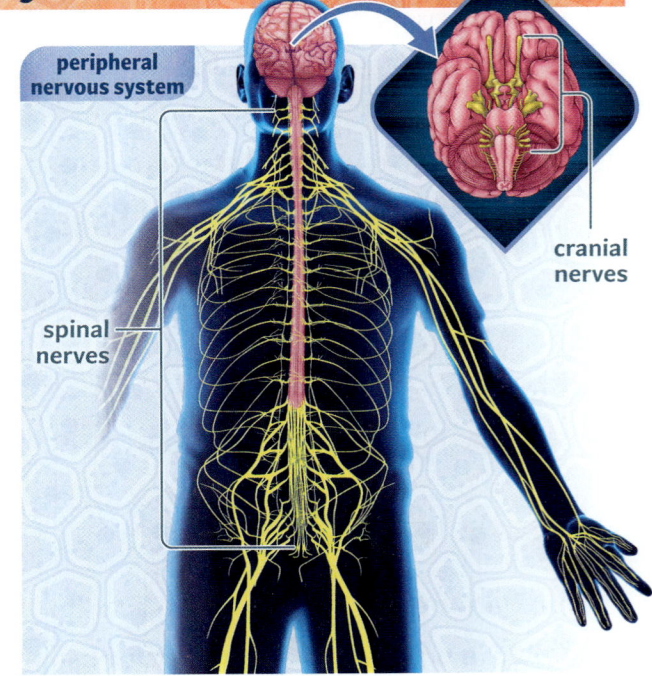

peripheral nervous system

cranial nerves

spinal nerves

What Are Nerves?

You have learned that every neuron (nerve cell) has three parts: the cell body, the dendrites, and the axon, or nerve fiber. Each nerve fiber is like a long, straight wire that transmits messages from the cell body to other neurons. A **nerve** is an *organ made of bundles of nerve fibers. Each nerve transmits messages between the central nervous system and one or more specific regions of the body.*

A nerve does not consist only of nerve fibers. Each nerve fiber is wrapped by insulating cells. The nerve also contains tissues that cushion the nerve fibers to protect them from damage. Still other tissues wrap around the parts of the nerve to keep them together.

Blood vessels run through the nerve to supply nutrients and remove waste.

Nerves must carry signals in two directions: from the CNS to the rest of the body and from the rest of the body to the CNS. But each nerve cell carries signals in only one direction. Therefore, *nerve fibers come in two types*: sensory nerve fibers and motor nerve fibers.

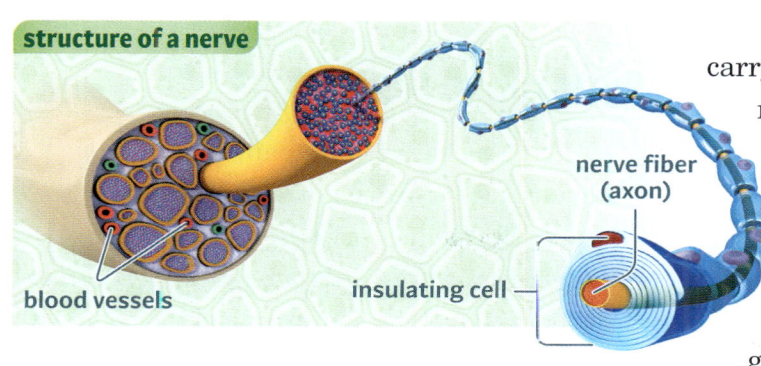

structure of a nerve

blood vessels

insulating cell

nerve fiber (axon)

Sensory Nerve Fibers

A **sensory nerve fiber** *carries signals from the body to the central nervous system.* These nerve fibers tell the CNS what conditions are like both inside and outside your body. Conditions inside your body include the tension, or stretching force, on your muscles; the rate of your heartbeat; and how much food is in your stomach. Conditions outside your body are detected by your senses—touch, smell, taste, sight, and hearing. Your body also detects sensations such as pain and temperature both inside and outside your body. These signals travel to your brain to be interpreted. Some signals, such as pain, can also trigger a reflex in the spinal cord.

Every signal carried by a sensory nerve fiber comes from a **sense receptor**, *a special cell or group of cells that detects a sensation and sends a message on a sensory nerve fiber.* Sense receptors in your internal organs help the brain control the automatic functions of your body. Your five senses come from sense receptors in your skin, nose, tongue, eyes, and ears.

Motor Nerve Fibers

A **motor nerve fiber** *controls some part of the body by delivering messages from the central nervous system.* We often think of motor nerve fibers as causing motion by

carrying messages to the muscles, but not all motor nerve fibers cause motion. Many of them control important automatic functions of your body. Motor nerve fibers tell the heart to slow down and speed up. Others tell various chemical-producing structures called glands when to make or stop making different chemicals.

Each motor nerve fiber carries a single message to an individual cell or group of cells. Depending on the nerve fiber, this message may tell muscle cells to contract, tell the heart to speed up, or tell a gland to stop producing a certain chemical. The brain chooses the specific motor nerve fiber for the message it wants to send and the cells the message needs to reach.

The end of a motor nerve fiber often branches out in several directions. Each branch delivers the same message to a different cell. A motion-controlling fiber with only a few branches tells only a few muscle cells to contract. The brain can send a message on this fiber to perform slow and gentle motions. Another fiber may have many branches and tell many muscle cells to contract. Sending a message on this fiber allows the brain to perform rapid and forceful motions.

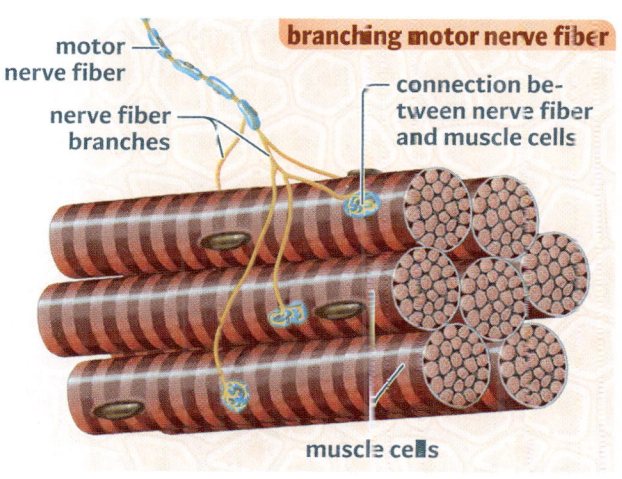

branching motor nerve fiber

motor nerve fiber

nerve fiber branches

connection between nerve fiber and muscle cells

muscle cells

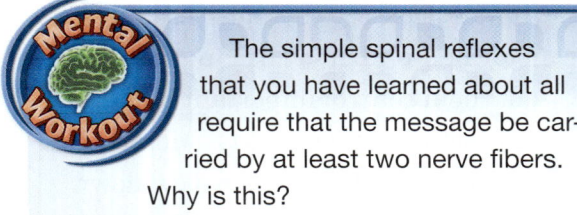

The simple spinal reflexes that you have learned about all require that the message be carried by at least two nerve fibers. Why is this?

Spinal Nerves

The nerves that branch from the central nervous system come in pairs. Each pair contains one nerve on the left side of the body and a matching nerve on the right side. You have a total of forty-three pairs of nerves. Most of these nerves are **spinal nerves**, *nerves that branch from the spinal cord and travel to the muscles and organs.* There are thirty-one pairs of spinal nerves.

Spinal nerves contain both sensory nerve fibers and motor nerve fibers. This means that each spinal nerve carries messages in both directions: from the organs to the CNS and from the CNS to the organs. Sensory nerve fibers in the spinal nerves carry sensations from the skin and muscles. They also carry pain sensations from various internal organs, such as your heart, stomach, and intestines. Motor nerve fibers in the spinal nerves carry messages to the muscles, causing motion. They also carry commands for the automatic function of some internal organs, especially those lower in the body.

Cranial Nerves

You also have twelve pairs of **cranial nerves**, *which branch directly from the brain.* Unlike the spinal nerves, *several of the cranial nerves contain only one type of nerve fiber* (sensory or motor). For example, the olfactory nerve contains sensory nerve fibers that carry messages from your nose to your brain; it does not have any motor nerve fibers that could transmit messages back to the nose. Most cranial nerves connect to parts of your head, face, and neck; but one also connects to the heart, stomach, and intestines to help control their automatic functions.

Stress Management

The way that your body responds to unfamiliar or difficult circumstances is **stress**. Stress is a normal part of life that can be positive or negative. Positive stress comes from adapting to new situations or overcoming challenges; it makes you physically, mentally, and emotionally stronger. Negative stress comes from too much stress or a wrong response to stress; it makes you overwhelmed and worn down. To benefit from stress, you must manage stress appropriately.

Managing stress begins by being ready for stress. A healthy diet and sufficient physical activity and rest will prepare your

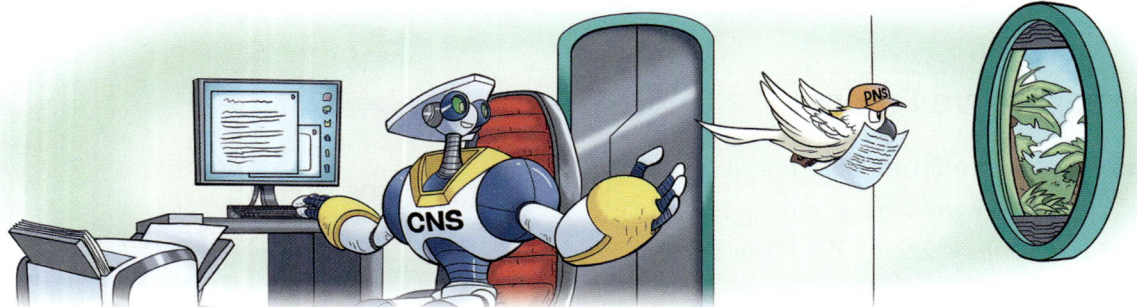

body and mind for challenges. Spending time with family and friends also prepares you for stress. Most importantly, spend time with God by yourself and with your family and church. Learn Scripture promises to apply when stress comes. Negative stress often tempts us to sin by not trusting God. Pray to be kept from this temptation, as Jesus teaches in the Lord's Prayer.

And lead us not into temptation, but deliver us from evil. **Matthew 6:13**

Avoiding all stress is not possible, but you can limit negative stress. For example, someone may dislike crowds. Going to a basketball game can be positive stress if he adapts to this uncomfortable situation. But if he is already stressed, the game can be negative stress that he should try to avoid. Volunteering to help others is good, but volunteering for too many things can become a burden instead of a joy. You do not have to say yes every time someone asks for help. But you must fulfill your own responsibilities, such as homework and chores, and honor your parents and other authorities. It is wrong to use avoiding stress as an excuse to shirk responsibility or disobey.

Plan to respond to stress in a healthy way that helps you grow. Avoid harmful responses such as ignoring the challenge, sulking, or ignoring your emotions. Stress can cause strong emotions; express emotions properly instead of in outbursts. Continue the strategies that helped you prepare for stress. Avoid overeating or bingeing on unhealthy foods. Use physical activity to clear your mind and emotions. Spend time with people who will encourage you. Read the Bible and pray for help to apply Bible promises.

The LORD sitteth upon the flood; yea, the LORD sitteth King for ever. The LORD will give strength unto His people; the LORD will bless His people with peace. **Psalm 29:10–11**

Taking time to pause and relax helps turn negative stress into positive stress. Find a quiet place to close your eyes and take slow, deep breaths. Focus your thoughts on something that comforts you. If possible, take a walk outside or listen to gentle music. Once you are relaxed, make a plan to deal with the challenge causing the stress. If the challenge is having too many activities, consider which are truly important. Maybe you can skip some or give some to someone else without shirking responsibility. Make a schedule to complete the rest. Also seek help from a parent, pastor, or other trusted adult if the challenge proves too difficult to manage yourself.

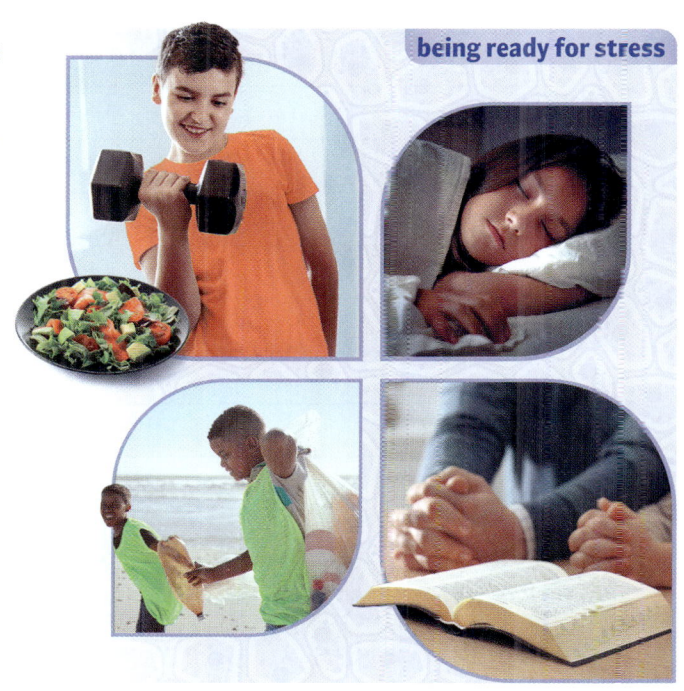

being ready for stress

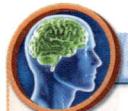

Fill in the Blank: *Write the correct word in the blank.*

1. An organ that transmits messages between the CNS and specific regions of the body is a(n) _____.

2. A nerve is made of bundles of _____.

3. Signals from the body to the CNS are transmitted by _____ nerve fibers.

4. A cell or group of cells that detects a sensation is a(n) _____.

5. Messages from the CNS are delivered to the body by _____ nerve fibers.

6. Nerves that branch from the spinal cord are called _____.

7. Cranial nerves branch from the _____.

8. The way that the body responds to unfamiliar or difficult circumstances is _____.

Think about It.

9. What are three specific steps that you can take in your own life to limit negative stress and to positively deal with unavoidable stress?

_____

_____

_____

_____

_____

_____

_____

_____

_____

_____

_____

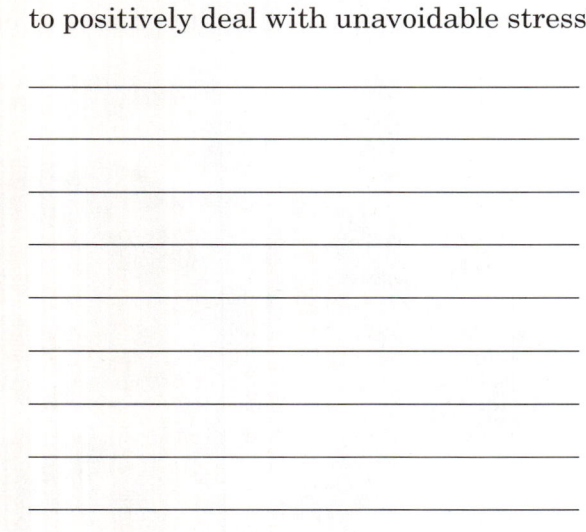
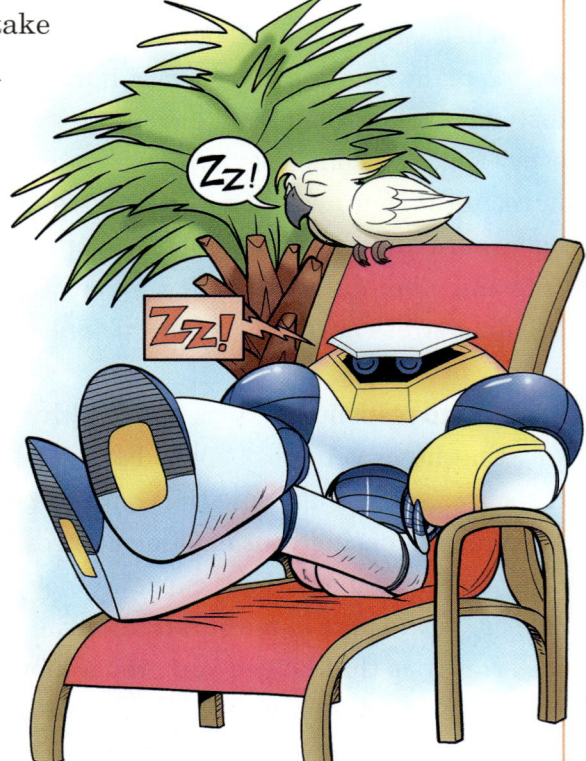

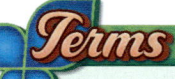

sclera: white of the eye

cornea: transparent front portion of the eye; lets light into the eye

pupil: round hole that lets light into the eye

iris: ring of muscles that surrounds the pupil and controls its size; colored part of the eye

lens: focuses light that enters the eye by refracting it; changes shape to focus on objects at different distances

retina: layer of nerve cells in the back of the eye; contains rod cells and cone cells

optic nerve: cranial nerve that carries messages of sight to the cerebrum

outer ear: division of the ear that consists of the cup-shaped structure on the side of the head and of the auditory canal

auditory canal: tube of the outer ear through which sound waves travel

eardrum: thin piece of tissue that separates the outer ear from the middle ear

middle ear: division of the ear that is a cavity inside the skull; contains three tiny bones: the hammer, the anvil, and the stirrup

inner ear: division of the ear that contains the cochlea and semicircular canals

cochlea: part of the ear that detects sound waves and sends them as messages to the brain

auditory nerve: nerve that carries messages of hearing from the cochlea to the brain

semicircular canals: three inner-ear structures that detect movements of the head; send information that the brain uses to help keep balance

ruptured eardrum: injury of a torn eardrum

3.4 Vision and Hearing

The senses of taste, touch, and smell each have many individual sense receptors. Every receptor individually detects sensations and sends messages to the brain for interpretation. Vision and hearing are more complex because of the wave properties of light and sound. Light waves and sound waves can be reflected and refracted, or bent. The waves can have different frequencies, which you see as different colors of light or hear as different pitches. Since vision and hearing are complex, they each have their own sense organs: the eyes and the ears.

The hearing ear, and the seeing eye, the LORD hath made even both of them.
Proverbs 20:12

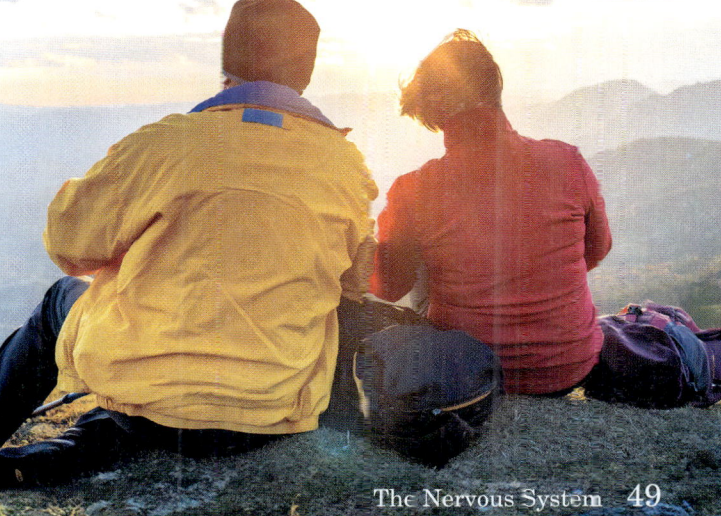

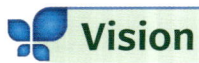 **Vision**

The Structure of the Eye

Each eye is a sphere filled with a jelly-like fluid covered by several layers. The outermost layer consists of the sclera and cornea. The **sclera** is the *white of the eye*; *it forms a tough covering that protects the delicate layers underneath.* The **cornea** is the *transparent front portion of the eye. All light that enters your eye comes through the cornea.*

Behind the cornea are the pupil and iris. The **pupil** looks like a black circle but is actually *a round hole that lets the right amount of light into the eye.* In a bright place, the eye gets more light than needed; your pupil shrinks to let less light in. In dim light, seeing your surroundings requires all the available light; your pupil enlarges to let in as much light as possible. *The size of the pupil is controlled by the* **iris**, *the colored part of the eye.*

The iris is a ring of muscles that surrounds the pupil. These muscles contract and relax to make the pupil larger and smaller.

Just behind the iris is a soft and flexible **lens**, which *focuses the light by refracting, or bending, it.* Muscles pull on the lens to change its shape. *Changing the shape of the lens lets you focus on objects at different distances.*

The light of the body is the eye: therefore when thine eye is single, thy whole body also is full of light; but when thine eye is evil, thy body also is full of darkness. Take heed therefore that the light which is in thee be not darkness. If thy whole body therefore be full of light, having no part dark, the whole shall be full of light, as when the bright shining of a candle doth give thee light. **Luke 11:34–36**

parts of the eye

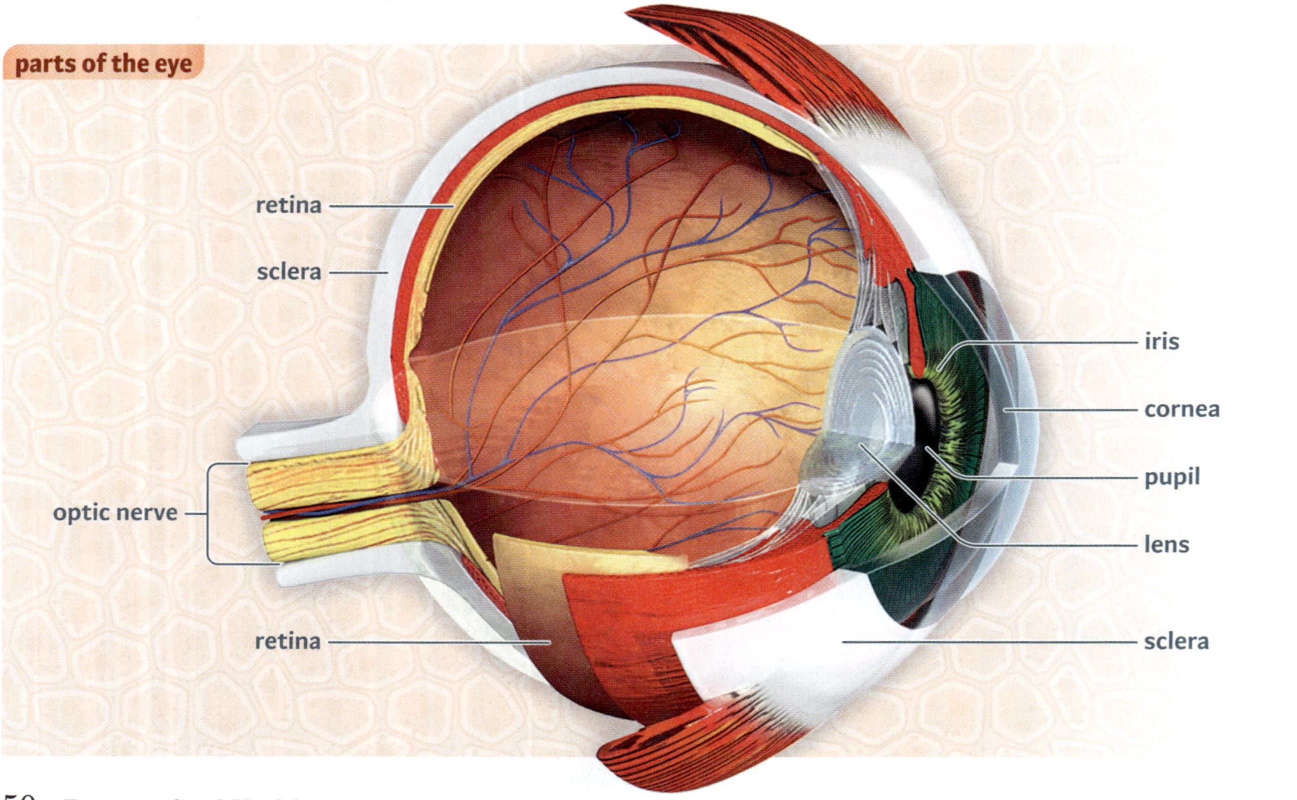

retina

sclera

optic nerve

retina

iris

cornea

pupil

lens

sclera

The lens focuses light onto a *layer of nerve cells* called the **retina**. The retina contains two main types of light-detecting cells. *Cone cells let you see colors*; different cone cells detect different colors of light. *Rod cells do not detect color but are extremely sensitive.* They let you see shapes even in very dim light.

The signals from the rod and cone cells travel through sensory nerve fibers to the back of the eye. There, they are bundled into the **optic nerve**, *the cranial nerve that carries messages of sight to your cerebrum*. Your cerebrum combines and interprets the messages from both eyes and tells your body how to respond to what you see.

Protecting Your Eyes

There are many healthy behaviors that can help protect your vision. The sun's ultraviolet rays, the same rays that cause sunburn, can damage your eyes. You should never look directly at the sun. *On a sunny day, wear sunglasses that block ultraviolet rays.*

Wear safety glasses or safety goggles during sports or other activities in which your eyes could be injured. Cleaning supplies and other dangerous chemicals can permanently harm your vision; wear chemical safety goggles, which protect against splashes, when using these chemicals.

Eyestrain can occur when you spend a long time focusing your eyes on something, most often the screens of electronic devices such as computers and cellphones. *To avoid eyestrain while using electronic devices, doctors recommend the 20-20-20 rule: every 20 minutes, look at an object 20 feet away for 20 seconds.*

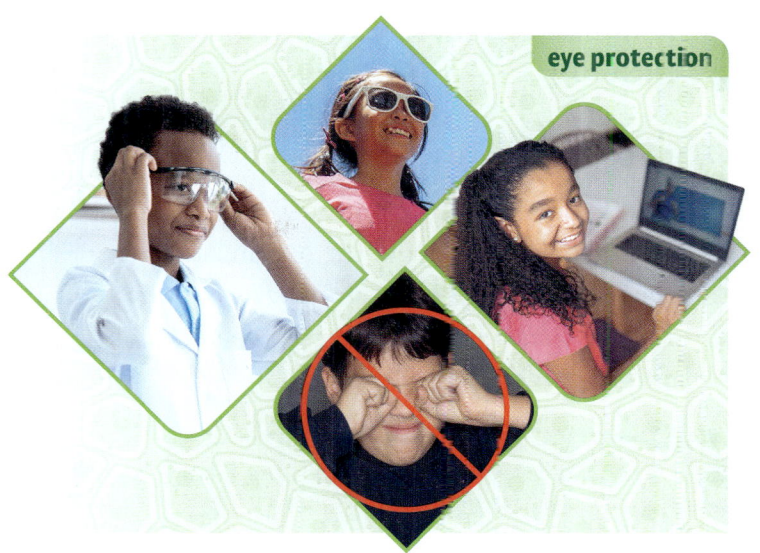

eye protection

To protect your eyes from infection, avoid rubbing or touching your eyes, especially with unwashed hands.

Eye Diseases

The most common eye diseases are nearsightedness, farsightedness, and astigmatism [ə·stĭg′mə·tĭz′əm]. *Nearsightedness* prevents focusing on distant objects, *farsightedness* makes it harder to focus on nearby objects, and *astigmatism* prevents focusing at any distance. Very little can be done to prevent these conditions, but an eye doctor, either an *optometrist* [ŏp·tŏm′ĭ·trĭst] or *ophthalmologist* [ŏf′thəl·mŏl′ə·jĭst], can prescribe glasses or contact lenses to correct the improper focus. An ophthalmologist can also perform surgery to treat some types of eye diseases.

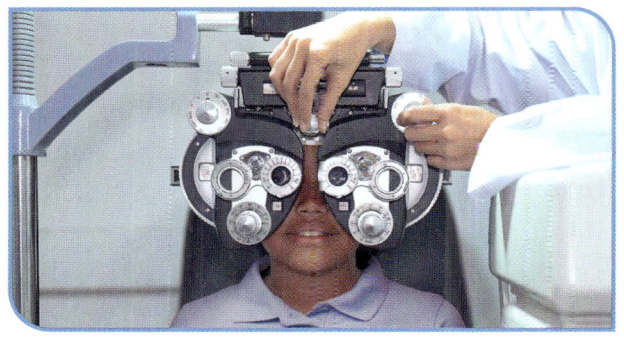

Hearing

The Structure of the Ear

The flexible structure on the side of your head is only a small part of the ear; most of the ear is buried inside the skull. *The ear has three main divisions: the outer ear, the middle ear, and the inner ear.*

For whosoever shall call upon the name of the Lord shall be saved. How then shall they call on Him in Whom they have not believed? and how shall they believe in Him of Whom they have not heard? and how shall they hear without a preacher? . . . So then faith cometh by hearing, and hearing by the Word of God. **Romans 10:13–14, 17**

Most of the **outer ear** is the *flexible, cup-shaped part visible on the side of your head.* God designed this structure perfectly for catching sound waves. *Once the sound waves are caught, they travel down a tube called the* **auditory canal**. *The auditory canal is also part of your outer ear.* The auditory canal produces *earwax* to trap and remove dust and dirt.

At the end of the auditory canal is the **eardrum**, *a thin piece of tissue that separates the outer ear and middle ear.* The eardrum is stretched tight, like a drum, and vibrates when sound waves strike it. These vibrations can then travel to your middle ear.

The **middle ear** is a *cavity inside the skull. In the middle ear are three tiny bones, the hammer, the anvil, and the stirrup, that transmit vibrations from the eardrum to the inner ear. A tube leads from the middle ear to the top of the pharynx.* This tube balances the air pressure on the two sides of the eardrum, making your ears "pop."

The **inner ear** *contains the cochlea and semicircular canals.* The **cochlea** is *the part of the ear that actually detects sound waves and sends them as messages to the brain. It is a spiral-shaped structure filled with liquid.* The bones of the inner ear transmit sound waves to the cochlea, making the liquid vibrate. Special sensory cells inside the cochlea detect the vibrations and generate messages. The **auditory nerve** *carries these messages of hearing to the brain.* The three **semicircular canals** in each ear do not take part in hearing but instead *detect movements of your head.*

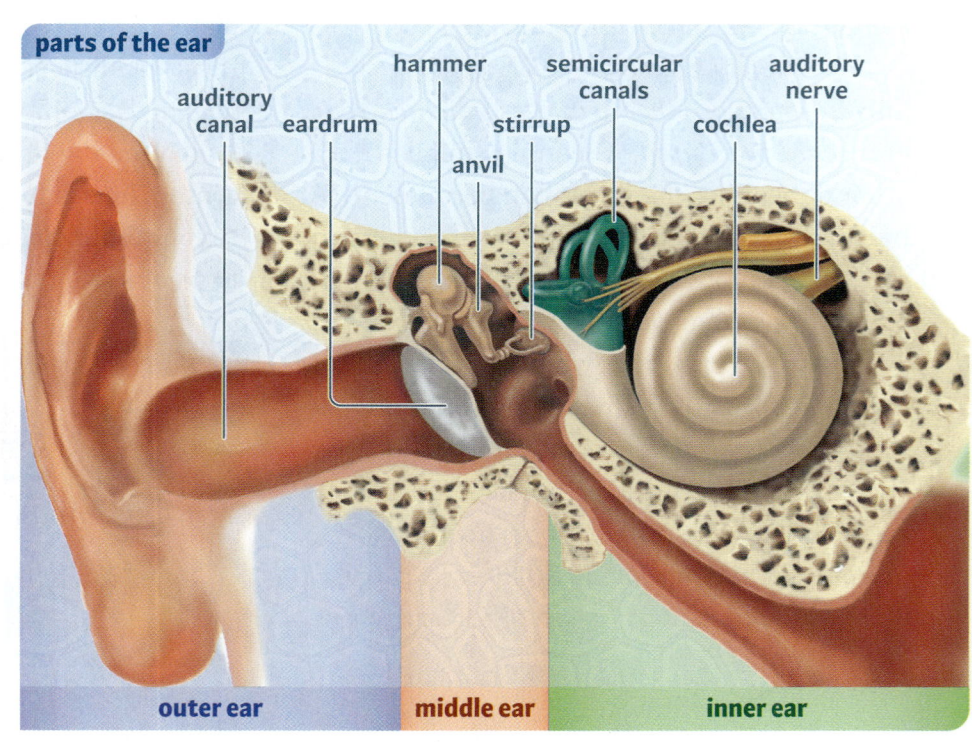

parts of the ear

auditory canal — eardrum — hammer — anvil — stirrup — semicircular canals — cochlea — auditory nerve

outer ear | middle ear | inner ear

Your brain uses the information from the semicircular canals to help keep your balance.

Protecting Your Ears

There are several ways to protect your hearing. Eardrum damage, very loud sounds, and infections can all harm your ears.

An eardrum can be damaged by objects; *the injury of a torn eardrum* is a **ruptured eardrum**. A ruptured eardrum can cause hearing loss and makes your ear more vulnerable to infection. *Protect your eardrums by keeping things out of your ears.* Do not use cotton swabs to clean earwax out of your ears. Ruptured eardrums usually heal on their own but occasionally require surgery.

Over time, *loud sounds can damage the sensory cells in your cochlea, causing permanent hearing loss.* This depends on the volume of the sound and on how long you listen to the sound. A single extremely loud sound and a long period of quieter, but still loud, sound can cause equal damage. Adjust the volume of music to a comfortable listening level. When using headphones or earbuds, set the volume to no louder than 50 to 60 percent of the maximum and take periodic breaks from listening. Wear earplugs or other hearing protection when you are near loud noises, such as lawnmowers, leaf blowers, or fireworks.

Infections of the outer ear can occur if water gets into your ears. This is especially common when you are swimming. To protect your outer ears, tilt your head to the side and let the water run out. Use a towel to gently dry the outside of your ear canal. You can also dry out your ears with a mixture of equal parts vinegar and rubbing alcohol.

A middle-ear infection occurs when fluid builds up in the middle ear and becomes infected. This type of infection occurs most often in children, usually when a respiratory disease, such as a cold or allergies, blocks the tube that connects the middle ear to the pharynx. Therefore, the best way to avoid these infections is to practice good disease-prevention habits. A middle-ear infection usually gets better on its own after a day or two.

Your primary care physician can treat many simple ear illnesses and injuries. For severe injuries or hearing loss, he will probably send you to an *ear, nose, and throat* (ENT) *doctor* or an *audiologist* [ȯ′dē·ŏl′ə·jĭst]. An ear, nose, and throat doctor is a physician who specializes in disorders of those three structures. ENT doctors can prescribe medicine and can perform surgeries, when needed. An audiologist diagnoses problems with hearing and balance, prescribes devices like hearing aids, and recommends other treatments.

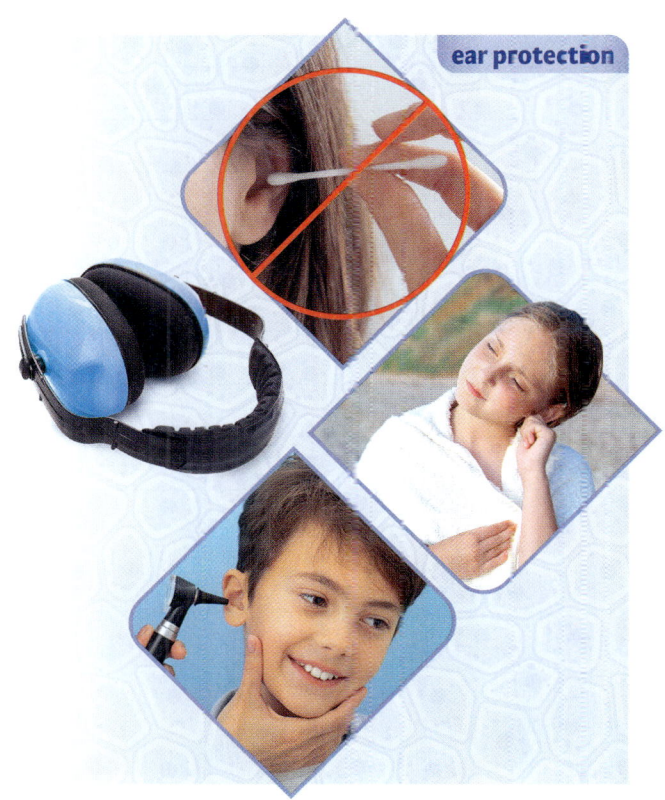

ear protection

Hearing Protection

LIVE IT OUT!

Suppose that your family is going running on a local trail and that you want to listen to music while you run. Use the following questions to make a health decision that will protect your hearing and the hearing of those around you.

1. List at least two options for listening to music on your run. For each option, consider factors like how you will listen to music (a portable speaker, headphones, etc.), the volume, and the style of music (instrumental, vocal, etc.). _____

_____

_____

_____

_____

2. For each option, explain how it will likely affect your health. _____

_____

_____

_____

_____

_____

_____

_____

_____

_____

_____

3. For each option, explain how it will affect others around you. _____

_____

_____

_____

_____

_____

_____

_____

_____

_____

_____

_____

_____

4. Choose one option to use for your run. Explain your choice. _____

_____

_____

_____

_____

_____

_____

Community HEALTH CORNER

Noise Pollution

Modern technology like cars, airplanes, lawnmowers, and factory machines can produce a great amount of unwanted sound, or *noise*. Excessive noise becomes noise pollution. Like any loud sounds, noise pollution can cause temporary or permanent hearing loss. But noise pollution can also affect other parts of the body. It has been linked to various diseases of the circulatory system. It can cause stress and poor sleeping. It can cause problems with thinking and learning. Noise pollution also harms animals, especially those that use echolocation (making sounds and listening for the echoes) to navigate or find prey.

You can do some things to reduce how noise pollution affects you. First, avoid loud noises when possible. Wear hearing protection when using loud equipment like lawnmowers and leaf blowers. You can also limit the effect of noise when you are trying to sleep or study. Turn off distracting background noises and music, and use earplugs or noise-canceling headphones if there are sounds that you cannot get rid of. Many people find quiet instrumental music, nature sounds, or white noise (sound that contains the entire pitch range of human hearing at a constant volume) to be relaxing for sleep. If you use background sounds to help yourself sleep, keep the volume low to prevent distraction and hearing damage.

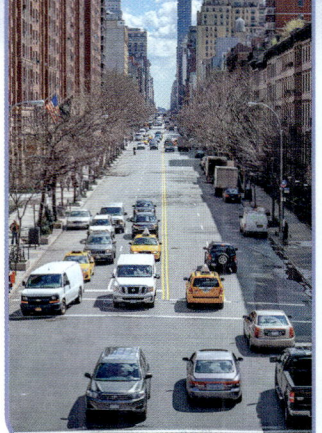
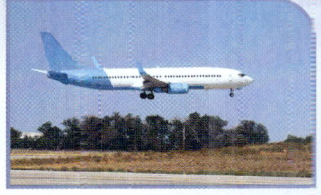
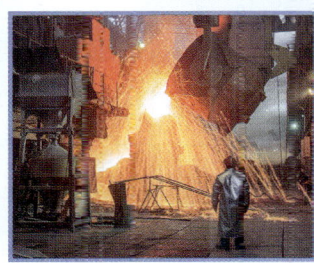

Because there are various sources of noise pollution, reducing noise pollution requires community efforts. Engineers can design cars, airplanes, and other machines in ways that reduce the noise produced. Walls or embankments (long hills) can be used to protect surrounding areas from the noise of highways and railroads. Businesses and individuals can also switch to quieter equipment; for example, electric cars and lawnmowers are much quieter than their gas-powered equivalents and therefore cause less noise pollution. Buildings can use materials that block unwanted sounds. What are some sources of noise pollution that affect your family and community? What are some ways that your community can work together to reduce these sources of noise pollution?

Identify: *Label the parts of the eye.*

1. _____
2. _____
3. _____
4. _____
5. _____
6. _____
7. _____

Short Answer: *Write the correct answer in the blank.*

8. What part of the eye forms a tough outer covering? _____

9. What part of the eye has muscles that change the size of the pupil? _____

10. What are the two main types of light-detecting cells in the retina? Which one allows you to see color? _____

11. What should you do to avoid eyestrain while using a computer, phone, or other device? _____

_____

12. What are the two types of eye doctors? _____

_____

13. What separates the outer ear from the middle ear? _____

14. Why are loud noises dangerous, especially when listened to for a long time? _____

_____

_____

Classify: *Write O for outer ear, M for middle ear, and I for inner ear.*

_____ 15. contains the hammer, the anvil, and the stirrup

_____ 16. includes the cochlea

_____ 17. includes the auditory canal

_____ 18. includes the semicircular canals

_____ 19. includes the cup-shaped structure on the side of the head

_____ 20. connected to the pharynx by a tube

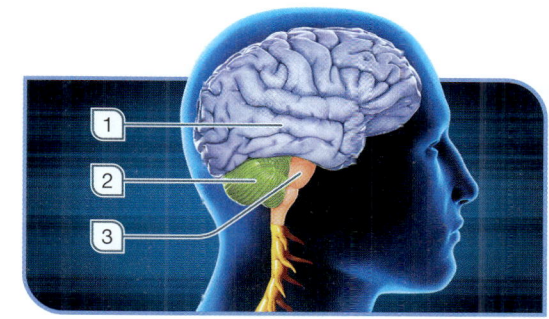

Concepts Review

Chapter 3

1 Neurology (3.1)

Fill in the Blank: *Write the correct word or phrase in the blank.*

1. Coordination and communication of the body parts is the job of the

   _____ system.

2. The medical study of the nervous system is called _____.

3. The abbreviation CNS stands for _____.

4. The nerves make up the _____ nervous system.

5. A neuron's nucleus and organelles are in the _____.

6. The long, straight part of a neuron that transmits messages to other cells is the

   _____.

2 Central Nervous System (3.2)

A. Identify: *Label the main parts of the brain.*

1. _____

2. _____

3. _____

B. Multiple Choice: *Write the letter of the correct answer in the blank.*

_____ 1. What part of the brain controls balance and the coordination of
   voluntary muscles?
   a. brain stem
   b. cerebellum
   c. cerebrum
   d. limbic system

_____ 2. To what part of the brain does the spinal cord attach?
   a. brain stem
   b. cerebellum
   c. cerebrum
   d. limbic system

_____ 3. What is a quick, automatic action that the body does in response to
   something else?
   a. axon
   b. desire
   c. reflex
   d. stress

(continued)

C. Write.

Explain how the brain's emotional reward system affects your desires. What should you do before acting on desires? _____

_____

_____

_____

_____

_____

_____

3 Peripheral Nervous System (3.3)

A. Short Answer: *Write the correct answer in the blank.*

1. What type of organ is made of a bundle of nerve fibers? _____

2. Which type of nerve fiber carries messages from sense receptors to the brain?

    _____

3. What is stress? _____

    _____

B. Think!

What are two differences between spinal nerves and cranial nerves? _____

_____

_____

_____

_____

4 Vision and Hearing (3.4)

A. True/False: *If the statement is true, write* true *in the blank. If the statement is false, replace the underlined word with a word that will make the statement true. Do not write* false *in any blank.*

_____ 1. The white of the eye is the <u>cornea</u>.

_____ 2. The round hole that lets the right amount of light into the eye is the <u>iris</u>.

_____ 3. Cone cells and rod cells are found in the <u>lens</u>.

_____ 4. Vision messages from the eye travel to the brain through the <u>optic</u> nerve.

_____ 5. The hammer, anvil, and stirrup are parts of the <u>inner</u> ear.

_____ 6. The ear structures that help you keep your balance are the <u>auditory</u> canals.

B. Short Answer: *Write the correct answer in the blank.*

1. What two parts form the outermost layer of the eye? _____

2. How does the lens of the eye let you focus on objects at different distances?

   _____

   _____

3. List three health behaviors that can help protect your vision. _____

   _____

   _____

   _____

   _____

   _____

4. Why should you <u>not</u> use cotton swabs to clean your ears?

   _____

   _____

   _____

   _____

   _____

continued

C. Identify: *Label the parts of the ear.*

1. _____
2. _____
3. _____
   _____
4. _____
5. _____
6. _____
7. _____
8. _____
9. _____

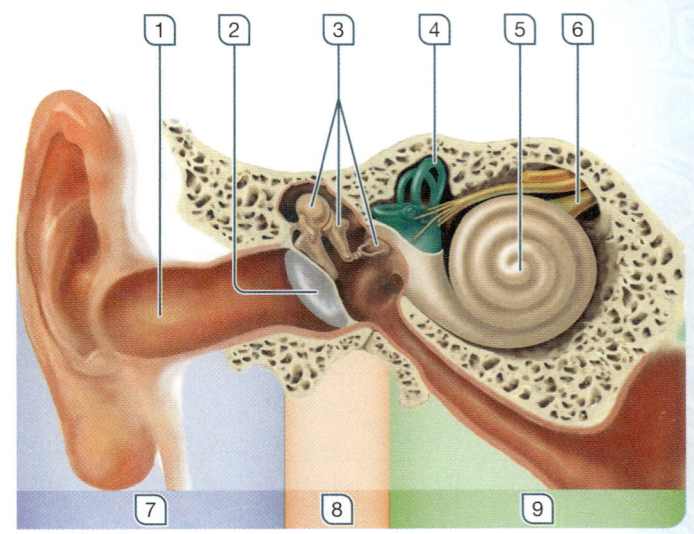

D. Think!

Georgia's older brother Daniel mowed the lawn using a gas-powered lawnmower. He did not wear any hearing protection while mowing. When he came inside, he complained that his ears were ringing. What harmful health behavior did Daniel practice? How can Georgia encourage him to practice good health behaviors? _____

_____
_____
_____
_____
_____
_____

5 Nervous System Review (3.1–3.4)

A. Concept Map: *Use the terms in the box to fill out the graphic organizer.*

brain	ears	nervous system	spinal cord
central nervous system	eyes	peripheral nervous system	spinal nerves
cranial nerves	nerves	sense organs	

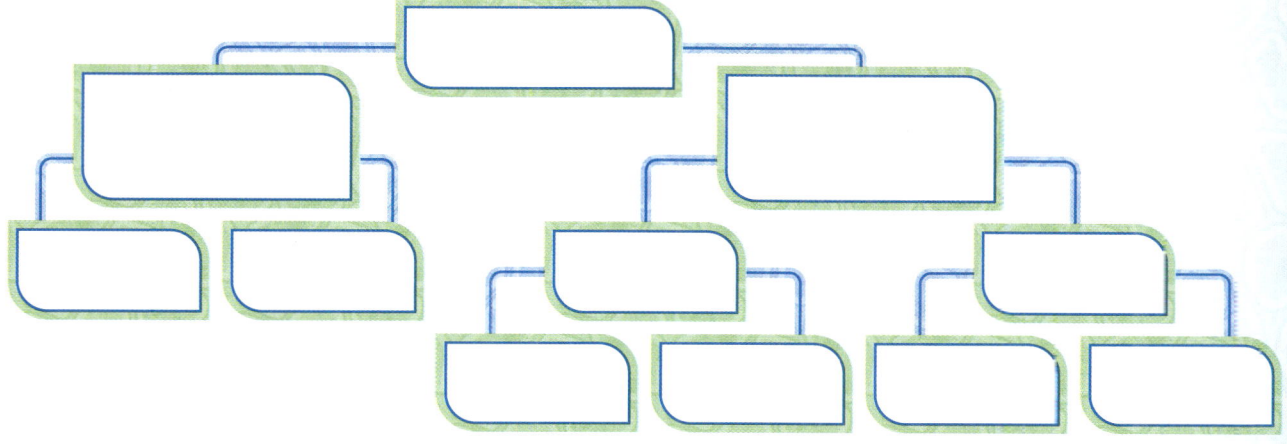

B. Puzzle: *Fill in the answers to find the phrase in the starred column.*

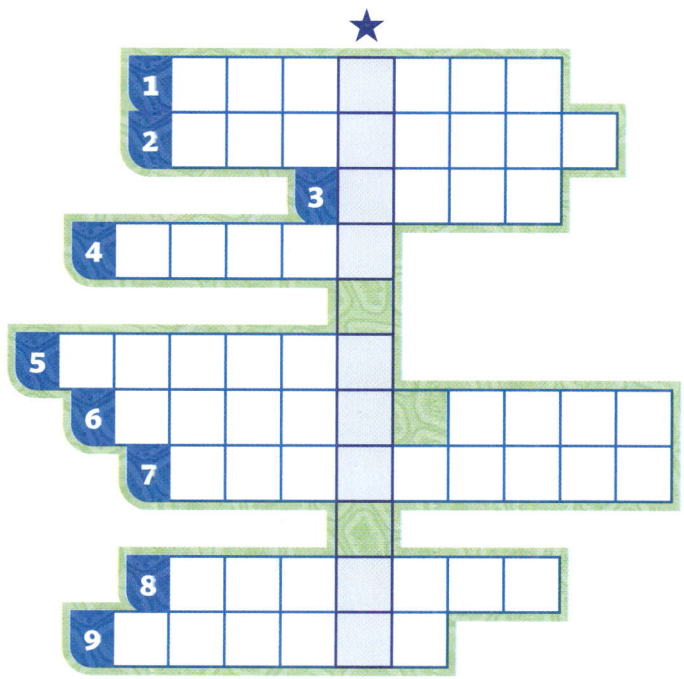

1. spiral-shaped structure of the inner ear
2. part of the brain that controls thinking and reasoning
3. long, straight part of a nerve cell
4. type of nerve fiber that controls some part of the body
5. layer of nerve cells in the back of the eye
6. part of the brain that controls involuntary functions
7. many short, branching parts that extend from a nerve cell's cell body
8. thin piece of tissue that separates the outer ear from the middle ear
9. nerve cell

★ James 1:22–25 says that we should do this with God's Word.

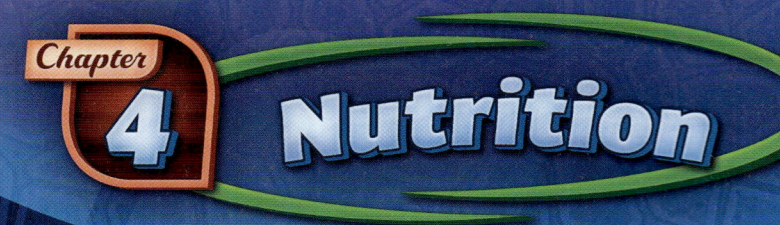

Chapter 4 — Nutrition

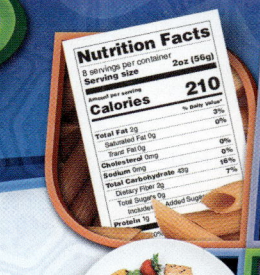

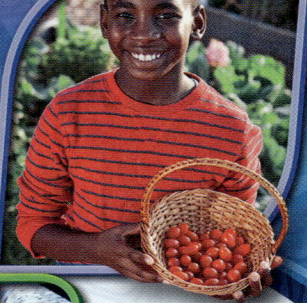

Terms

nutrients: substances in food that the body uses to grow, have energy, and stay healthy

macronutrients: nutrients that the body needs in relatively large amounts; can be used by the body as sources of energy

carbohydrates: group of macronutrients that includes sugars and starches; the body's main source of energy

simple carbohydrates: sugars; have molecules that are small and relatively simple

complex carbohydrates: large molecules made of many connected sugar molecules; also called starches

fiber: carbohydrates that the body cannot break down and absorb

protein: macronutrients that provide material for body growth and repair

fats: nutrients that help the body to store energy, make cell parts, and use certain vitamins

saturated fats: fats that are usually solid at room temperature

unsaturated fat: fats that are liquid at room temperature; found in oils

hydrogenated oil: unsaturated vegetable oil that has had hydrogen atoms added to make the oil more solid

4.1 Macronutrients

All movement of your body requires energy. Your cells also need various materials to grow, repair themselves, and produce substances. Your body gets most of the materials it needs through the food you eat. *The substances in food that your body uses to grow, have energy, and stay healthy* are **nutrients**. Your body needs just the right amount of each nutrient. Healthy eating habits ensure that your body gets the nutrients it needs but does not get more nutrients than it can use.

Nutrients are divided into two main groups: macronutrients and micronutrients. **Macronutrients** are *nutrients that your body needs in relatively large amounts. Macronutrients are also the nutrients that your body can use as sources of energy.* The three main types of macronutrients are carbohydrates, proteins, and fats.

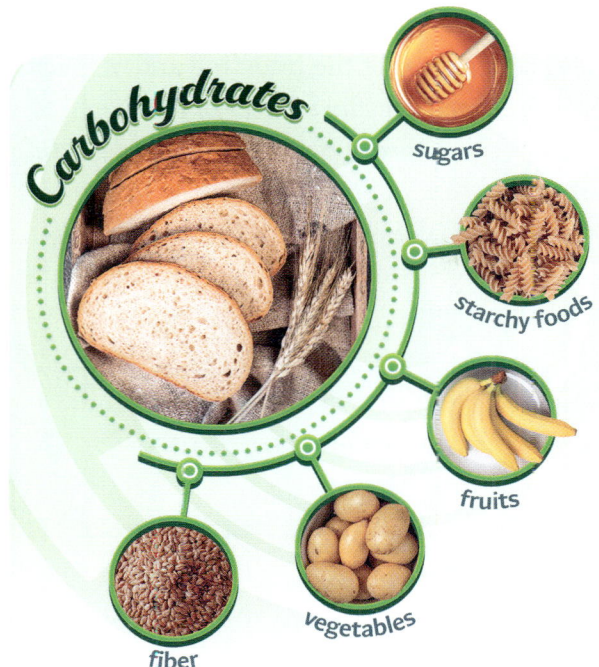

Carbohydrates
- sugars
- starchy foods
- fruits
- vegetables
- fiber

Carbohydrates

Carbohydrates are *a group of macronutrients that includes sugars and starches. Carbohydrates are your body's main source of energy.* Do you enjoy sugary foods such as honey, syrups, cookies, and fruits? What about the starchy foods like potatoes, bread, noodles, and rice? All of these foods contain carbohydrates.

Sugars are called **simple carbohydrates** *because their molecules are small and relatively simple.* Common sugars that you may eat are *glucose* (found in honey and most plant foods), *fructose* (found in fruits and vegetables), *lactose* (found in milk), *maltose* (found in wheat, corn, rice, and oats), and *sucrose* (table sugar; found in sugar beets and sugarcane). Processed foods, such as many prepackaged snacks and frozen meals, and candy also contain large amounts of simple carbohydrates, often as high-fructose corn syrup.

Your body can easily digest and absorb simple carbohydrates. *Simple carbohydrates give your body quick energy that does not last.*

You may feel energetic after eating a candy bar but then feel tired again after a few hours. You may have mood changes, feel exhausted, and have difficulty concentrating. This condition is sometimes called a sugar crash. Because of your body's response to simple carbohydrates, it is unhealthy to eat too much of them. Sugary treats are enjoyable in moderation but are not the best fuel for daily energy. Foods like fruits, vegetables, milk, and grains contain some simple carbohydrates, but they mostly consist of other types of nutrients.

Complex carbohydrates *have large molecules made of many connected sugar molecules.* Complex carbohydrates are also called *starches.* Starches are found in all fruits and vegetables. *Especially rich sources of starches are grains and root vegetables, including potatoes, sweet potatoes, and carrots.*

Before your body can use complex carbohydrates, it must break them down into simple carbohydrates. This means that *complex carbohydrates give your body a steady supply of energy that lasts for a long period of time.* Complex carbohydrates are the best fuel for daily energy because they give you long-lasting energy.

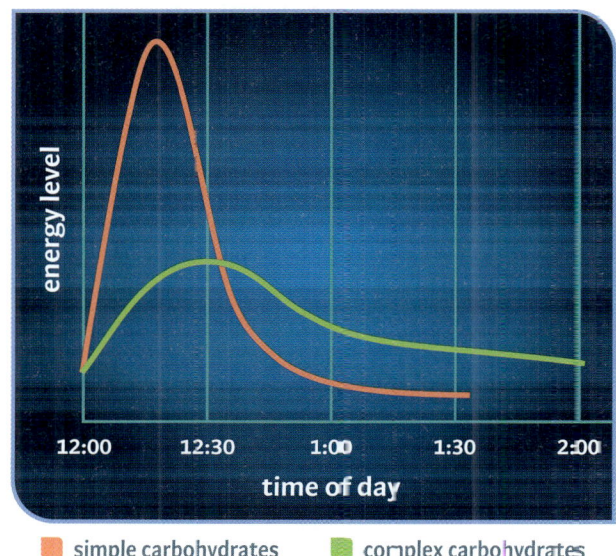

■ simple carbohydrates ■ complex carbohydrates

Fiber *consists of carbohydrates that your body cannot break down and absorb. Although fiber does not provide any energy, it is still an important nutrient for health.* Fiber helps clean out the digestive tract. It also reduces the risk of cancer of the intestine and of heart disease. *Some healthy sources of fiber are oatmeal; whole-grain bread; legumes, including peas, beans, and lentils; flaxseed; cauliflower; broccoli; and blackberries.*

Build-It-Yourself Baked Potato Bar

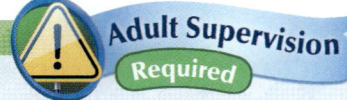
Adult Supervision Required

Baked potatoes are a good source of complex carbohydrates. This recipe lets four people customize this healthy meal option to their own preferences.

Be aware of allergies or sensitivities before you handle or eat food.

Ingredients:

- four medium-sized russet potatoes
- bell peppers, chopped
- jalapeño peppers, sliced
- lettuce, shredded
- green onions, chopped
- red onions, chopped
- tomatoes, diced
- cheese, shredded*
- cooked black beans
- cooked chicken, shredded
- plain Greek yogurt

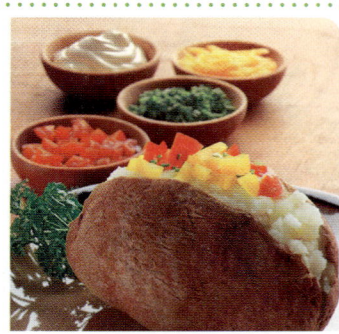

*For variety, have several types of shredded cheese available.

Directions:

1. Clean the potatoes with a vegetable scrubber or kitchen sponge.

2. Poke each potato several times with a fork to make holes in the skin.

3. With an adult's help, microwave the potatoes on high for 12 minutes. If they are not tender, microwave them for another minute.

4. While the potatoes cook, put each topping in a bowl with a serving spoon. Keep cold toppings refrigerated until you are ready to serve the potatoes.

5. With an adult's help, use a knife to slice each potato lengthwise.

6. Set up a serving line with the potatoes at the start and the toppings laid out attractively.

7. Enjoy with your family.

Build on TRUTH

Your health includes both body and spirit. Your body needs physical food, but you must not neglect to feed your spirit on the Word of God. The health of your spirit depends on hearing the Word of God and receiving it in repentance and faith.

Man doth not live by bread only, but by every word that proceedeth out of the mouth of the LORD doth man live.
Deuteronomy 8:3

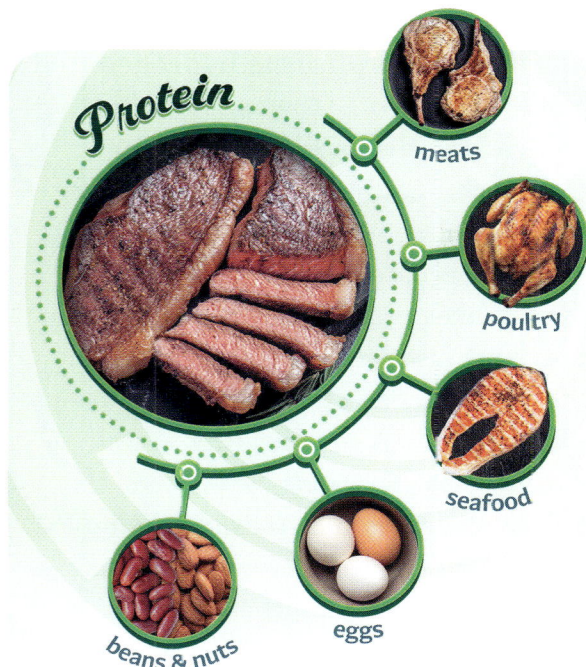

Protein

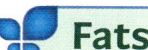
meats

poultry

seafood

eggs

beans & nuts

Protein

Proteins are *macronutrients that provide material for body growth and repair.* Every cell of your body uses proteins to repair and replace worn out components. *Proteins are also used to build and repair muscles.* If you are growing rapidly, you need extra protein. Protein also helps keep your body well; if you are sick, your body needs extra protein to fight the infection and heal itself. Whenever you are involved in strenuous or long-endurance activities, you also need additional protein. Although your body can also use protein for energy, a healthy diet gets most of the body's energy from carbohydrates and fats. This leaves protein available to be used for growth and repair. *Some foods high in protein are meats, poultry, seafood, eggs, beans, and nuts.*

You need to eat protein foods every day. Your body can use the protein better when it is divided among three meals, rather than being eaten all at one time. *You need some protein food at every meal.* Your breakfast should contain protein to sustain your active body throughout the day. While you are in school, protein foods help keep your mind alert so that you can think better. Proteins that you eat at your evening meal are used at night while you sleep to repair and build your body cells. You do most of your growing while you are asleep.

Fats

Lipids [lĭp′ĭdz] *are macronutrients that do not dissolve in water. The main lipids that we eat* are **fats**, *which help the body store energy, make cell parts, and use certain vitamins. Oils are fats that are liquid at room temperature.* Fats and oils provide about twice as much energy as carbohydrates; however, carbohydrate foods should be your primary source of energy because they are converted into energy more quickly than fats.

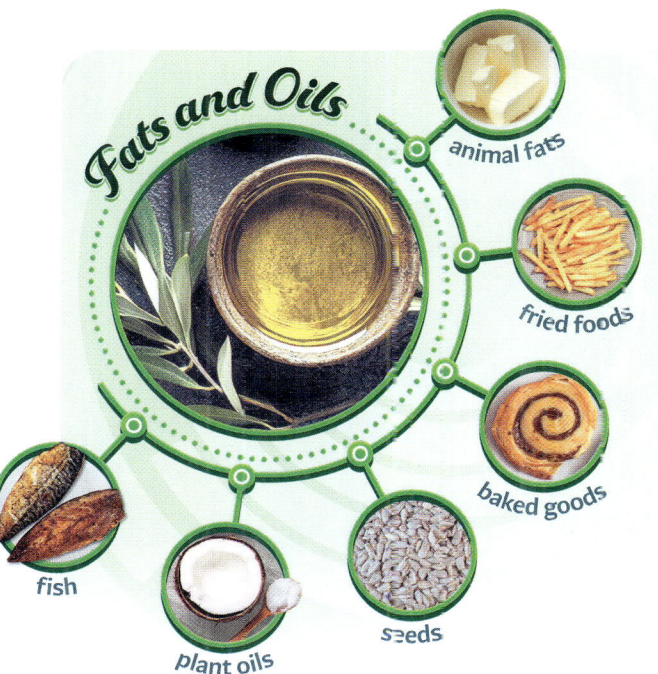

Fats and Oils

animal fats

fried foods

baked goods

seeds

plant oils

fish

There are two main kinds of fats: *saturated fats and unsaturated fats*. **Saturated fats** are *usually solid at room temperature*. They are found in foods from animals, such as beef, pork, poultry, and butter. Coconut oil and palm oil are plant sources of saturated fat. Sometimes saturated fats are used to make fried foods, like french fries, or baked goods, such as pastries and cookies. Saturated fats should be eaten only in moderation. Too much saturated fat in the body is not healthy. Saturated fats raise the amount of *cholesterol* (another lipid) in your blood. Although your body needs some cholesterol, *your liver makes all the cholesterol you need*. The extra cholesterol caused by saturated fats can lead to health problems, including heart disease and stroke. Remember that layers of cholesterol can gradually build up in the arteries and restrict blood flow, a condition called *atherosclerosis*.

Oils mostly contain **unsaturated fats**, which *are liquid at room temperature*. Unsaturated fats are generally healthier than saturated fats; *most of the fat you eat should be unsaturated fats*. Good sources of unsaturated fats are plant seeds, vegetable oils, and fish.

Hydrogen atoms can be added to unsaturated vegetable oils to make the oils more solid; this process produces **hydrogenated** [hī′drə·jə·nāt′əd] **oil**. The more hydrogen that is added, the harder the oil becomes and the more saturated it becomes. Margarine and vegetable shortening are made from hydrogenated oil. Processed foods like cookies, cakes, crackers, granola bars, and candy bars also contain hydrogenated oil.

Too much of any type of fat, even unsaturated fat, can be unhealthy. *If you frequently eat fried foods, fatty meats, cinnamon rolls, cakes, pies, cookies, or candy bars, you are eating too much fat.* To have a healthy fat intake, limit the amount of fried foods that you eat. Choose foods that are sautéed, steamed, grilled, or air fried instead of foods fried in fat or oil. Pan frying is healthier than deep frying because less oil is used. Regardless of the cooking method, choose lean meats when possible—either naturally lean meats such as chicken and turkey or lean cuts of meats such as beef and pork. Trim excess fat off of chops and steaks. When cooking or baking, use vegetable oils when possible; limit your use of animal fats like butter and lard and hydrogenated oils like margarine and shortening. Avoid processed foods, which often contain unhealthy amounts of sugar, salt, and hydrogenated oil.

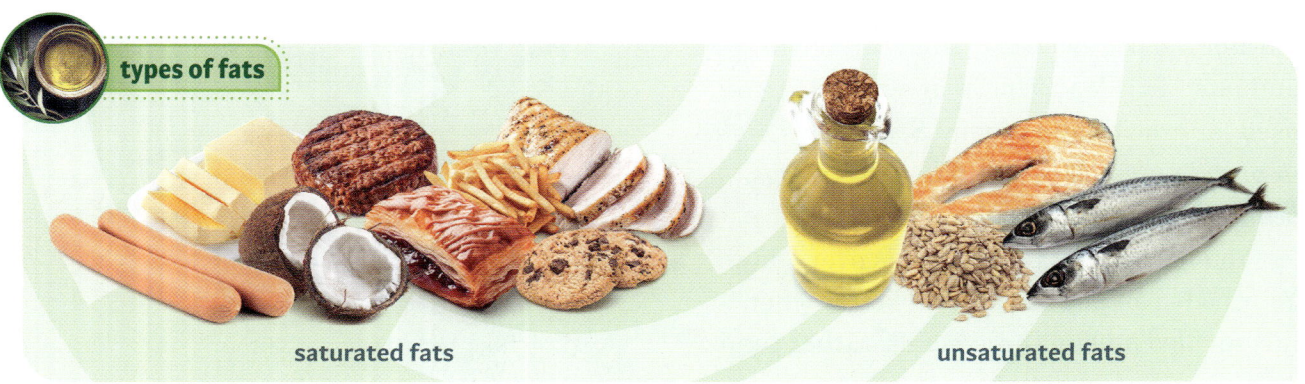

types of fats

saturated fats

unsaturated fats

Dietitian

Your local community offers resources to support healthy eating habits. Medical professionals can work with you and your parents to make wise decisions about nutrition. Dietitians are medical professionals who work with the community to evaluate individual nutritional needs, develop nutrition plans, and meet nutritional goals. Dietitians can serve their community in many ways. A clinical dietitian helps with the nutritional needs of people in places like hospitals and nursing homes, while a management dietitian might oversee meal planning in institutions like cafeterias. If you need someone to help with your personal nutritional goals, you will need to find a consultant dietitian. Other dietitians perform research or work for the government.

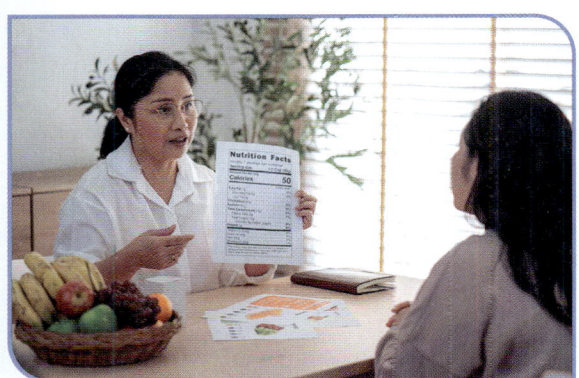

Know ye not that ye are the temple of God, and that the Spirit of God dwelleth in you? **1 Corinthians 3:16**

LIVE IT OUT!

Identifying Macronutrients

List five of the foods that you have eaten in the last 24 hours. For each food, place a check mark ✓ in the box for each type of nutrient it contains a large amount of.

Food	Sugar	Starch	Fiber	Protein	Saturated Fat	Unsaturated Fat
_____	☐	☐	☐	☐	☐	☐
_____	☐	☐	☐	☐	☐	☐
_____	☐	☐	☐	☐	☐	☐
_____	☐	☐	☐	☐	☐	☐
_____	☐	☐	☐	☐	☐	☐

Are there any foods that you can replace with healthier options? If so, which ones?

_____

_____

_____

Classify: *Write* C *for carbohydrates,* P *for proteins, and* F *for fats.*

_____ 1. present in unhealthy amounts in fried foods

_____ 2. used for growth and repair

_____ 3. sugars and starches

_____ 4. good sources include meats, poultry, seafood, eggs, beans, and nuts

_____ 5. help your body to store energy, make cell parts, and use certain vitamins

_____ 6. the body's main source of energy

_____ 7. the main lipids that we eat

Short Answer: *Write the correct answer in the blank.*

8. What are macronutrients? _____

_____

9. What are the three main types of carbohydrates? Which type provides long-lasting energy? _____

_____

10. Why is fiber important to the body? _____

_____

_____

11. What are the two main types of fats? Which type should most of the fat you eat be?

_____

12. Why are vegetable oils processed to make hydrogenated oil? _____

_____

Think about It.

13. Your parents have scheduled a big family yard-work day. What can you eat for breakfast to help you work well? Why? _____

_____

_____

_____

_____

_____

4.2 Micronutrients

Besides macronutrients, you also need **micronutrients** in your diet. Micronutrients are *substances that are needed by the body in small amounts to help protect the body systems and help them work properly.* The two types of micronutrients are vitamins and minerals.

Vitamins

Vitamins are *micronutrients manufactured by living things in their body cells; vitamins support the normal function and development of the body's systems.* Although vitamins do not supply energy, many help the body use energy. Some act as *antioxidants* [ăn′tē·ŏk′sĭ·dənts], *substances that protect cells from damage by harmful molecules.* You must eat a variety of foods to get the vitamins your body needs.

Vitamins are divided into two groups. **Water-soluble vitamins** are *easily eliminated from the body and must be eaten every day.* Vitamin C and the B-complex vitamins are water-soluble vitamins. **Fat-soluble vitamins** can be stored in your body. They include vitamins A, D, E, and K. The fat from food helps your body absorb these vitamins and circulate them throughout the body.

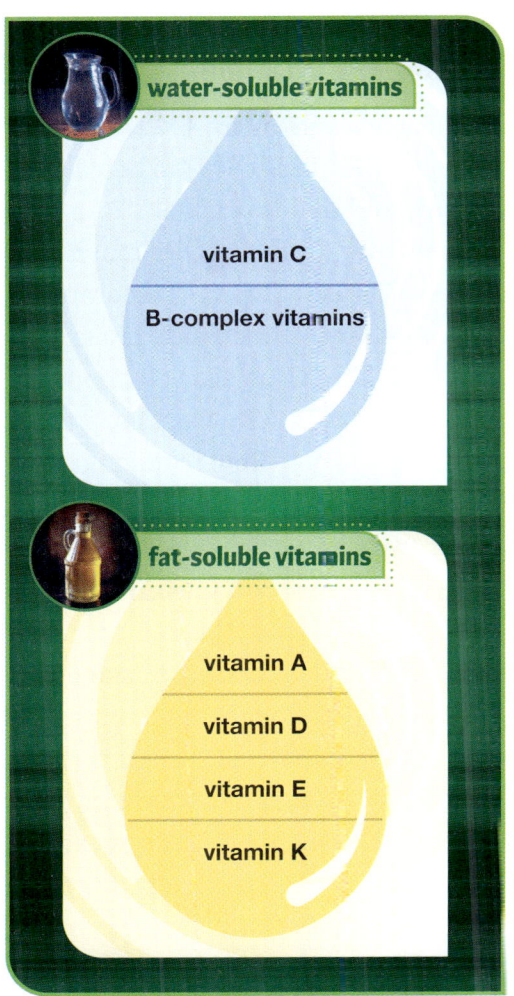

water-soluble vitamins

vitamin C

B-complex vitamins

fat-soluble vitamins

vitamin A

vitamin D

vitamin E

vitamin K

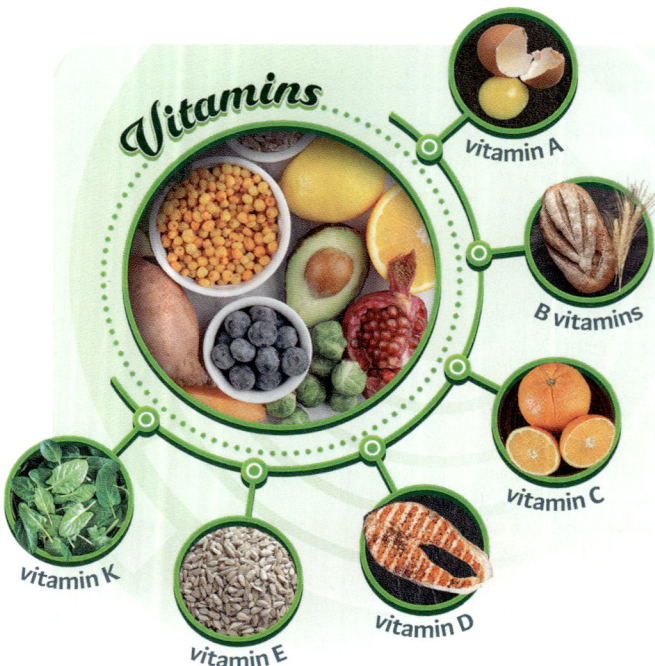

Vitamins

vitamin A

B vitamins

vitamin C

vitamin D

vitamin E

vitamin K

Fat-Soluble Vitamins

Vitamin A in the form the body uses is found only in animal foods, but *your body can also make* **vitamin A** *from* **carotene** [kăr′ə·tēn′]*, a chemical found in green or deep-yellow fruits and vegetables.* Salmon, egg yolks, butter, carrots, spinach, and bell peppers are good sources of vitamin A or carotene. *Vitamin A helps keep your eyes and skin healthy. Your immune system and skeletal system also depend on vitamin A for fighting infections and maintaining healthy bone growth.* Some evidence suggests that foods rich in carotene can help prevent cancer.

Your body makes **vitamin D** *when rays of sunlight fall on your skin*, but you also need to eat foods that contain this vitamin. *Receiving enough vitamin D builds strong bones and teeth. A lack of vitamin D can cause rickets, a disease in which the bones soften and may even bend*, producing irregular growth and deformities. Vitamin D is also needed to absorb the minerals calcium and iron. Because of its importance, vitamin D is added to milk and some milk products. Fish and egg yolks are natural sources of vitamin D.

Vitamin E *protects cells from damage and helps the body use nutrients from food.* Burns and wounds can be healed when vitamin E is applied. Vitamin E is also an antioxidant. Some good sources of vitamin E are sunflower seeds, almonds, peanuts, hazelnuts, mangoes, avocados, and dark, leafy greens.

Water-Soluble Vitamins

The body uses **vitamin C** *to resist and fight infection.* Vitamin C also helps the body repair and maintain itself. It is an antioxidant that protects cells from harmful molecules. Citrus fruits, such as oranges, lemons, limes, and grapefruits, are excellent sources of vitamin C, as are bell peppers, broccoli, cauliflower, strawberries, pineapples, and papayas. Raw fruits and vegetables contain more vitamin C than canned, cooked, or frozen ones.

The eight **B-complex vitamins**, *or B vitamins, help to digest food and use it for energy.* They also help make healthy cells and tissues. Your circulatory and nervous systems need B vitamins to function well. Liver is the only single food containing all the B vitamins; you can also get all of them by eating a variety of whole-wheat foods, oatmeal, poultry, fish, nuts, eggs, and dairy foods.

types of vitamins

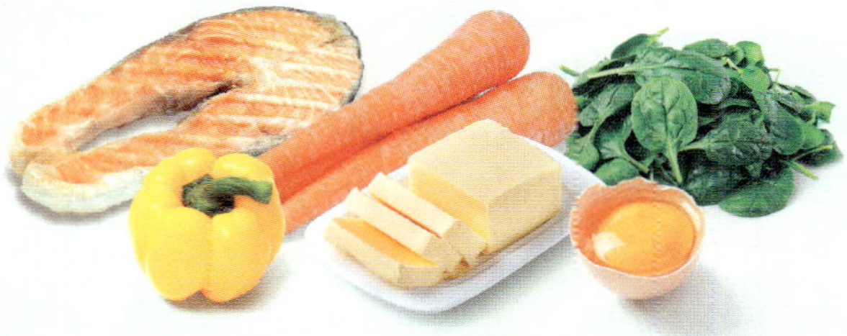

vitamin A
keeps eyes and skin healthy

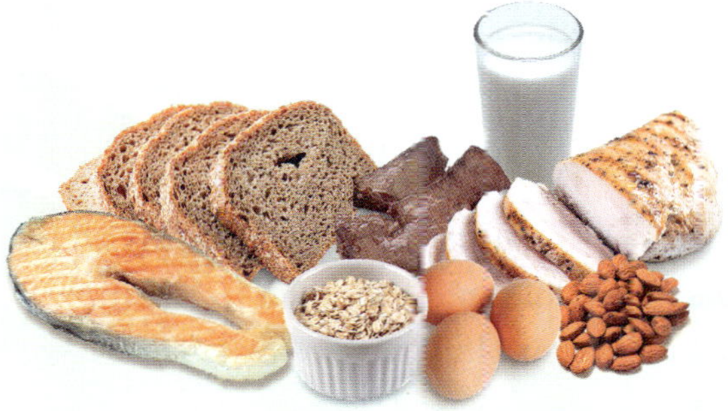

B vitamins
helps the body use food for energy

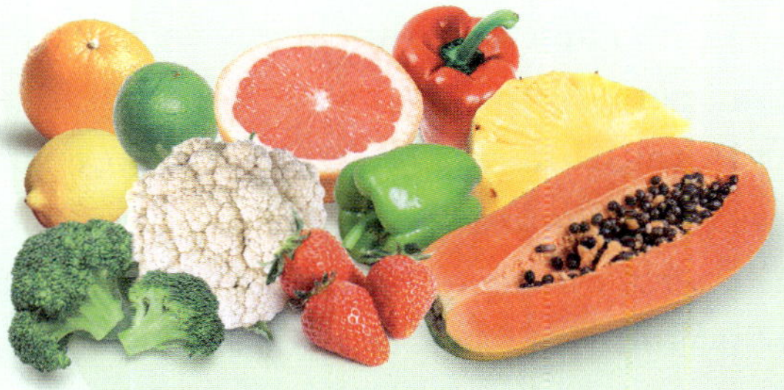

vitamin C
resists and fights infection

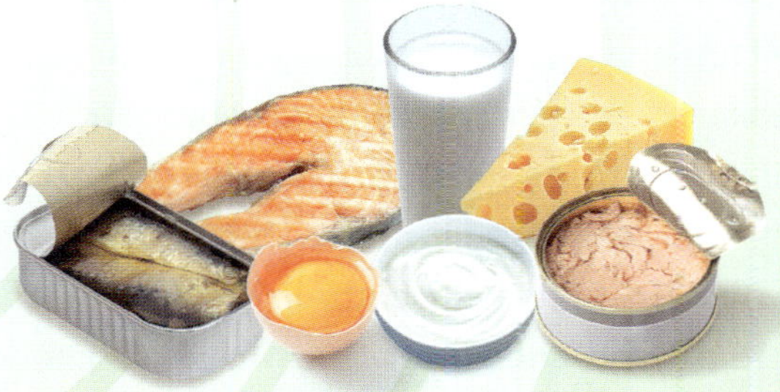

vitamin D
builds strong bones and teeth

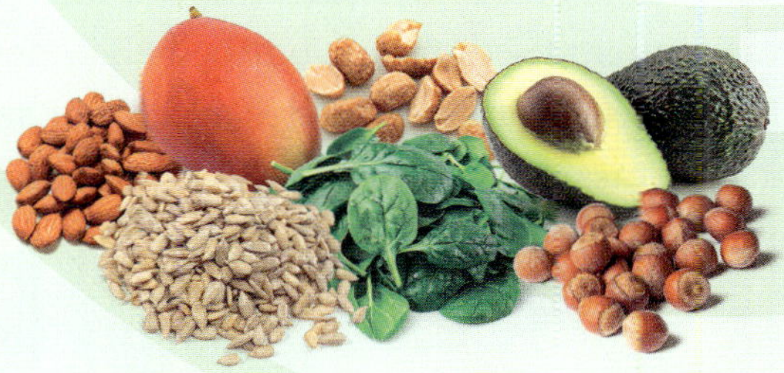

vitamin E
protects cells from damage

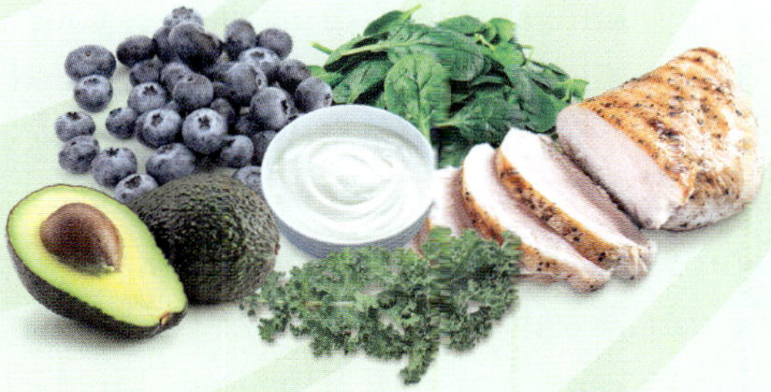

vitamin K
helps blood to clot

When you get a cut or scrape, **vitamin K** *stops the bleeding by helping your blood to clot.* The body can make some vitamin K, but it is also important to get this vitamin from foods. Dark, leafy greens are the best sources; some other food sources are chicken, avocados, and blueberries. Yogurt contains no vitamin K but contains bacteria that make vitamin K in your large intestine.

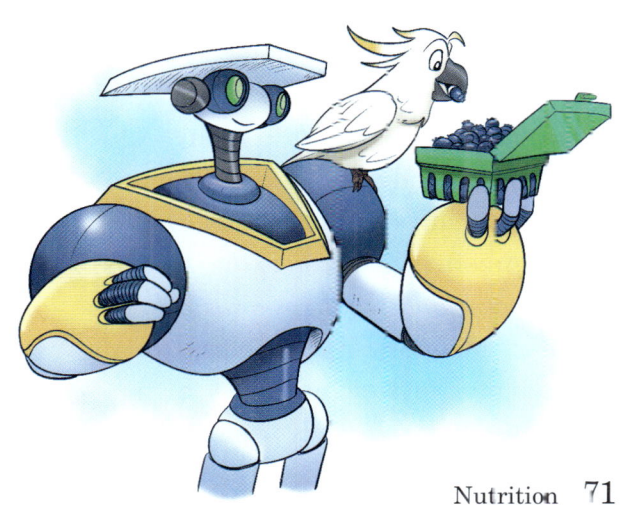

Minerals

Minerals are *chemical elements that are needed as micronutrients*. Plants get minerals from the soil. Your body gets minerals when you eat parts of a plant or food from animals that have eaten plants. *Minerals help regulate the body systems.*

Calcium *is the most common mineral found in our bodies*. The best sources of calcium are milk and milk products, including buttermilk, yogurt, and most types of cheese. Other sources are dark, leafy greens; canned salmon or sardines with bones; dried figs; dried beans and peas; some nuts; soybeans; and broccoli. Most of the calcium in your body is in your teeth and bones, but your blood also needs calcium. Your muscles use calcium to maintain normal muscle tone and strong muscular contractions. *Calcium is also necessary for the normal functioning of the nerves.* If your body does not get enough calcium, your blood will take calcium from your bones. *A lack of calcium may eventually result in osteoporosis* [ŏs′tē·ō·pə·rō′sĭs], *a disease in which the bones become fragile and easily fractured.* Exercise also helps strengthen your bones. Getting sufficient calcium from the foods you eat and exercising regularly can help prevent osteoporosis when you are older.

Phosphorus [fŏs′fər·əs] *helps give rigidity, or hardness, to your bones and teeth.* It is abundant in many foods, but the body cannot use it unless you also get sufficient calcium.

Magnesium *affects how the nervous system works and regulates muscle contractions.* Magnesium also helps regulate the circulatory system and lower high blood pressure. Your body needs additional magnesium for strenuous or long-endurance activities. Whole grains; beans; almonds; potatoes; berries; and dark, leafy greens are good sources of magnesium.

Sodium *helps regulate water balance in your body.* You probably get all the sodium that you need from table salt and other sodium-containing compounds used to prepare or preserve foods. In fact, most people get too much sodium. Canned foods, processed meats, and packaged foods are usually high in sodium. Too much sodium keeps your body from using potassium.

Potassium *helps regulate the movement of muscles, including the heart, and helps deliver nerve messages.* If you do not eat enough potassium-rich foods, or if too much sodium keeps your body from using the potassium, you will feel tired and grouchy. You will not be able to think well or do good work at school. A lack of potassium also affects the heart. To keep potassium and sodium in your body balanced, eat more fruits and vegetables and fewer salty foods. Potassium-containing foods include oranges, bananas, whole-grain breads, nuts, and meats.

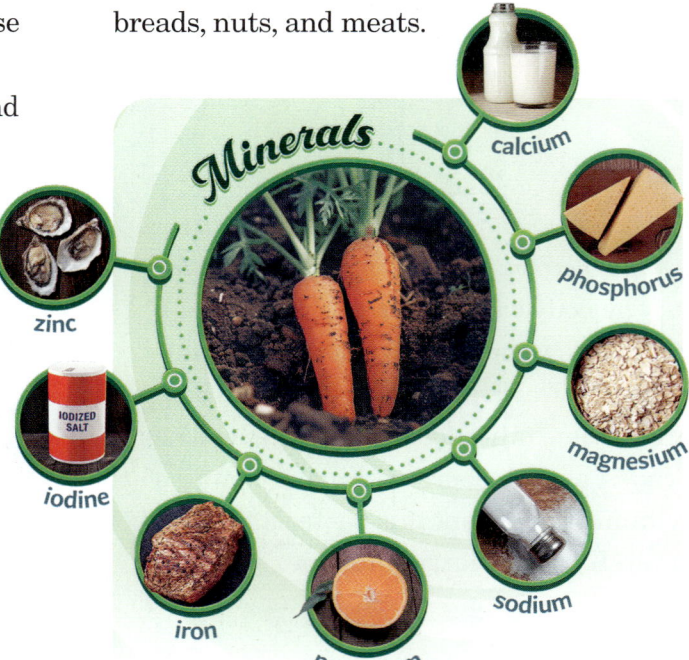

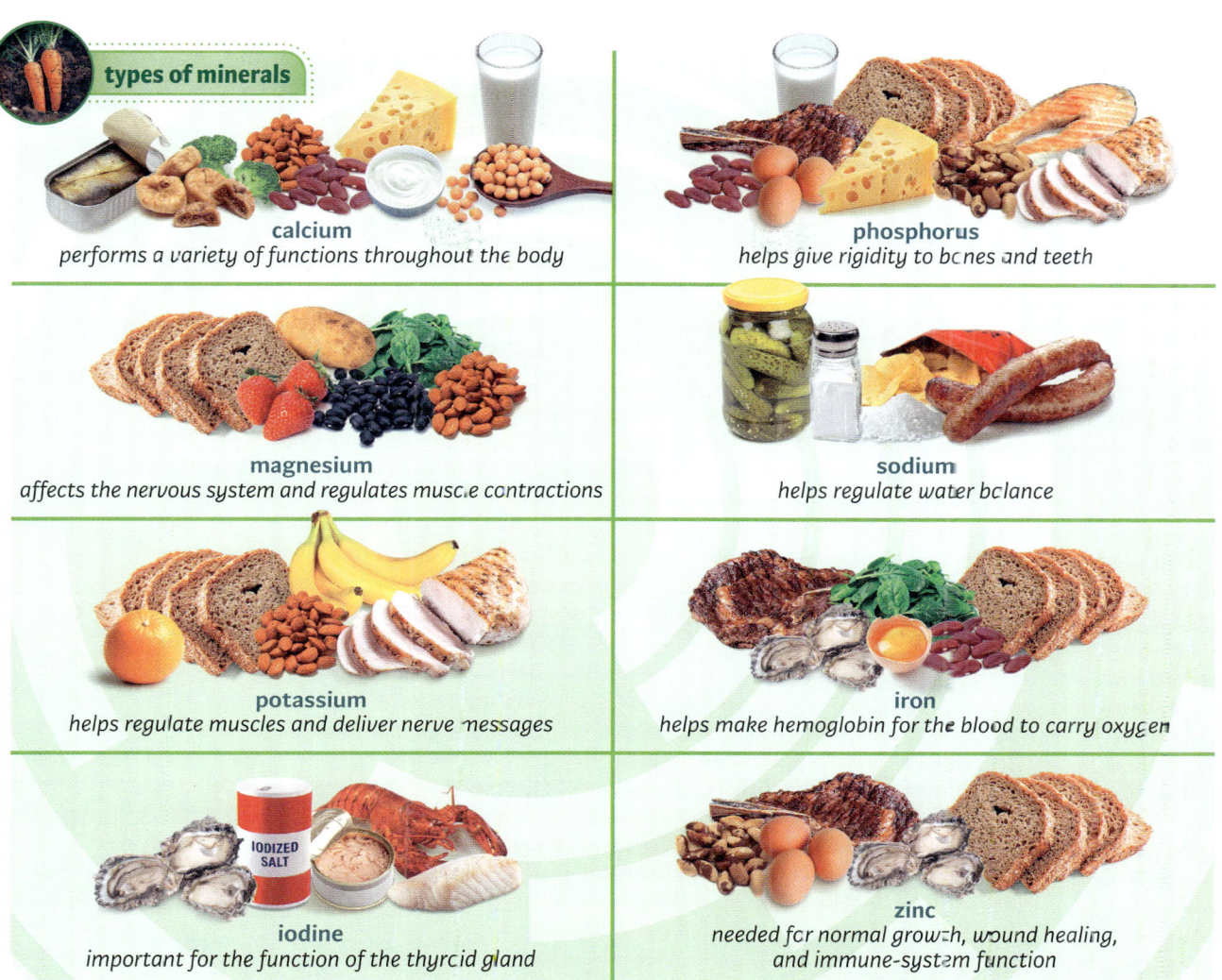

types of minerals

calcium
performs a variety of functions throughout the body

phosphorus
helps give rigidity to bones and teeth

magnesium
affects the nervous system and regulates muscle contractions

sodium
helps regulate water balance

potassium
helps regulate muscles and deliver nerve messages

iron
helps make hemoglobin for the blood to carry oxygen

iodine
important for the function of the thyroid gland

zinc
needed for normal growth, wound healing, and immune-system function

Iron *helps the body make hemoglobin, the oxygen-carrying protein in red blood cells.* A lack of iron will keep the body from being able to make enough hemoglobin; this will make you feel weak and tired. *A condition in which a person's blood cannot carry enough oxygen is known as anemia* [ə·nē′mē·ə]. Meat, shellfish, dark-green leafy vegetables, egg yolks, beans, and whole grains contain iron. The acids from such foods as buttermilk, yogurt, and citrus fruits and juices help your body absorb iron.

At the front of your neck is the thyroid gland, which affects how you grow and how your body functions. *The thyroid gland needs* **iodine** *to do its job properly.* A lack of iodine may cause the thyroid gland to enlarge; *the enlarged thyroid gland produces a swelling in the neck called a goiter. Iodine also helps in proper bone and brain development during pregnancy and infancy.* Iodine is often added to table salt; if you use only *iodized salt, your* body will get the iodine it needs. Fish and other seafood are also good sources of iodine.

A small amount of **zinc** *is needed for normal growth, wound healing, and immune-system function.* The best source of zinc is shellfish, but zinc is also found in meat, eggs, whole grains, and nuts. Iron, iodine, and zinc are called **trace elements** because *the body needs extremely tiny amounts of these minerals.*

Nutrients Your Body Needs

Nutrient	Good Sources	Function
Macronutrients		
Carbohydrates	Fruits, vegetables, whole-grain breads and cereals, brown rice, seeds, nuts, dried beans, honey	Give energy for physical activity Help heat your body Allow your body to use protein for growth and repair Help your body use fats
Fiber	Whole-grain breads and cereals, bran, raw fruits and vegetables, fruits with seeds (figs, berries), nuts	Helps clean out the digestive tract and eliminate waste materials
Protein	Lean meats, fish, poultry, eggs, milk, buttermilk, powdered milk, yogurt, cheese, soybeans, yeast, wheat germ, legumes, nuts	Enables your body to grow Builds muscles Fights infection Repairs your body Helps your body function properly
Fats	Cooking oil, butter, margarine, mayonnaise, cheese, whole milk, egg yolks, nuts, peanut butter, seeds, wheat germ *Limit consumption of saturated fats and hydrogenated oils, such as butter, margarine, mayonnaise, cheese, whole milk, and egg yolks.*	Carry vitamins A, D, E, and K to all parts of your body Give an extra supply of energy Help keep your body warm Help keep your skin from becoming dry and flaky Help keep you from feeling hungry
Vitamins		
Vitamin A	Egg yolks, milk, fish-liver oils, liver, butter, enriched margarine, dark green vegetables, deep yellow fruits and vegetables	Helps keep your skin healthy and smooth Helps you see well Helps the development of bones and tooth enamel Helps protect against colds and infections
B Vitamins	Liver, yeast, wheat germ, brown rice, milk, meat, whole-grain breads and cereals, nuts, most vegetables	Help your body use protein to build new tissue Help change food into energy Help the digestion of your food Help your body grow at a normal rate Help keep your blood healthy Help keep your gums healthy and prevent tooth decay Help keep the skin around your eyes and mouth smooth and healthy Help your heart and nervous system work properly
Vitamin C	Citrus fruits, berries, papaya, cantaloupe, tomatoes, broccoli, raw cabbage, Brussels sprouts, green pepper	Helps your body resist and fight infection Helps heal cuts, scrapes, burns, and broken bones Helps keep your gums healthy Develops strong bones and teeth Helps prevent allergies Helps form the material that holds the body cells together Helps prevent fatigue
Vitamin D	Milk fortified with vitamin D, liver, fish-liver oils, sardines, salmon, tuna, egg yolks	Helps your body use minerals to build strong bones and teeth Helps prevent tooth decay

Nutrient	Good Sources	Function
Vitamin E	Vegetable oils, wheat germ, whole-grain breads and cereals, sunflower seeds, almonds, peanuts, hazelnuts, mango, avocado, dark-green leafy vegetables, egg yolks, liver, bean sprouts, cabbage, yeast	Keeps nutrients from being destroyed by oxygen in your body Helps your body use vitamin A Increases the amount of vitamin A that can be stored in your liver Helps change food into energy Helps keep your heart and skeletal muscles healthy Helps burns heal faster
Vitamin K	Yogurt, alfalfa sprouts, dark-green leafy vegetables, avocado, blueberries, cabbage, cauliflower, chicken, egg yolks, liver, soybean oil	Helps your blood clot properly

Minerals

Nutrient	Good Sources	Function
Calcium	Milk, buttermilk, yogurt, frozen yogurt, most cheeses, canned salmon and sardines (with bones), shellfish, dark-green leafy vegetables (except spinach, chard, and beet greens), broccoli, soybeans, dried dates and figs, barley	Builds strong bones and teeth Helps broken bones mend Prevents tooth decay Regulates muscle contractions Helps you relax
Iodine	Seafood, iodized salt	Helps your thyroid gland function properly
Iron	Liver, lean meat, shellfish, dark-green leafy vegetables, egg yolks, soybeans, dried peas and beans, dried fruits, wheat germ, whole-grain breads and cereals	Helps the body make hemoglobin Prevents fatigue
Magnesium	Whole grains, soybeans, dried peas and beans, nuts, dark-green leafy vegetables, potatoes, fruits, yeast	Helps change food into energy Helps your body absorb calcium Helps your circulatory system work properly Regulates muscle contractions Helps you relax
Phosphorus	Milk, cheese, meat, fish, poultry, eggs, whole-grain breads and cereals, legumes, nuts	Works with calcium to build strong bones and teeth Helps regulate many body functions Helps store and release energy
Potassium	Fruits, vegetables, soybeans, mushrooms, wheat germ, whole-grain breads and cereals, nuts, yeast, lean meats	Keeps your heartbeat regular Helps your nervous system work properly Helps you think clearly
Sodium	Table salt *Most people get more than enough sodium from salt and other sodium-containing compounds used in food preparation or as preservatives, especially in processed foods. Too much sodium in the diet is harmful to health.*	Helps regulate water balance Helps your nervous system work properly
Zinc	Shellfish, lean meat, poultry, eggs, whole grains, nuts	Helps repair your body Helps heal wounds Helps your immune system

Liquids

Nutrient	Good Sources	Function
Liquids	Water, milk, 100% fruit juice, vegetable juice *To avoid unhealthy amounts of macronutrients, most liquid intake should be plain or flavored water. Drink milk and juice mainly for vitamins and minerals, not for liquid content.*	Help control body temperature Carry nutrients throughout your body Help digest food Help change food into energy Help to produce blood, saliva, and digestive juices Carry wastes from your body

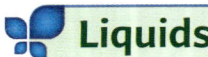

Liquids

Water is an important part of what you take into your body. More than half of your body is water because *every cell of the body needs water*. Water protects body organs and tissue, helps maintain normal body temperature, enables joints to bend smoothly, and protects the nervous system. The brain and spinal cord are protected and cushioned by fluids. Water also helps the body use nutrients and remove waste.

Drink water throughout the day when you feel thirsty. Milk and 100% juice are good sources of liquids, but too much will give you more macronutrients than your body can use. Avoid soft drinks and juice drinks that are not 100% juice, since they often have few nutrients but large amounts of sugar. Many soft drinks also contain *caffeine, a substance that causes your body to lose water*.

Comprehension Check 4.2

Matching: *Write the letter of the correct answer in the blank.*

_____ 1. helps the body resist and fight infection

_____ 2. helps the body use food for energy

_____ 3. keeps skin and eyes healthy

_____ 4. builds strong bones and teeth

_____ 5. protects cells from damage

A. vitamin A
B. B-complex vitamins
C. vitamin C
D. vitamin D
E. vitamin E
F. vitamin K

Multiple Choice: *Write the letter of the correct answer in the blank.*

_____ 6. Which mineral builds strong bones and teeth?
    a. calcium   b. iron   c. magnesium   d. potassium

_____ 7. Which mineral helps the nervous system and regulates muscle contractions?
    a. iodine   b. iron   c. magnesium   d. zinc

_____ 8. Which condition can be caused by a lack of iron in the diet?
    a. anemia   b. goiter   c. osteoporosis   d. rickets

_____ 9. Which condition can be caused by a lack of iodine in the diet?
    a. anemia   b. goiter   c. osteoporosis   d. rickets

Short Answer: *Write the correct answer in the blank.*

10. What term refers to vitamins that protect your cells from damage by harmful molecules? _____

11. What types of food contain carotene? _____

_____

12. What mineral is needed to prevent osteoporosis? _____

13. What is the best source of liquids when you are thirsty? _____

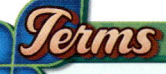
calorie: measure of the amount of energy stored in food

metabolism: the process by which the body produces and uses energy from food

Recommended Dietary Allowance (RDA): the typical daily amount of a nutrient that a healthy individual needs, considering age and other factors

Nutrition Facts label: tool that tells the most important nutritional information for every kind of packaged food

serving size: the portion of a food that an adult will usually eat in one sitting

percent Daily Value (% Daily Value or %DV): how much one serving of a food contributes to a nutrient's total daily amount

added sugar: sugar that is not naturally present in a food but has been added in its preparation

food allergy: situation in which the immune system overreacts to a food protein that has entered the bloodstream

allergen: protein or other substance that causes an allergic reaction

anaphylaxis: most severe allergic reaction; affects the whole body by causing difficulty breathing, a drop in blood pressure, and swelling of various body parts

---

4.3 Nutrient Needs

Energy for Activity

The food you eat provides your body with energy for growth and action. *The amount of energy that is stored in food is measured in* **calories**. Foods that contain a lot of energy are high-calorie foods; foods producing little energy are low-calorie foods. Do you remember which nutrients give you energy? You get energy from carbohydrates, proteins, and fats.

The amount of energy that you need from the food you eat each day depends on the amount of energy you use. Some factors that affect how much energy you use are your size, how fast you are growing, how active you are, and whether you are a boy or a girl. As a general rule, from the ages of nine to twelve, boys require about 200 more calories per day than girls. If you are growing rapidly or are involved in strenuous activities,

your body needs extra calories. The harder and longer your muscles are used, the more high-calorie foods you need to provide the extra energy.

The *process by which your body produces and uses energy from food* is called **metabolism** [mǐ·tăb′ə·lǐz′əm]. Your rate of metabolism is lowest when you are sleeping or resting. Activity raises your rate of metabolism because you are using up more energy. The faster your rate of metabolism, the more calories you use.

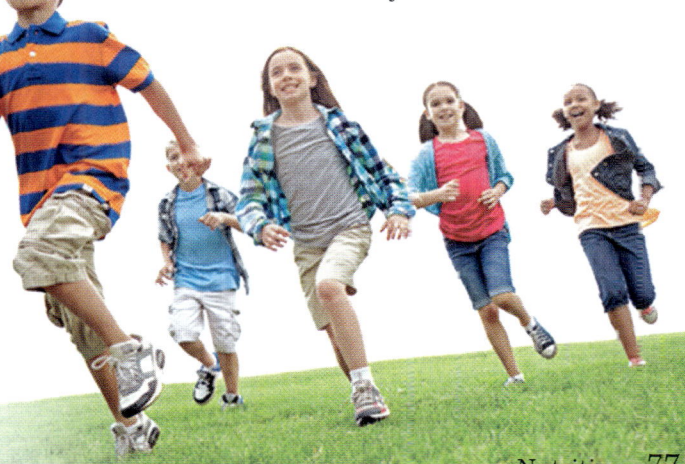

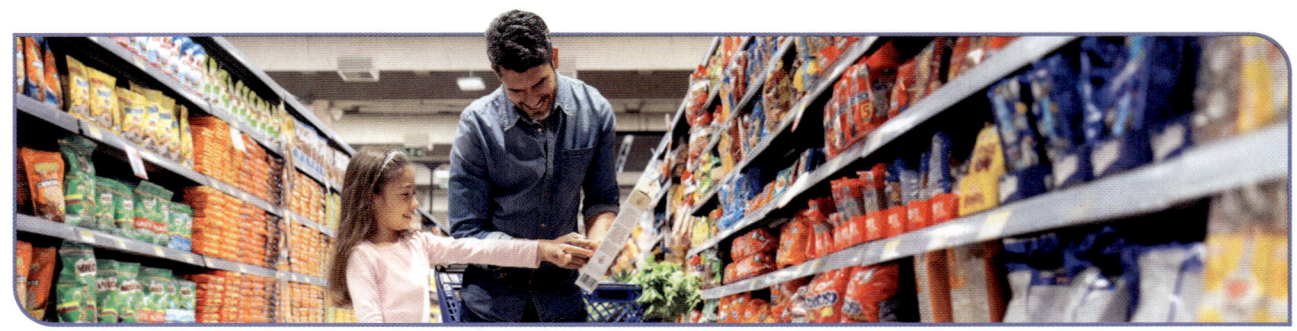

Recommended Dietary Allowance

Besides needing energy for activities, you need the right amount of each nutrient daily. Nutrition experts use scientific understanding of nutrition to set the **Recommended Dietary Allowance**, or *RDA*, for each nutrient. *The RDA is the typical daily amount of a nutrient that a healthy individual needs, considering age and other factors.* For example, the RDA for protein indicates that a person between the ages of nine and thirteen needs about 34 grams of protein each day. As he or she goes through the teen years and reaches adulthood, protein needs will increase to about 56 grams per day for a young man and 46 grams per day for a young woman.

Reading Food Labels

Nutrition Facts Label

Have you ever chosen a box of cereal by looking at the pictures on the box? Advertisers try to sell, or market, their product by making you want to buy it. Using cartoon characters, including toys, and promising prizes are marketing strategies used by manufacturers. Why do they do this? Their goal is to influence you to buy their products. Imagine the cereal aisle in your grocery store as a contest for your attention. Each box is shouting, "Pick me! Pick me!" Food advertisements are often common in media such as the internet and television; some of these advertisements are disguised by a character mentioning or eating some brand of food. It is the job of advertisers to sell products; it is your job to make healthy choices. Instead of making choices because of eye-catching advertisements, make healthy choices based on facts.

No matter how food is advertised, facts are provided that will help you make healthy decisions. If you look on the side of a cereal box, you will find the Nutrition Facts label. The **Nutrition Facts label** is *a tool that tells the most important nutritional information for every kind of packaged food.* It was designed to be easily read and understood.

At the top of the Nutrition Facts label is the **serving size**, the *portion of the food that an adult will usually eat in one sitting. The serving size does not tell how much of the food is a healthy amount to eat,* just how much people typically do eat. You will notice that in most cases, a serving size is only part of the whole package. All the other values in the Nutrition Facts are based on eating one full serving. Being aware of your portions requires knowing how much you are eating and how that portion will affect your body. You may decide to eat half a serving, a full serving, or a different food.

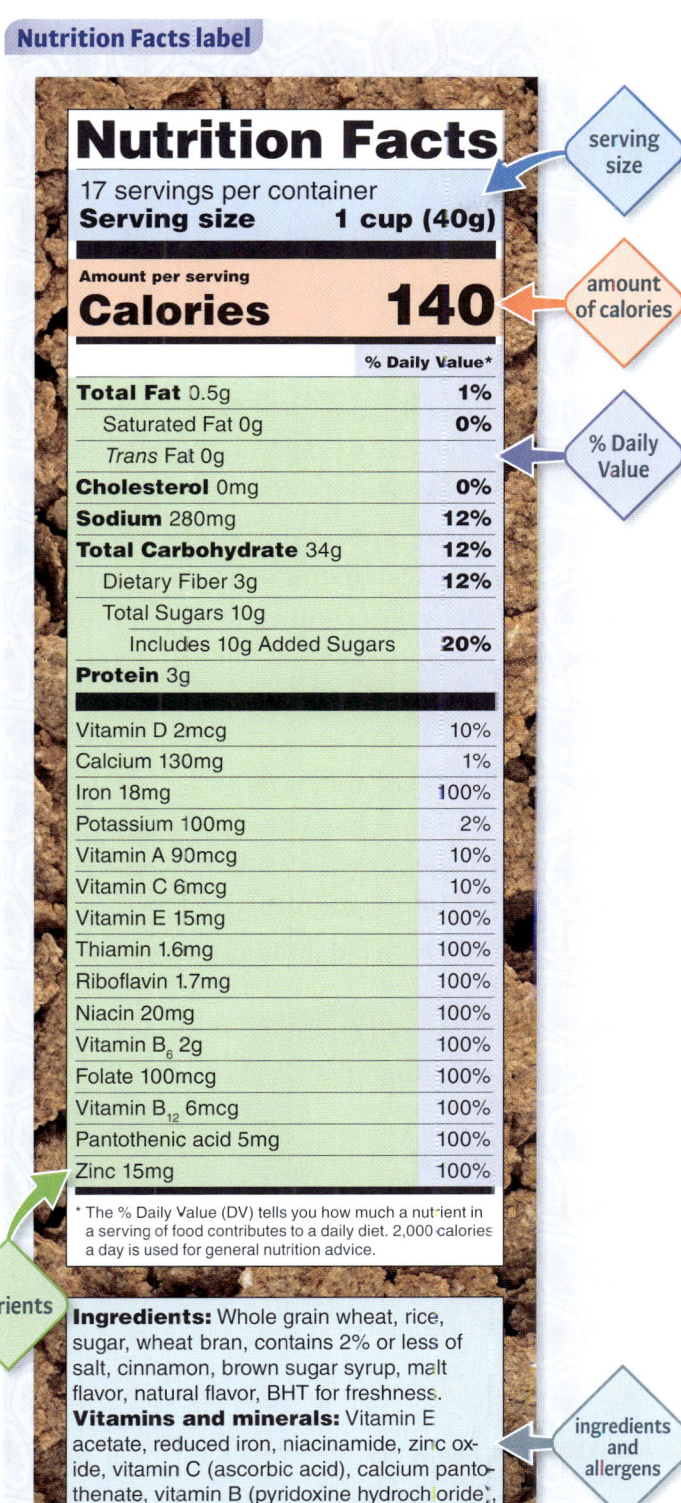

Nutrition Facts label

Nutrition Facts

17 servings per container

Serving size   1 cup (40g)

Amount per serving

Calories   140

	% Daily Value*
Total Fat 0.5g	**1%**
Saturated Fat 0g	**0%**
Trans Fat 0g	
Cholesterol 0mg	**0%**
Sodium 280mg	**12%**
Total Carbohydrate 34g	**12%**
Dietary Fiber 3g	**12%**
Total Sugars 10g	
Includes 10g Added Sugars	**20%**
Protein 3g	
Vitamin D 2mcg	10%
Calcium 130mg	1%
Iron 18mg	100%
Potassium 100mg	2%
Vitamin A 90mcg	10%
Vitamin C 6mcg	10%
Vitamin E 15mg	100%
Thiamin 1.6mg	100%
Riboflavin 1.7mg	100%
Niacin 20mg	100%
Vitamin B$_6$ 2g	100%
Folate 100mcg	100%
Vitamin B$_{12}$ 6mcg	100%
Pantothenic acid 5mg	100%
Zinc 15mg	100%

* The % Daily Value (DV) tells you how much a nutrient in a serving of food contributes to a daily diet. 2,000 calories a day is used for general nutrition advice.

Ingredients: Whole grain wheat, rice, sugar, wheat bran, contains 2% or less of salt, cinnamon, brown sugar syrup, malt flavor, natural flavor, BHT for freshness. **Vitamins and minerals:** Vitamin E acetate, reduced iron, niacinamide, zinc oxide, vitamin C (ascorbic acid), calcium pantothenate, vitamin B (pyridoxine hydrochloride), vitamin B (riboflavin), vitamin B (thiamin hydrochloride), folic acid, vitamin A palmitate, vitamin B, vitamin D.

serving size

amount of calories

% Daily Value

nutrients

ingredients and allergens

Next, *the Nutrition Facts label lists the energy (in calories) in one serving of the food.* A balance between food intake and activity is important to avoid extra calories. Your body stores extra calories as fat. This fat can result in unnecessary weight gain. Fat can also build up around the heart, which can increase the risk of heart disease. The calorie value does not indicate what nutrients are in the food. You should get your needed calories from a variety of healthy foods to ensure that you are getting the nutrients you need.

Most of the Nutrition Facts label is the nutrient information. *This section lists the amount of macronutrients and selected micronutrients in each serving.* For each nutrient, the label lists the actual amount in grams (g), milligrams (mg; $\frac{1}{1,000}$ gram), or micrograms (mcg; $\frac{1}{1,000,000}$ gram). More importantly, the label also lists the **percent Daily Value** (% Daily Value or %DV) of each nutrient. *A nutrient's percent Daily Value indicates how much one serving of the food contributes to the nutrient's total daily amount, based on the RDA. The food is low in the nutrient if the percent Daily Value is 5% or less, while it is high in the nutrient if the percent Daily Value is 20% or greater.* If one serving of a food contains 2% of the Daily Value (DV) of calcium, that food is low in calcium. If one serving of the food contains 23% of the Daily Value (23% DV) of sodium, that food is high in sodium. Using the percent Daily Value will help you get the fiber, vitamins, and minerals needed for good health. It will also help you limit the fat (especially saturated fat), sodium, and sugar you include in your diet.

One thing to especially be aware of in the nutrient information is **added sugar**. *Added sugar is sugar that is not naturally present in a food but has been added in its preparation.* Suppose that you are eating applesauce. The apples used to make applesauce naturally contain some sugar; this natural sugar is balanced by the fruit's fiber, vitamins, and minerals. In regular applesauce, more sugar is added when cooking the apples; this sugar adds calories without providing other nutrients. This added sugar is indicated on the Nutrition Facts label. *Because added sugar can contribute to a variety of health problems, you should limit the amount of foods with added sugar that you eat.* For example, you can choose applesauce that has no sugar added but contains only the sugar that was naturally present in the apples. *It is recommended that no more than 10% of your daily calorie intake be added sugar.*

Ingredients and Allergens

Below or next to the Nutrition Facts label, *the ingredients are listed in order based on amount.* That means that if sugar is the first ingredient, there is more sugar in that product than any other ingredient. Foods that have sugar as one of the first three ingredients are usually high in added sugars.

The ingredients list is also important for people with food allergies. A **food allergy** *occurs when your immune system, the body system that defends against infections, overreacts to a food protein that has entered your bloodstream. A protein or other substance that causes an allergic reaction* is an **allergen**. The reaction can be relatively mild, such as

swelling or an itchy rash called hives. Other allergic reactions can be more severe. *The most severe allergic reaction* is **anaphylaxis** [ăn′ə•fə•lăk′sĭs]. Anaphylaxis *affects the whole body by causing difficulty breathing, a drop in blood pressure, and swelling of various body parts.* It is a life-threatening medical emergency that requires immediate treatment.

Although there are many foods that people can be allergic to, *the nine most common food allergens are milk, eggs, fish, crustaceans (such as shrimp and crabs), peanuts, tree nuts, wheat, soybeans, and sesame.* In the United States, the ingredients listing of packaged food must indicate if any of these nine allergens are present. The allergen may be in the ingredients list, for example "milk," "egg yolk," or "flour (wheat)." Other times, a sentence below the ingredients list will state what allergens are present. If you have food allergies or are preparing food for someone with food allergies, always check the ingredients carefully to avoid an allergic reaction.

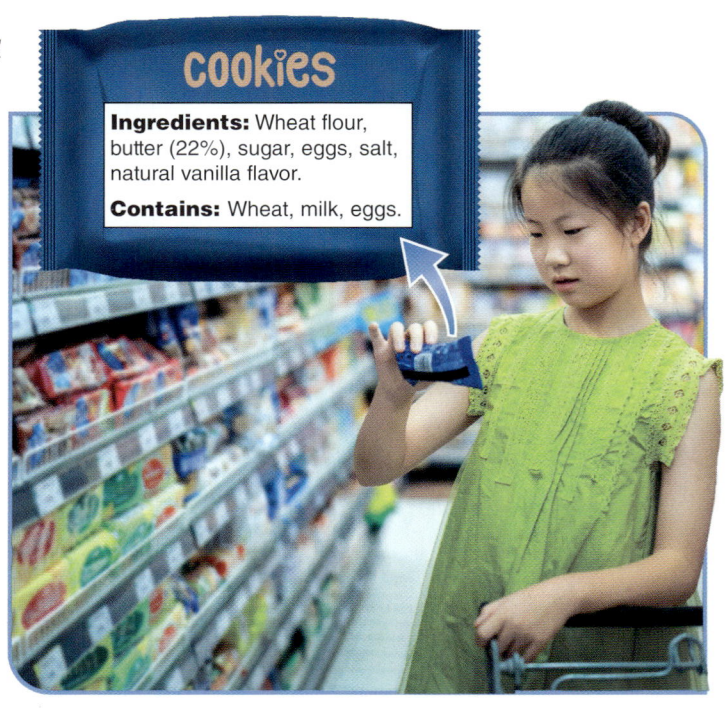

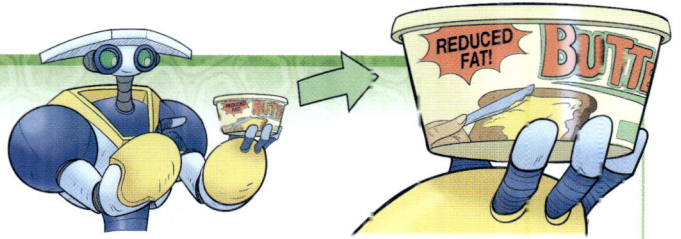

Evaluating Nutrition Claims

You will see nutrition claims in many places. Food packages will often have statements that a food is "reduced fat" or "high fiber" or "has no added sugar." You may also see claims in science articles, on the internet, or in other media that certain foods can help prevent or treat certain diseases. To be a good steward of your health, you need to evaluate nutrition claims to determine whether they are trustworthy and accurate.

In the United States, federal law requires that nutrition claims on food packages be accurate and backed by scientific evidence. A food labeled as "reduced fat" must actually have less fat than other similar foods. This can make it easier to choose healthy foods, but you should still check the Nutrition Facts label. The manufacturer points out the reduced fat because doing so helps sell the product. The Nutrition Facts will tell you if a reduced-fat food contains unhealthy amounts of fat, sodium, or added sugars. Healthy eating requires considering the amounts of all nutrients, not just one nutrient that the manufacturer decided to emphasize on the package.

When you see a nutrition claim in a science article, on the internet, or in other media, do not simply accept the claim as trustworthy and accurate. Instead, consider if it is from a reliable source, is current, and is unbiased. Beware of health claims that are based on stories or personal experiences instead of on scientific research. Someone may claim, "You should eat lots of bananas to get rid of a cold. I had a cold for several days, but then I ate five bananas and was better the next day." This story provides no evidence that eating bananas will cure someone else's cold. In fact, there is no reason to believe that eating bananas cured this person's cold. Someone with a cold will usually get better after a few days, with or without eating bananas.

One common type of nutrition claim says that eating or avoiding some specific food will prevent or cure a disease such as cancer, heart disease, or diabetes. Such a claim might be based on someone's personal experience or on misunderstanding the conclusions of scientific research. A person's diet is just one of many factors that can affect cancer, heart disease, and diabetes. An overall healthy lifestyle, including a healthy diet, can reduce the chance of developing these diseases, but there is no scientific evidence that any food or combination of foods can prevent or cure them.

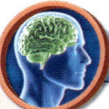

Comprehension Check 4.3

True/False: *If the statement is true, write* true *in the blank. If the statement is false, replace the underlined word(s) with a word or phrase that will make the statement true. Do not write* false *in any blank.*

_____ 1. The amount of energy that is stored in food is measured in <u>allergens</u>.

_____ 2. The process by which the body produces and uses energy from food is <u>digestion</u>.

continued

_____ 3. The Recommended Dietary Allowance is the typical amount of a nutrient that a healthy individual needs <u>weekly</u>.

_____ 4. The portion of a food that an adult will usually eat in one sitting is the <u>percent Daily Value</u>.

_____ 5. The second thing on the Nutrition Facts label is the <u>energy in calories</u>.

_____ 6. If the percent Daily Value of fiber for a food is 4%, that means that the food is <u>high</u> in fiber.

_____ 7. The most severe type of allergic reaction, which is a life-threatening medical emergency, is <u>anaphylaxis</u>.

Short Answer: *Use the Nutrition Facts label to answer the questions below. Write the correct answer in the blank.*

8. What is the serving size of this food? _____

9. How much energy does a serving of the food provide? _____

10. Is this food a good source of dietary fiber? How do you know? _____

_____

11. What micronutrients are listed on the Nutrition Facts label? _____

_____

Think about It.

12. You are helping to plan a birthday party at the park for one of your friends. List three things you can do to protect your guests from food-allergy reactions. _____

_____

_____

_____

_____

_____

_____

Nutrition Facts

10 servings per container

Serving size   1/4 cup (40g)

Amount per serving

Calories   130

	% Daily Value*
Total Fat 0g	0%
Saturated Fat 0g	0%
Trans Fat 0g	
Cholesterol 0mg	0%
Sodium 10mg	0%
Total Carbohydrate 34g	12%
Dietary Fiber 2g	1%
Total Sugars 28g	
Includes 0g Added Sugars	0%
Protein 1g	

Vit. D 0mcg 0%	•	Calcium 30mg 0%
Iron 1mg 4%	•	Potas. 300mg 6%

* The % Daily Value (DV) tells you how much a nutrient in a serving of food contributes to a daily diet. 2,000 calories a day is used for general nutrition advice.

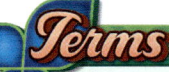
balanced diet: diet containing all the nutrients necessary to keep you healthy

MyPlate: tool, prepared by the U.S. Department of Agriculture, that helps you choose a variety of foods to obtain the nutrients that your body needs each day; divides foods into fruits, vegetables, protein, grains, and dairy

vegan: type of diet in which a person does not eat meat or animal products

grains: the seeds and fruits of certain types of grass plants

perishable food: food that can spoil easily and must be kept refrigerated or frozen; includes most foods containing meat, eggs, or dairy products

nonperishable food: food that does not require refrigeration or freezing; includes fresh fruits and vegetables, most foods in unopened cans and bottles, baked goods, and most types of dried foods

cross-contamination: transfer of harmful microorganisms from one object to another

4.4 Choosing Healthy Eating

MyPlate

Your eating habits are an important factor that affects your health. To grow and function properly, your body must be well nourished. You should have a **balanced diet**—*a diet containing all the nutrients necessary to keep you healthy*. Most foods contain several nutrients, but no one food supplies all the nutrients that you need. Therefore, *it is important to eat a variety of foods*.

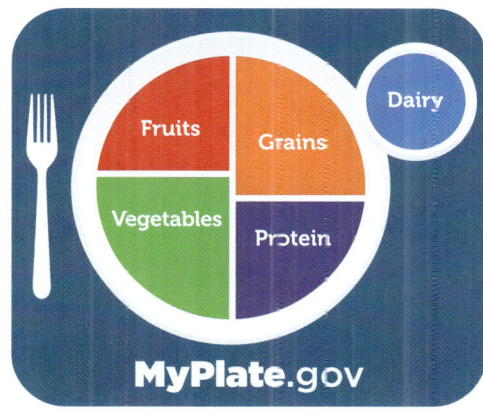

MyPlate is *a tool, prepared by the U.S. Department of Agriculture, that helps you choose a variety of foods to obtain the nutrients that your body needs each day. MyPlate divides foods into five main groups: fruits, vegetables, protein, grains, and dairy.* MyPlate can help you develop a healthy diet that is appropriate for your individual needs and dietary preferences.

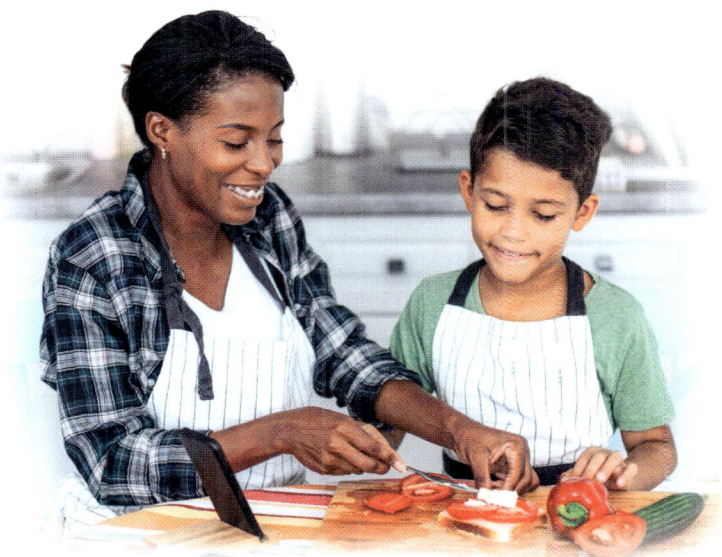

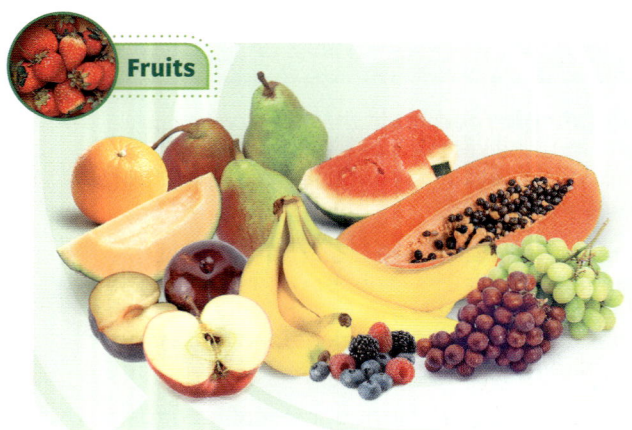

Fruits

Fruits

Fruits are rich in vitamins, minerals, and fiber. God gave many fruits a natural "wrapper"—a skin, rind, or peel—that makes them easy to take with you. Berries have less sugar than many other fruits; add fresh or frozen berries to plain yogurt or granola. Some other fruits that you can enjoy are oranges, bananas, papayas, cantaloupes, apples, pears, grapes, watermelons, and plums.

At your age, *you should eat 1½ to 2 cups of fruit every day.* One cup of 100% fruit juice or applesauce or ½ cup of dried fruit counts the same as one cup of fresh, frozen, or canned fruit.

Vegetables

Like fruits, *vegetables are rich in vitamins, minerals, and fiber.* Since different-colored vegetables contain different nutrients, there are different groups of vegetables. Vegetables in the beans, peas, and lentils group, including black beans, chickpeas, and kidney beans, are also good sources of protein. (Despite their names, green beans and green peas are not in this group.) Eating a variety of vegetables ensures that you get the vitamins and minerals you need.

At your age, *girls need 1½ to 3 cups of vegetables every day; boys need 2 to 3½ cups.* Because raw leafy vegetables (such as lettuce in a salad) are loosely packed, 2 cups counts the same as 1 cup of other vegetables. Together, *fruits and vegetables should be about half of your plate.*

Vegetable Types

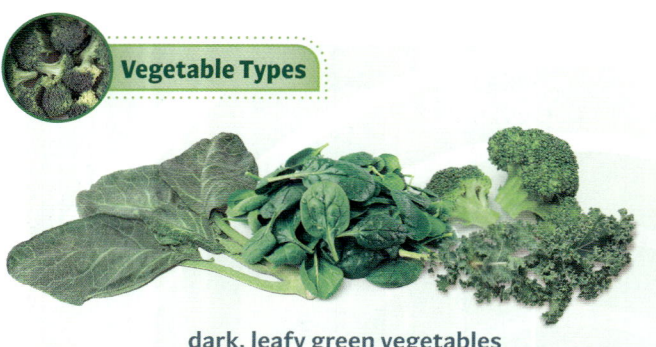

dark, leafy green vegetables

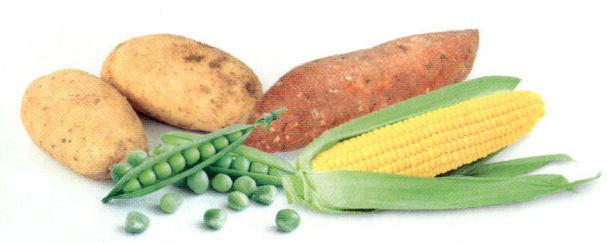

starchy vegetables

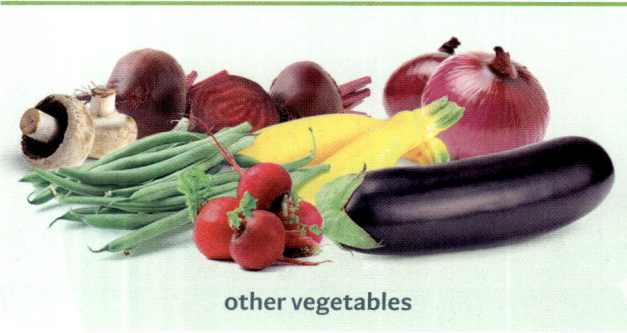

other vegetables

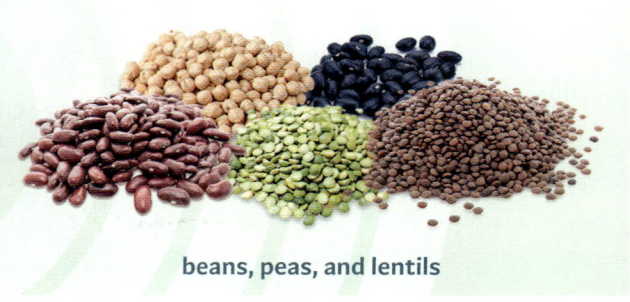

beans, peas, and lentils

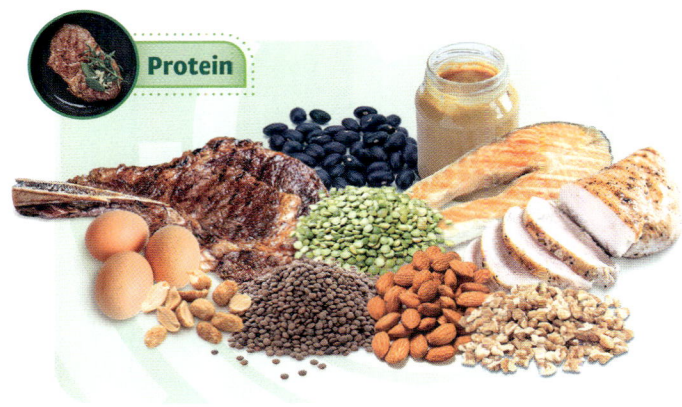

Protein

Protein

Foods in the protein group are rich in the protein that your body needs to maintain its cells and build muscle. Meats, poultry, seafood, and eggs are animal foods in this group. *Vegetables in the beans, peas, and lentils group are protein foods.* Peanuts, walnuts, almonds, and other nuts are also plant sources of protein.

At your age, *girls daily need protein foods equivalent to between 4 and 6 ounces of meat; boys need protein foods equivalent to between 5 and 6½ ounces of meat.* Some food portions equivalent to 1 ounce of meat are one egg; ¼ cup of cooked beans; ½ ounce of nuts; and 1 tablespoon of peanut butter. *When eating meats, lean meats are best because they have less fat, especially saturated fat, than other meats.*

Some people choose to have a **vegan** [vē′gən] diet, in which they *do not eat meat or animal products.* A person with a vegan diet can get enough protein by eating plant-based protein foods.

Grains

Grains are *the seeds and fruits of certain types of grass plants.* Grain seeds have three parts: a starchy inner *endosperm*, which gives the young plant food; a young plant called the *germ*; and an outer layer called the *bran.* The germ is especially rich in nutrients, and the bran has valuable fiber and nutrients. Some grains are refined, or processed, in a way that removes the bran and germ. *Whole grains and whole-grain flours are the healthiest choices because they contain the bran and germ.*

Oats (including oatmeal), popcorn, and quinoa are always whole grains. Brown and wild rice are whole grains, but white rice is refined. Grains such as wheat and cornmeal are often refined; check the ingredients list for "whole grain." "Enriched" flour or cornmeal is a refined grain that has had some vitamins and minerals (but not fiber) added back.

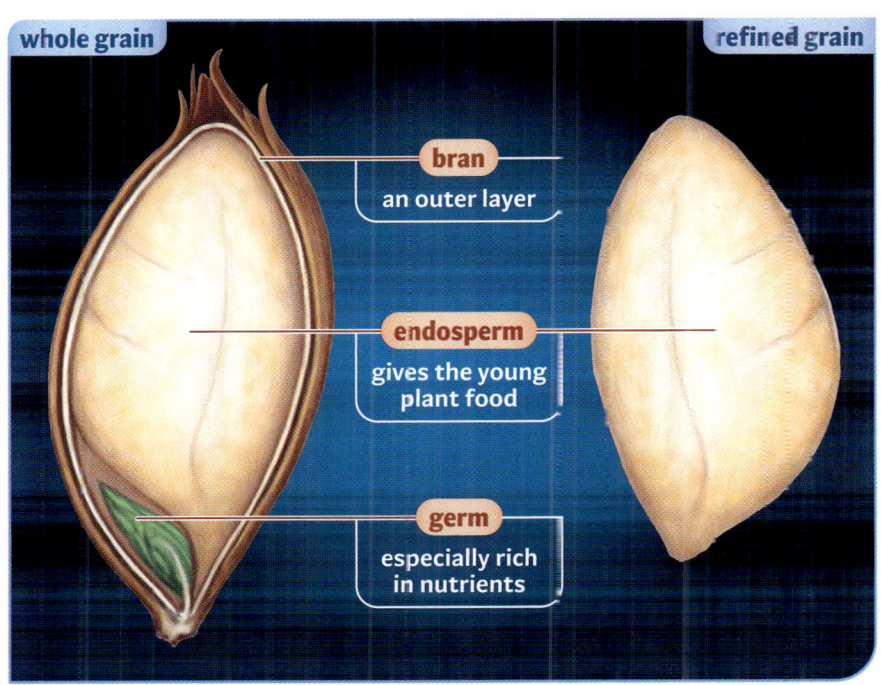

whole grain · refined grain

bran
an outer layer

endosperm
gives the young plant food

germ
especially rich in nutrients

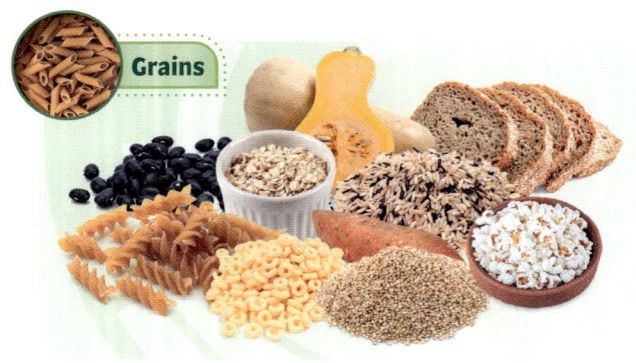

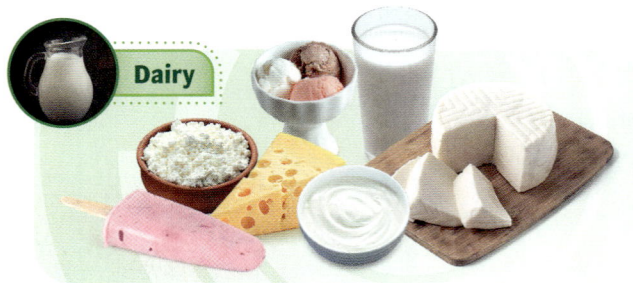

At your age, *girls should eat 5 to 7 ounces of grains daily; boys should eat 5 to 9 ounces of grains.* Some 1-ounce portions of grains are ½ cup of cooked oatmeal, rice, or pasta; one slice of bread; and 1 cup of breakfast cereal (or 1¼ cup of puffed cereal). *At least half of your grains should be whole grains.*

Some people cannot eat certain grains because of food allergies or intolerances. Someone who cannot eat one specific grain can choose foods containing other grains. Someone who cannot eat grains at all must depend on foods such as sweet potatoes, squash, and beans for carbohydrates and fiber.

Dairy

Dairy includes milk and most foods made from milk, including yogurt and cheese. Desserts such as ice cream, frozen yogurt, and sherbet are also in the dairy group but should be limited because they have high sugar. *Dairy provides the body with calcium and vitamin D* to build strong bones and teeth. Dairy products also contain protein and other nutrients.

Preteens, teenagers, and adults should have 3 cups of dairy daily. Count 1 ounce of American cheese; 1½ ounces of cheddar, mozzarella, Swiss, or Parmesan cheese; ⅓ cup of shredded cheese; or 2 cups of cottage cheese or feta as 1 cup of dairy. Since God designed

cows' milk for calves, its original fat content is too rich for most people. Low-fat or nonfat milk, yogurt, and cheese are usually a better choice. *People who have dairy allergies, cannot digest dairy products well, or choose a vegan diet can meet their dairy needs using fortified soy milk and soy yogurt.*

Making Nutrition Decisions

You can use MyPlate guidelines to make healthy food choices for yourself. Consider what foods you eat and how they fit into your nutritional needs. *Also consider where you can substitute healthier foods or ingredients.* For example, you can reduce saturated fat in a hamburger by replacing regular ground beef with lean ground beef or ground turkey or with a vegetable protein such as a black-bean burger. You can use this same reasoning when you are eating out; consider how many calories each item has (often printed on the menu), what food groups it contains, and how it fits into your overall needs.

You can work with others in your family, school, or community to make healthy nutrition decisions. Your parents probably buy most of the food your family eats. You can help them select healthy alternatives to foods that are high in added sugar and saturated fat. Your family can also discuss what foods each person likes and what healthy options are available. Work together to plan meals that contain a proper balance of nutrients and that everyone will enjoy.

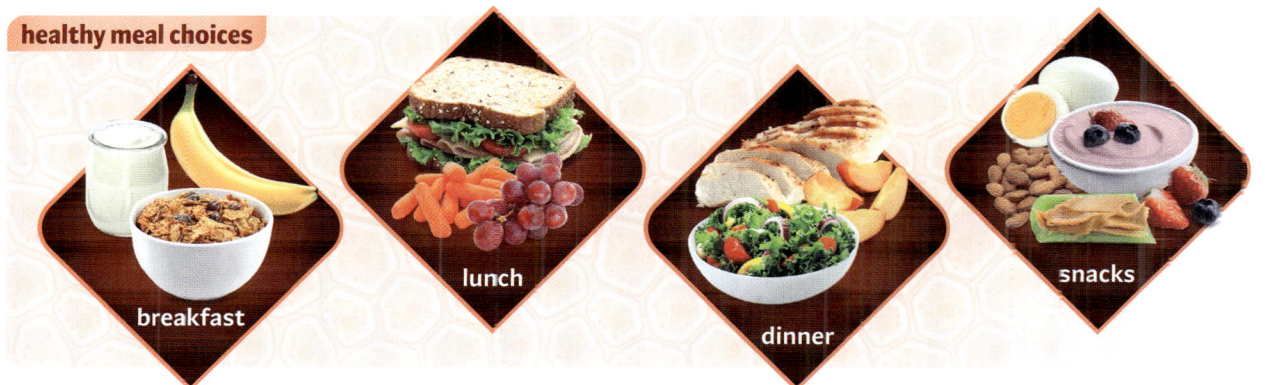

breakfast

lunch

dinner

snacks

Making Nutrition Decisions

LIVE IT OUT!

Think about the most recent meal that you have eaten. List all the foods that you ate; identify which MyPlate food group(s) are present in each food. Remember that some foods may have ingredients from more than one food group.

Food	Food Groups

Is this a balanced meal according to MyPlate guidelines? Explain your answer. _____

_____

_____

Can you change this meal to make it healthier? _____ If so, how? _____

_____

_____

_____

Food Safety

Besides good food choices, healthy eating requires storing and preparing food properly. Improper storage and preparation allows the growth of harmful microorganisms that can make you sick if you eat the food.

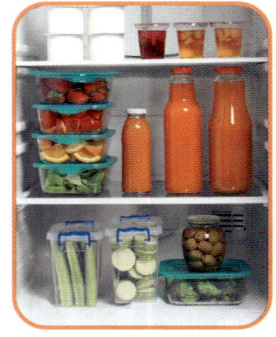

Storing Food

Perishable foods *spoil easily and must be refrigerated or frozen. Most foods containing meat, eggs, or dairy products are perishable.* These foods should be refrigerated or frozen until you are ready to eat or cook them. Meats and most dairy products can be frozen if they need to be stored for longer. *It is best to thaw frozen meats and dairy products by placing them in the refrigerator.* You may defrost frozen meats in a microwave if you will cook them immediately. *Do not thaw perishable foods at room temperature.*

Nonperishable foods *do not require refrigeration or freezing. Nonperishable foods include fresh fruits and vegetables, nuts, most foods in unopened cans and bottles, baked goods (including bread), and most types of dried foods (including jerky and other dried meats).* These foods last for days or weeks without refrigeration; unopened canned goods can last for months or years.

Preparing Food

Always wash your hands before, during, and after preparing food. Hand washing helps prevent **cross-contamination**, the *transfer of harmful microorganisms from one object to another.* Hand washing is especially important after handling raw meat or eggs. Do not use the same utensils for raw meats and vegetables unless you wash them thoroughly between foods. Raw meats must be cooked to the correct internal temperature; a meat thermometer can help ensure the meat is fully cooked. Wash fresh fruits and vegetables to remove dirt from their surfaces. *When serving food, keep hot foods above 140°F; keep cold dishes containing perishable foods below 40°F.* Refrigerate leftovers within two hours and reheat them well before serving.

Community HEALTH CORNER

Disordered Eating

Any eating behavior that harms your body's health and development is disordered eating. Someone with an eating disorder may eat hurriedly, often skip meals, be very picky about food, or eat more food than is healthy (even if he is not hungry). Some eating disorders occur because the person sees himself as overweight, although he may be a healthy weight. This can lead him to try to lose weight by taking diet pills, forcing himself to vomit, or exercising even when tired or sick.

Disordered eating is a complex problem that can result in physical illness, discouragement, and poor social relationships. If you think that you or a friend may have an eating disorder, do not try to deal with it on your own. Instead, speak to a parent or other trusted adult. Many communities have resources available to help those with disordered eating; a parent or trusted adult can direct you or your friend to the appropriate treatment and guidance for overcoming disordered eating.

Comprehension Check 4.4

Matching: *Write the letter of the correct answer in the blank.*

_____ 1. rich in vitamins and minerals

_____ 2. protein food

_____ 3. contains bran, endosperm, and germ

_____ 4. provides calcium and vitamin D

_____ 5. transfer of harmful bacteria

A. celery, broccoli, oranges
B. cross-contamination
C. dairy
D. meats, eggs, beans
E. whole grain

True/False: *If the statement is true, write* true *in the blank. If the statement is false, replace the underlined word(s) with a word or phrase that will make the statement true. Do not write* false *in any blank.*

_____ 6. A fifth grader should eat <u>4 to 5</u> cups of fruit every day.

_____ 7. Together, vegetables and <u>grains</u> should be about half your plate.

_____ 8. Beans, peas, and lentils can count as either vegetables or <u>dairy</u> foods.

_____ 9. People who do not eat dairy products can meet their dairy needs using products made from <u>soy</u> milk.

_____ 10. Foods that must be refrigerated or frozen are called <u>spoiling</u> foods.

_____ 11. It is best to thaw frozen meats in the <u>refrigerator</u>.

_____ 12. When serving hot food, keep it above <u>160°F</u>.

Think about It.

13. To make chicken salad, Emma has purchased a can of cooked chicken, a bottle of mayonnaise (made from oil, egg yolk, and vinegar), a bag of sliced almonds, and a bag of dried cranberries. Does Emma need to refrigerate any of these ingredients? Does she need to refrigerate the chicken salad once she has made it? Explain your answers. _____

_____
_____
_____
_____
_____

1 Macronutrients (4.1)

Short Answer: *Write the correct answer in the blank.*

1. What term refers to substances from food that the body uses to grow, have energy, and stay healthy? _____

2. Why are carbohydrates, protein, and fats called macronutrients? _____

_____

3. What are two food sources of simple carbohydrates? of complex carbohydrates?

_____

_____

_____

_____

4. Why is fiber important? _____

_____

5. What is the main benefit that protein provides to the body? _____

_____

6. Why are saturated fats harmful to your body? _____

_____

7. What type of fats are liquid at room temperature? _____

2 Micronutrients (4.2)

A. Matching: *Write the letter of the correct answer in the blank.*

_____ 1. helps the immune system resist and fight infection

_____ 2. helps in the digestive processes

_____ 3. helps maintain good eyesight and healthy skin

_____ 4. helps build strong bones and teeth

_____ 5. helps protect the cells from damage and helps the body use nutrients from food

_____ 6. helps in blood clotting to prevent loss of blood

A. vitamin A

B. B-complex vitamins

C. vitamin C

D. vitamin D

E. vitamin E

F. vitamin K

B. Matching: *Write the letter of the correct answer in the blank.*

_____ 1. helps build strong bones and teeth

_____ 2. helps the way the nervous system works and regulates muscle contraction

_____ 3. helps regulate water balance in the body

_____ 4. helps deliver nerve messages

_____ 5. helps the body make hemoglobin

_____ 6. supports the thyroid for growth and development

A. calcium

B. iodine

C. iron

D. magnesium

E. phosphorus

F. potassium

G. sodium

C. True/False: *If the statement is true, write* true *in the blank. If the statement is false, replace the underlined word(s) with a word or phrase that will make the statement true. Do not write* false *in any blank.*

_____ 1. Micronutrients manufactured by living things in their body cells are <u>minerals</u>.

_____ 2. Vitamins that protect cells from harmful molecules are <u>trace elements</u>.

_____ 3. The substance from fruits and vegetables that the body uses to make vitamin A is <u>carotene</u>.

_____ 4. A lack of calcium can cause the bones to become fragile and easily fractured, a disease called <u>rickets</u>.

3 Nutrient Needs (4.3)

A. Fill in the Blank: *Write the correct word in the blank.*

1. The amount of energy stored in foods is measured in _____.

2. The typical amount of a nutrient that a person needs daily is the _____, or RDA.

3. A tool that tells the important nutritional information for a packaged food is the _____ label.

4. The portion of a food that an adult will usually eat in one sitting is the _____.

5. The number indicating how much a food contributes to a nutrient's daily amount is the _____.

6. Added sugar should be no more than _____% of your daily calorie intake.

7. A food protein or other substance that causes an allergy is an _____.

8. The most severe type of allergic reaction is called _____.

continued

B. Think!

Based on the Nutrition Facts labels provided, which beverage is the healthier choice? Explain your answer. _____

_____

_____

_____

_____

_____

_____

_____

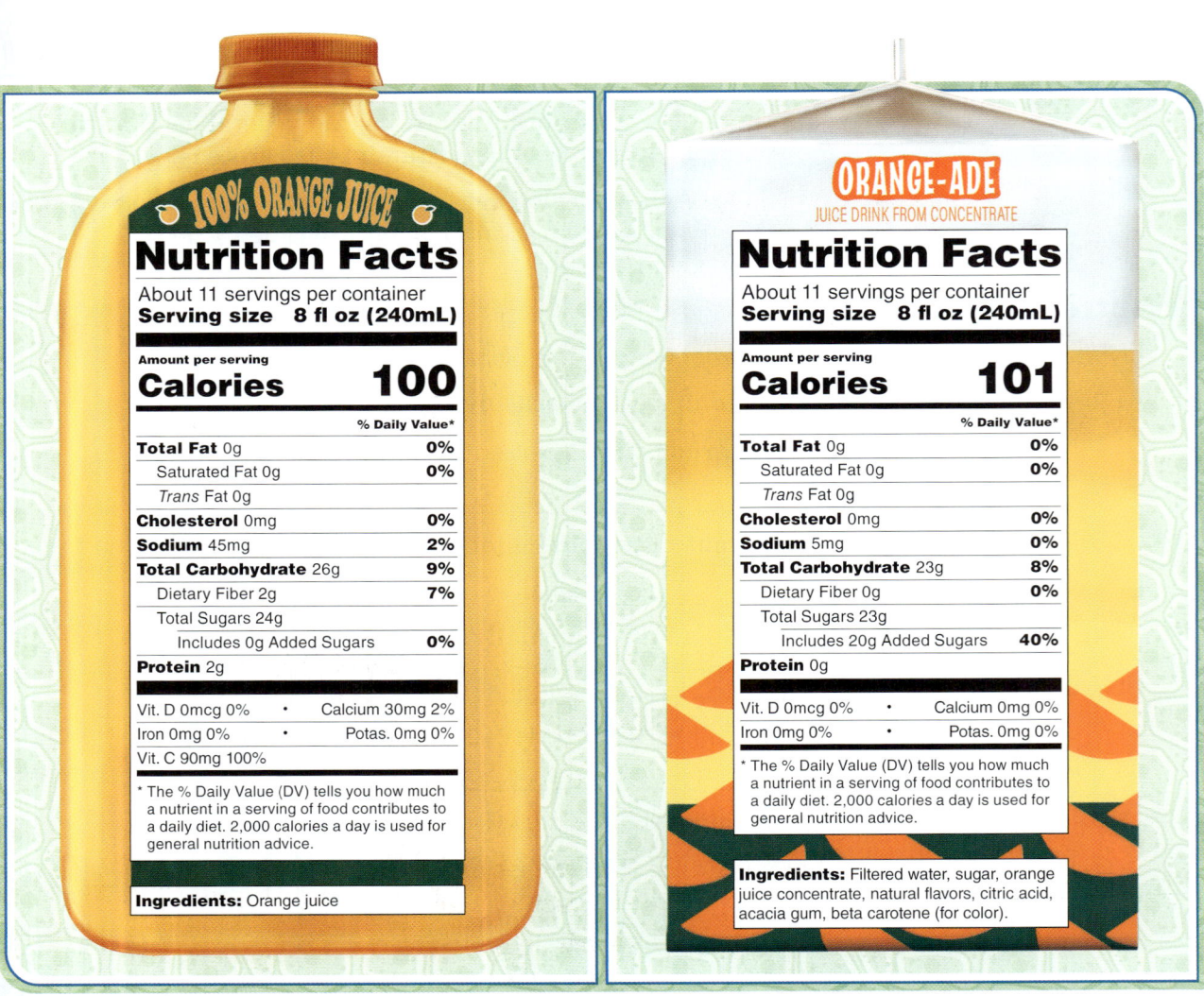

4 Choosing Healthy Eating (4.4)

A. Matching: *Write the letter of the correct answer in the blank. Answers may be used more than once.*

_____ 1. divided into groups based on color

_____ 2. includes meats and nuts

_____ 3. seeds of grass plants

_____ 4. can be classified as whole or refined

_____ 5. have 3 cups every day

_____ 6. provides calcium and vitamin D

A. dairy

B. fruits

C. grains

D. protein

E. vegetables

B. Classify: *Write the first letter of each MyPlate food group present in the food: F for fruits, V for vegetables, P for protein, G for grains, and D for dairy. Remember that some ingredients are in more than one food group.*

_____ 1. a dish of black-eyed peas (cowpeas)

_____ 2. spaghetti topped with a tomato-based meat sauce and Parmesan

_____ 3. parfait made with vanilla yogurt, blueberries, and granola

_____ 4. puffed rice breakfast cereal with skim milk

C. Think!: *Does the statement describe proper food-safety practices? If yes, explain why. If no, explain what should be done.*

1. Freya bought milk and eggs at the grocery store; then she left them in her trunk for two hours while she went clothes shopping. _____

   _____

2. While making a strawberry smoothie, Lillian rinsed off the strawberries before adding them to the blender. _____

   _____

3. River left a package of frozen pork chops in the sink for several hours to thaw.

   _____

   _____

4. After cutting raw chicken, Amir got a fresh knife before cutting broccoli.

   _____

   _____

5. David left a loaf of bread in the kitchen cabinet until he was ready to eat it.

   _____

   _____

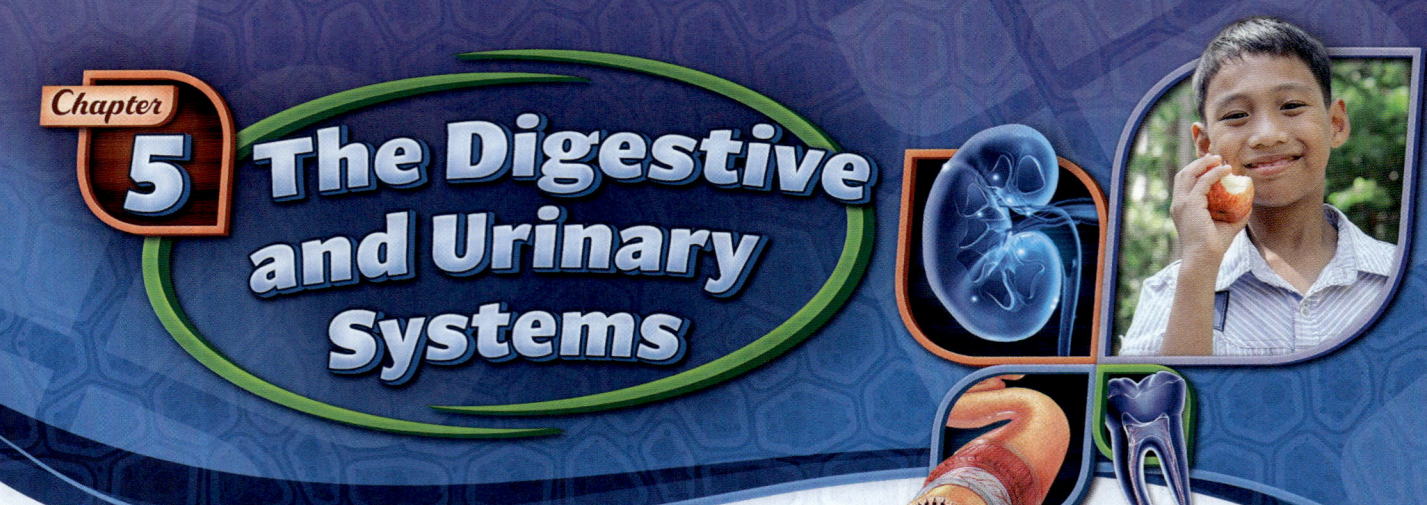

The Digestive and Urinary Systems

Terms

digestion: the process of breaking down food into a form that the body can use

digestive system: body system that performs digestion

alimentary canal: long, muscular tube through which food travels in the digestive system; includes the mouth, esophagus, stomach, small intestine, and large intestine

saliva: digestive juice in the mouth

salivary glands: digestive glands in the mouth that produce saliva

enzyme: any of the special chemicals that perform chemical reactions within the body

esophagus: muscular tube that carries food from the pharynx to the stomach

stomach: digestive organ that is a small elastic bag made of bands of muscles; breaks down and stores food

5.1 Digestion Begins

In the last chapter, you learned how nutrients in the food you eat give you energy, help you grow, and keep your body systems healthy. Before your body can use any food, it must first break the food down into a form that it can use. *The process of breaking down food into a form that the body can use is* **digestion**. God designed the organs of the **digestive system** to work together to perform digestion. *Food travels through the digestive system in a long, muscular tube* called the **alimentary** [ăl′ə·měn′tə·rē] **canal**. *The organs that form the alimentary canal are the* *mouth, esophagus* [ĭ·sŏf′ə·gəs], *stomach, small intestine, and large intestine.* The digestive system also includes several organs that produce substances needed for digestion.

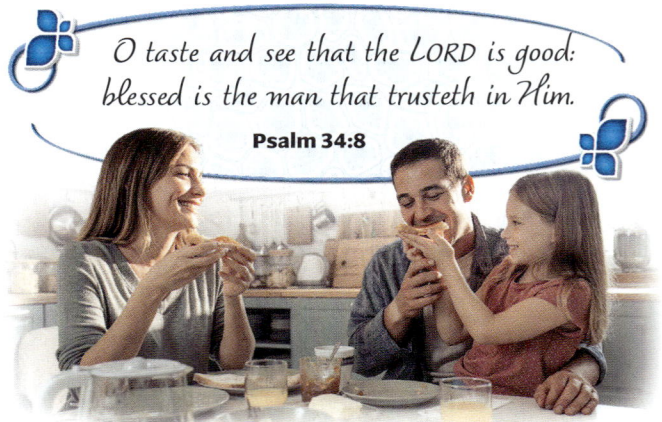

O taste and see that the LORD is good: blessed is the man that trusteth in Him.
Psalm 34:8

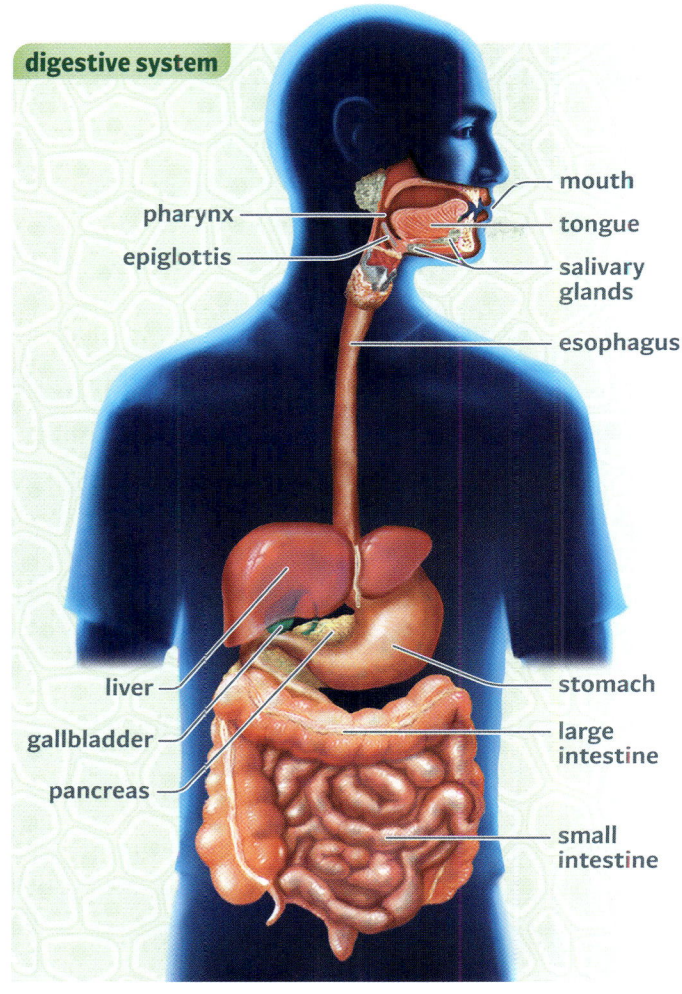

digestive system

- pharynx
- epiglottis
- mouth
- tongue
- salivary glands
- esophagus
- liver
- gallbladder
- pancreas
- stomach
- large intestine
- small intestine

out, and bicuspids grow in to replace them. The name *bicuspids* contains the prefix *bi-*, meaning "two." *This name indicates that bicuspids have two cusps, which they use to tear and crush the food. In the back part of your mouth are the molars, which grind your food into tiny pieces.* Most adults have three pairs of molars on each side of the jaw. The pair that is farthest back are called *wisdom teeth.* Your wisdom teeth will probably grow in when you are between seventeen and twenty-five years old.

Your teeth must be hard in order to cut, tear apart, crush, and grind food. If you eat a well-balanced diet, your teeth will get the calcium, phosphorus, and vitamins they need to grow strong and healthy. Do you brush your teeth after every meal? Do you clean between your teeth with dental floss or dental tape? Because the work of your teeth is important for proper digestion, it is essential that you care for them.

🟣 Chewing

Your alimentary canal begins with your mouth. The food that enters your mouth is broken into small pieces by chewing. You have four different types of teeth, each of which has a different job. All four types are needed to chew your food well. *Your front teeth, or incisors* [ĭn·sī′zərz], *bite and cut your food.* The teeth next to the incisors *are called cuspids* [kŭs′pĭdz] *because they have one cusp, or point. Cuspids tear apart coarse fruits, vegetables, and meats.* Next to the cuspids you have either *primary molars* or *bicuspids* [bī·kŭs′pĭdz]. Sometime between the ages of nine and twelve, your primary molars fall

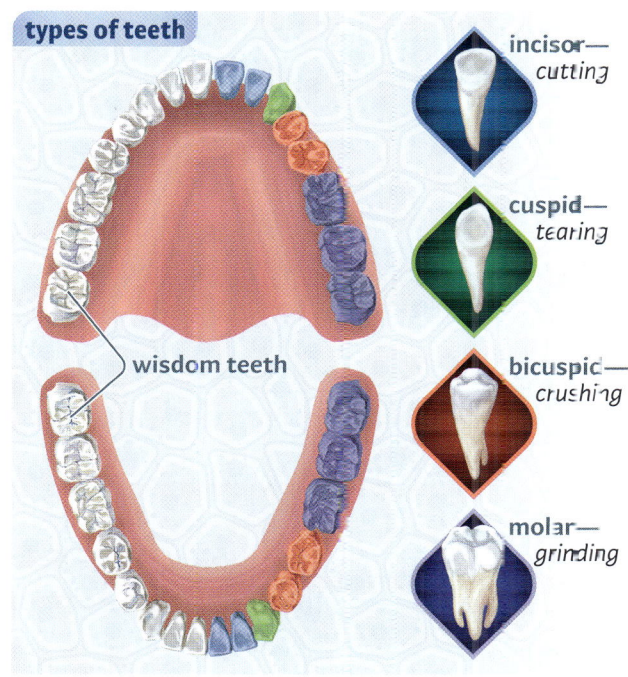

types of teeth

- wisdom teeth
- incisor— *cutting*
- cuspid— *tearing*
- bicuspid— *crushing*
- molar— *grinding*

You should chew every mouthful of food thoroughly to break the food into fine bits—dry foods require longer chewing than soft, creamy foods. As you chew, the food mixes with *a colorless digestive juice* called **saliva**. The saliva flows from the six **salivary** [săl′ə·věr′ē] **glands** *located under your tongue and in your upper and lower jaws*. Saliva and other digestive juices contain **enzymes** [ĕn′zīmz], *special chemicals that perform chemical reactions within the body*. Before you even swallow the food, the enzymes in saliva begin digesting carbohydrates by quickly breaking starches into smaller sugars.

The mixing of saliva with the food increases the taste of the food, and the pleasing taste makes the gastric juice in your stomach begin to flow. Therefore, well-chewed food is easier to digest, since it is crushed into tiny pieces and there is more digestive juice to work on it. You should be sure to always chew and swallow the food in your mouth before you take a drink. If you take a drink while food is in your mouth, you will probably wash down food that is not thoroughly chewed.

Swallowing

As you chew, *your tongue helps mix the food with saliva*. Just before you swallow, your tongue forms the chewed food into a ball and pushes it to your *pharynx* (throat). *While you swallow, your epiglottis* [ĕp′ĭ·glŏt′ĭs], *a tiny flap of cartilage*, closes the opening to your *trachea* (windpipe). This prevents food from traveling down the wrong tube and blocking the flow of air into your lungs. *From your pharynx, the softened food passes to the stomach through a long tube* called your **esophagus**. Food does not fall down the esophagus but is forced through the esophagus by muscle contractions. It takes only four or five seconds for the food to be forced through the esophagus and into the stomach. Drinks can travel down your esophagus in even less time. These muscle contractions allow food to move through your esophagus to your stomach even if you are standing on your head.

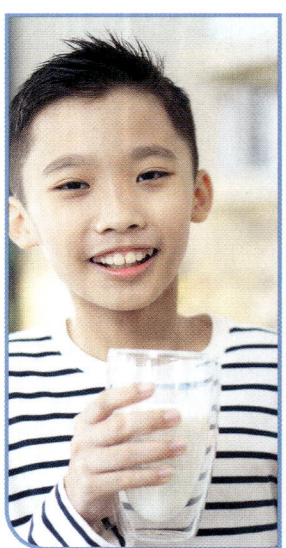
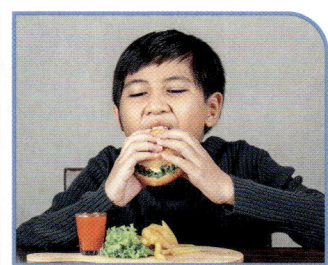
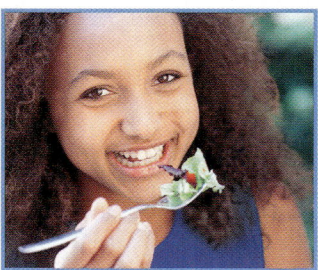

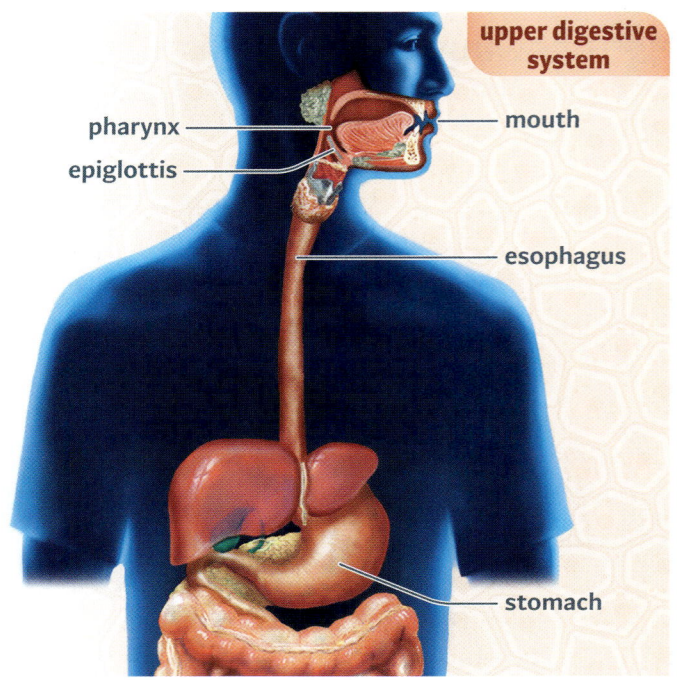

upper digestive system

pharynx — — mouth
epiglottis —

— esophagus

— stomach

🔹 Churning

Your **stomach** is *a small elastic bag made of bands of muscles.* Because the stomach is elastic, it can stretch to hold the food that enters it from the esophagus. *The major purpose of the stomach is to break down and store food.* The stored food is released a little at a time into the small intestine for further digestion. The stomach's lining contains thousands of tiny glands that make *gastric juice. Gastric juice softens foods, kills bacteria, and starts digesting protein foods like meat and eggs.* Gastric juice contains a strong acid that helps stomach enzymes do their work. The powerful muscles of the stomach mash, press, and squeeze the softened food and digestive juices together. *The churning of the stomach forms food and gastric juice into a thick liquid called chyme* [kīm].

Nutrients from food pass through the stomach at different rates. Water is absorbed into the bloodstream without any change. Vitamins and minerals are dissolved and then absorbed into the blood. Starches and sugars from carbohydrates are broken down quickly and usually stay in the stomach only a short time. Protein foods remain in the stomach for a longer period. Fried foods and poorly chewed food are difficult for the digestive juices to break down. Fats and oils leave the stomach even more slowly than proteins; they may remain in the stomach for up to six hours.

Community HEALTH CORNER

The Stomach at Work

In 1822 at an army post in northern Michigan, Dr. William Beaumont (1785–1853), a young army surgeon, was called upon to care for an 18-year-old who had been struck by an accidental shotgun blast. The shot, which went through Alexis St. Martin's left side, tore a gaping hole in his stomach. With Dr. Beaumont's care, St. Martin recovered, but the hole in his stomach never completely closed. A flap of loose tissue covered the hole, and Dr. Beaumont could move this flap to watch the stomach at work.

From observing St. Martin's stomach, Dr. Beaumont learned that the stomach finishes its work more quickly with some foods than with others. Do you remember which foods stay in the stomach the longest? Which foods leave the stomach first? Dr. Beaumont noted the importance of saliva and the work of the teeth in digestion. He also learned that food digests better when meals are eaten regularly and when the stomach has a chance to rest between meals. Whenever St. Martin was unhappy or worried, the digestive juice in his stomach did not flow as freely

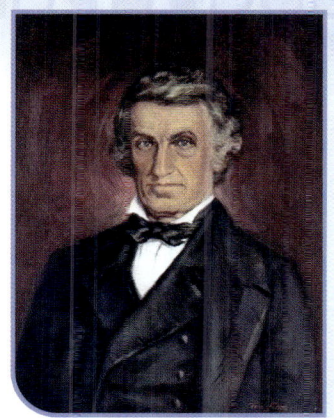

Dr. William Beaumont

as usual, and with less gastric juice, the stomach could not do its work as well as it should. However, when St. Martin was happy, gastric juice poured out to mix with the food. Another thing Dr. Beaumont observed was that alcoholic drinks made the stomach red and sore-looking. Again, the stomach did not work as well as it should.

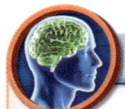

Matching: *Write the letter of the correct answer in the blank.*

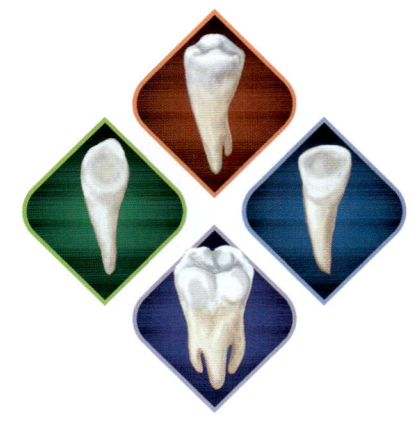

A. bicuspids   C. incisors
B. cuspids   D. molars

_____ 1. front teeth that bite and cut food

_____ 2. sharp teeth that tear apart food

_____ 3. back teeth that grind food into tiny pieces

Short Answer: *Write the correct answer in the blank.*

4. What is the process of breaking down food? _____

5. What is the muscular tube through which food travels? _____

6. What is the digestive juice in the mouth called? _____

7. What is the tube connecting the mouth and stomach? _____

8. What is the main purpose of the stomach? _____

_____

Identify: *Label the parts of the upper digestive system.*

9. _____

10. _____

11. _____

12. _____

13. _____

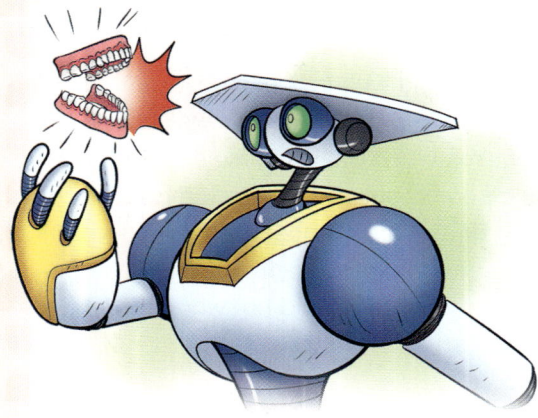

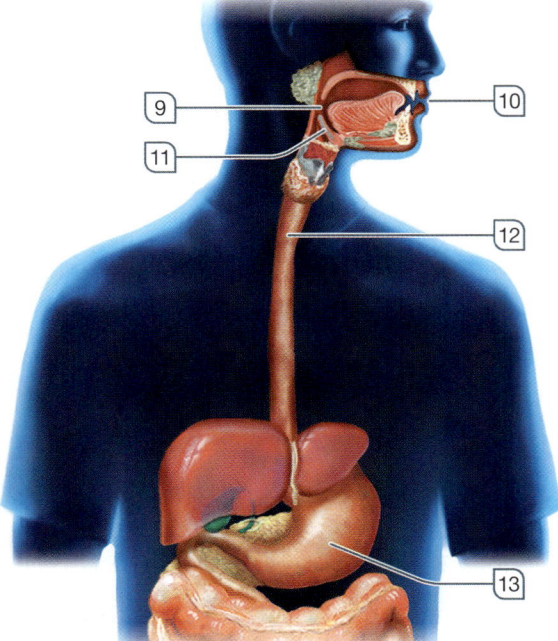

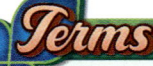

Terms

small intestine: twenty-foot-long tube of muscle and other tissues that is coiled up just below the stomach; digests most food and absorbs most nutrients

absorption: process by which digested nutrients are taken into the bloodstream

villi: hair-like projections in the small intestine through which food is absorbed (villus, *sing.*)

large intestine: the last organ of the alimentary canal; prepares undigested food to be removed from the body as waste

liver: the largest organ inside the body; recycles red blood cells to produce bile salts, stores and processes nutrients, and filters blood

bile: a greenish digestive juice produced by the liver; performs emulsification of fats

pancreas: digestive organ located between the stomach and small intestine; produces pancreatic juice and insulin

insulin: hormone, or chemical messenger, made in the pancreas; helps the body remove excess sugar from the blood

5.2 Digestion Continues

You have learned about how food travels from the mouth, through the esophagus, and into the stomach. These organs start the process of digestion. The remaining organs of the alimentary canal continue this process by breaking down food, absorbing nutrients, and removing undigested materials from the body.

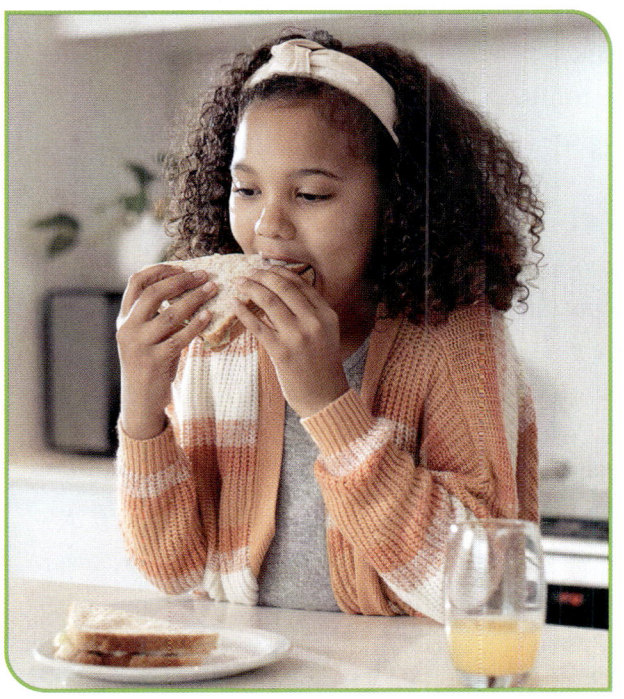

 **Absorption**

As the food becomes soft enough, continuous muscle contractions in your stomach squeeze small amounts of chyme into the **small intestine,** *a twenty-foot-long tube of muscle and other tissues that is coiled up just below the stomach.* God designed the stomach to send food into the small intestine at just the right rate for the small intestine to do its job.

Your small intestine produces intestinal juice from millions of tiny glands. This intestinal juice begins to flow as partly digested food moves into your small intestine. Other digestive juices from the liver and pancreas pour into your small intestine through *ducts, or tubes.* These digestive juices complete the digestion of carbohydrates and proteins that was started in your mouth and stomach. They also digest the fats and oils. *Most of the food you eat is digested in your small intestine.*

Another important function of your small intestine is **absorption,** the *process by which digested nutrients are taken into the* *bloodstream*. Although some nutrients are absorbed in other organs of the alimentary canal, most nutrients from the food you eat enter your bloodstream from your small intestine. *The inside wall of the small intestine is covered by millions of tiny, hair-like projections* called **villi** [vĭl′ī]. These villi are in the path of the digested food as it moves along. *Nutrients from digested food are absorbed as they pass through the thin walls of a villus* [vĭl′əs] *and into capillaries inside the villus.* Your blood then transports these life-giving substances to all parts of your body.

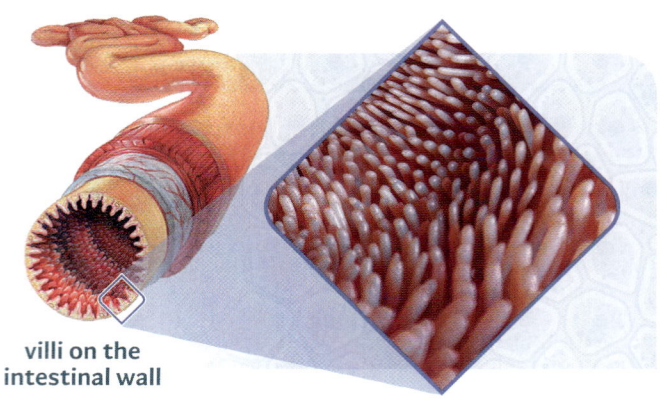

villi on the intestinal wall

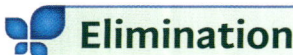

When cells in the small intestine are absorbing nutrients, they use more oxygen and give off more carbon dioxide than they do when they are at rest. What does this tell you about their activity?

Elimination

By the time food reaches the end of your small intestine, most of the nutrients that can be used have been absorbed into your bloodstream. The rest of the food is sent to *the last organ of the alimentary canal*, the **large intestine**. The large intestine is twice as wide as your small intestine but only about five feet long. Like the rest of the alimentary canal, it is made of muscles that move food through it. *The main job of the large intestine is to prepare undigested food to be removed from the body as waste.*

By the time food reaches the large intestine, it is mostly fiber and water. *Fiber, the rough parts of some fruits, vegetables, and grains, consists of complex carbohydrates that humans cannot digest.* Although fiber is not used for energy, it has the important role of cleaning the intestinal walls and helping food move through the large intestine. The fiber is stored temporarily in the large intestine before being removed as waste. Water and any remaining minerals are absorbed in the large intestine. The large intestine contains helpful bacteria that produce vitamins from undigested food; these vitamins are also absorbed into the bloodstream.

When waste material reaches the end of the large intestine, it is in a solid form that is ready for *elimination, the removal of waste substances by the body*. These wastes are eliminated by the movement of muscles in the large intestine, called a bowel movement. From the time you eat food until your body eliminates the undigested portion usually takes between 24 and 48 hours.

Your diet affects the function of your large intestine. If you drink too little water, eat too little fiber, or drink too many beverages containing caffeine, the undigested food will not move through the large intestine as it should. Since the food remains in the large intestine too long, too much water is removed from the food. *The dryness of the food can cause constipation, a condition in which a person has bowel movements less often than he should.* Long-term constipation can cause a variety of other health problems and needs to be treated by a physician.

Organs That Aid Digestion

So far, we have discussed the organs of the alimentary canal, which carry food through the body. Some other digestive organs are not part of the alimentary canal. Although food does not move through them, they are important because they help the small intestine with digestion and absorption. God marvelously designed each part of the digestive system to work together.

Liver and Gallbladder

Your **liver**, the *largest organ inside your body*, is located just below the diaphragm. It is partially surrounded by your ribs and is connected to the alimentary canal by a duct. *One important job of the liver is recycling red blood cells.* Every second, millions of red blood cells finish their work in your body and die. Your liver filters out these dead cells and recycles their components. It uses some of these components to produce a *greenish digestive juice* called **bile**. Bile contains important substances called bile salts, which help in the digestion of fats and oils. In the small intestine, *bile separates oil droplets so that they can be mixed with digestive juices, a process called emulsification* [ĭ·mŭl′sə·fĭ·kā′shən]. Bile also carries some waste material out of your body. Each day, your liver produces about one quart of bile. *A sack-like pouch called the gallbladder stores the bile and delivers it to the small intestine as needed.*

Your liver also stores and processes nutrients and filters blood. It removes minerals, vitamins, and extra sugar from the blood and stores these nutrients until the body needs them. It makes vitamin A from the carotene found in deep yellow and dark green vegetables. Blood from the stomach and small intestines passes through your liver before returning to the heart; the liver removes poisons that formed in the small intestine during digestion.

Pancreas

Another *organ that aids in digestion* is your **pancreas**, which is *located between your stomach and small intestine. Your pancreas produces pancreatic* [păng′krē·ăt′ĭk] *juice.* This juice pours through a duct into your small intestine and digests carbohydrates, proteins, and fats. Pancreatic juice also neutralizes the acid in gastric juice, making the inside of the small intestine *neutral, neither acidic nor basic.* Without this neutralization, the digestive juices in your small intestine would not be able to function.

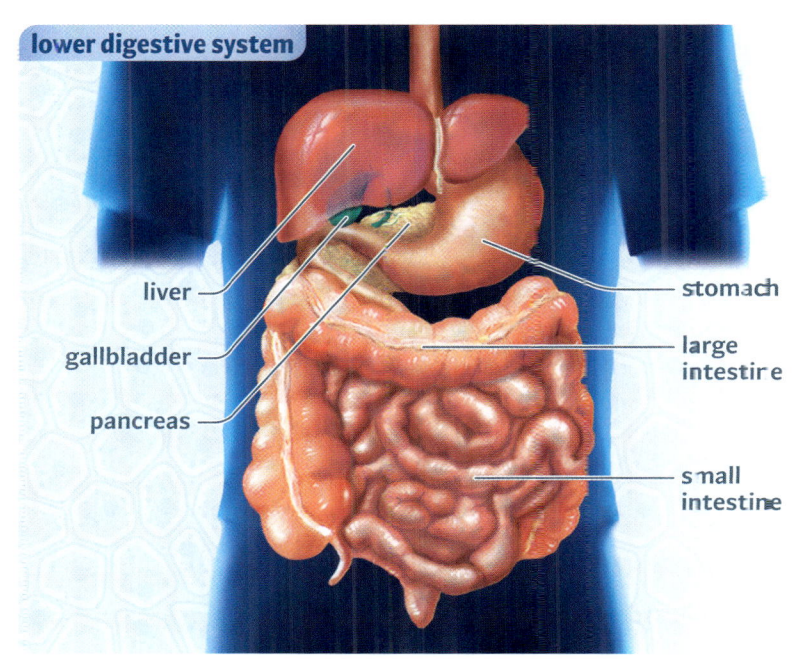

lower digestive system

liver —
gallbladder —
pancreas —
— stomach
— large intestine
— small intestine

The pancreas also makes **insulin***, a hormone, or chemical messenger, that helps your body remove excess sugar from the blood.* During digestion, your small intestine absorbs more sugar than the body can immediately use for heat and energy. Too much sugar in your blood is dangerous to your health; the body removes the extra sugar from the blood and stores it in the liver. *An error in how the body produces or responds to insulin causes the disease diabetes.*

Community HEALTH CORNER

Gastroenterologist

Your digestive system is marvelously designed to break down food so that your body can get the nutrition you need. Sometimes, your digestive organs do not work properly because of a disease. If you experience severe stomach pain or unexplained weight loss, you may need to see a gastroenterologist [găs′trō·ĕn′tə·rŏl′ə·jĭst]. A gastroenterologist is a physician who has received special training in the treatment of the digestive organs.

A gastroenterologist can use an endoscope to look at the insides of your digestive organs. An endoscope is a tiny camera on the end of a thin tube, which can be sent down your alimentary canal. With an endoscope, the doctor can view the insides of your organs, take pictures, and even perform small procedures to fix problems. After the examination, the gastroenterologist will develop a treatment plan and prescribe medicine.

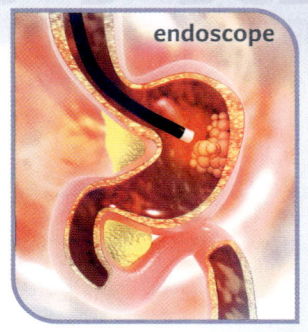

endoscope

Many disorders of the digestive system are caused by poor nutrition. One of the best ways to keep your digestive organs healthy is by eating a nutritious diet. You can also encourage your family and friends to make wise choices about the foods they eat.

Hands-On Health

Acid Attack

Materials needed:
- 3 cups or clear containers
- white vinegar or lemon juice
- crackers, crushed
- data sheet (from *Activity Book*)
- kitchen scale
- various foods high in protein or fats, crushed or chopped: nuts, dry beans, baking chips, etc.

You can observe the effects of acid on different types of foods by following these procedures:

1. Fill three cups with the same amount of white vinegar or lemon juice.

2. Weigh out equal amounts of each type of food.

3. Place each food into its own cup.

4. Record your observations.

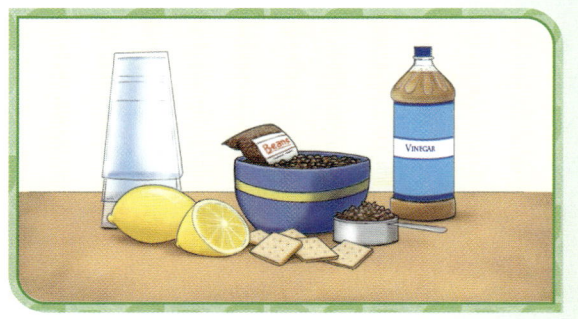

Multiple Choice: *Write the letter of the correct answer in the blank.*

_____ 1. What is the process by which digested nutrients are taken into the bloodstream?

    a. constipation   c. elimination

    b. absorption   d. emulsification

_____ 2. What organ prepares undigested food to be removed from the body?

    a. gallbladder   c. pancreas

    b. large intestine   d. small intestine

_____ 3. Which digestive juice contains salts that help break down fats and oils?

    a. bile   c. intestinal juice

    b. gastric juice   d. pancreatic juice

_____ 4. What organ stores bile?

    a. gallbladder   c. pancreas

    b. liver   d. small intestine

_____ 5. Which of the following is a function of the pancreas?

    a. absorption   c. recycling red blood cells

    b. producing insulin   d. storing extra sugar

Short Answer: *Write the correct answer in the blank.*

6. What are the two important functions of the small intestine? _____

_____

7. What are the tiny, hair-like projections that cover the inside of the small intestine?

_____

8. List three functions of the liver. _____

_____

_____

Think about It.

9. What would happen if your pancreas stopped working properly? _____

_____

_____

_____

_____

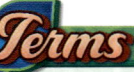
5.3 Hydration and Excretion

The Importance of Water

As you have learned, *water is important for your body's function.* Your body loses about two quarts of water every day through breathing, perspiring, and removing wastes. **Hydration**, *replacing water that has been lost from the body*, is therefore needed for survival. If you do not drink enough liquids, your blood draws water from your body tissues, and your skin becomes dry. The large intestine removes more water than usual from undigested food, causing constipation. If you were without water for several days, your body would completely cease to function.

You probably do not get enough hydration unless you drink water or juice between meals. Chewing gum can cause you to not feel thirsty and thus to not drink enough water. If you breathe through your mouth instead of through your nose, you will get used to your mouth feeling dry. In cold weather, you may not drink enough liquids because you do not feel thirsty. You need to drink sufficient water, even if you do not feel thirsty, to help prevent colds and diseases.

Hydration is especially important in hot weather because your body can quickly lose water through perspiration. During moderate exercise in normal summer weather, you lose from one to two pints of water an hour. Drinking liquids, such as soft drinks, that contain caffeine can cause your body to lose water even faster. As you lose water, your body can no longer regulate its temperature. Losing excessive amounts of water can result in fainting and heatstroke. To prevent fatigue, you should replace water that is lost in perspiration as soon as possible.

You can also lose water quickly during an illness that causes fever, vomiting, or diarrhea. If a person with one of these conditions cannot take water or other fluids by mouth, he may require hospitalization to have fluid pumped directly into his bloodstream.

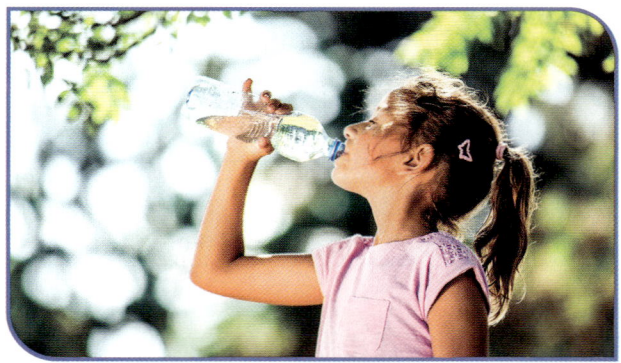

The Excretory System

Excretion is the *removal of unneeded substances from the body. Excretion is performed by the excretory* [ĕk′skrĭ·tôr′ē] *system.* Many organs in the excretory system are also part of other body systems. The large intestine performs excretion by eliminating undigested food. Your liver aids excretion by filtering wastes from the blood. Your sweat glands help remove various substances that were dissolved in the blood.

The Urinary System

One part of the excretory system is the **urinary system**, *or renal system, which removes liquid waste products and regulates the amount of water in the body.* Unlike the large intestine, liver, and sweat glands, the organs of the urinary system have excretion as their main function. *The main organs of the urinary system are the kidneys and bladder.*

The **kidneys** are *two bean-shaped organs that filter the blood.* They are located on either side of your spine in your upper back, behind your liver and stomach. As blood passes through the kidneys, blood plasma and dissolved substances pass out of the capillaries and into the kidneys' filtration system. This system returns water and other useful materials back to the bloodstream. The brain tells the kidneys how much water to return to the blood; in this way, the body maintains a proper amount of water.

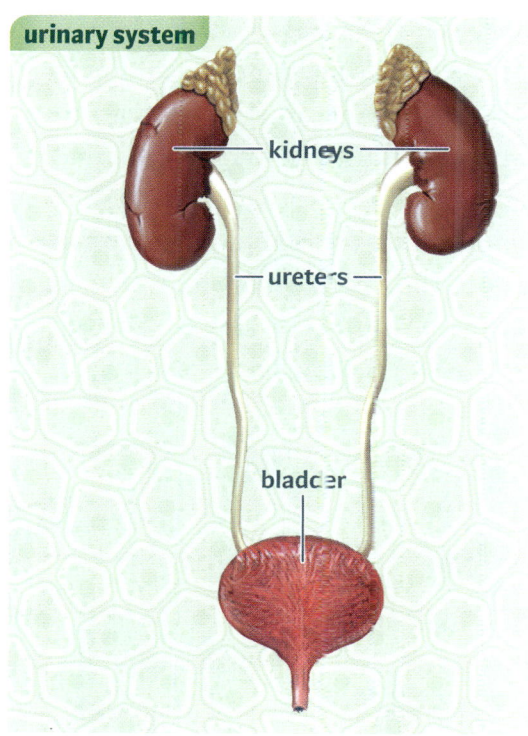

urinary system

kidneys

ureters

bladder

The fluid remaining in the kidneys after filtration is urine. Urine contains various waste products that were dissolved in the bloodstream. The main waste product in urine is urea [yŏŏ·rē′ə], which the liver forms by breaking down protein parts and releases into the bloodstream. *The kidneys release urine into ureters* [yŏŏ·rē′tərz], *ducts that carry urine down to the bladder.* The **bladder** is an *expandable pouch that stores urine.* When the bladder is full, the *urine leaves the bladder and exits the body through a canal called the urethra* [yŏŏ·rē′thrə].

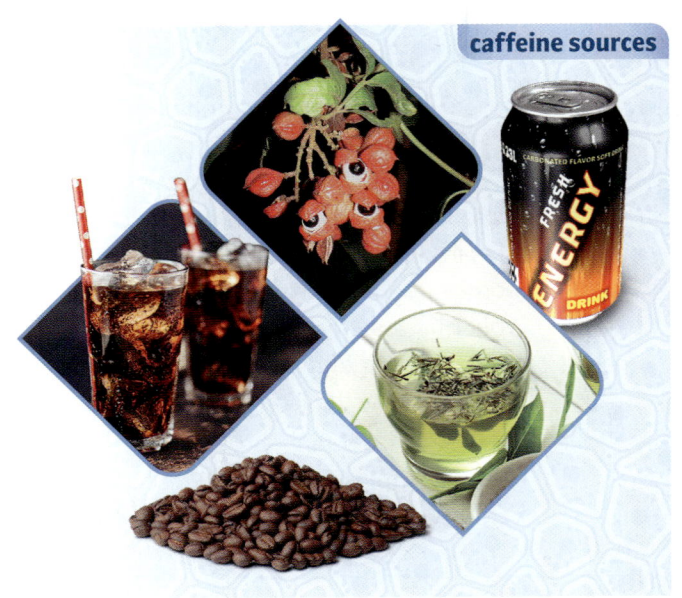

caffeine sources

Caffeine and the Urinary System

What is your favorite drink? Do you enjoy drinking soft drinks or energy drinks? Many people drink coffee or tea every day. These drinks contain **caffeine**, *a drug that is naturally found in the leaves or fruits of some plants.* You might enjoy drinks with caffeine because they make you feel as if you have more energy than you really have. Caffeine can also help reduce symptoms of asthma, headaches, and low blood pressure. However, caffeine can harm the body if it is consumed in large amounts.

Caffeine affects the body in many ways. It stimulates the nervous system, which can cause restlessness and sleeping problems. The heart begins beating faster, causing high blood pressure. *Caffeine also forces the kidneys to give up more water, increasing the amount of urine produced and the amount of water lost by the body.* Once the effects of caffeine wear off, you may feel tired and develop a bad headache. This causes you to want to drink even more caffeine. Besides caffeine, energy drinks and soft drinks usually contain large amounts of added sugar, which can be harmful for your body.

You should limit the amount of caffeine that you drink each day. Instead, choose drinks like water, juice, or milk. You can also encourage your friends and family to make healthy choices about the drinks that they consume.

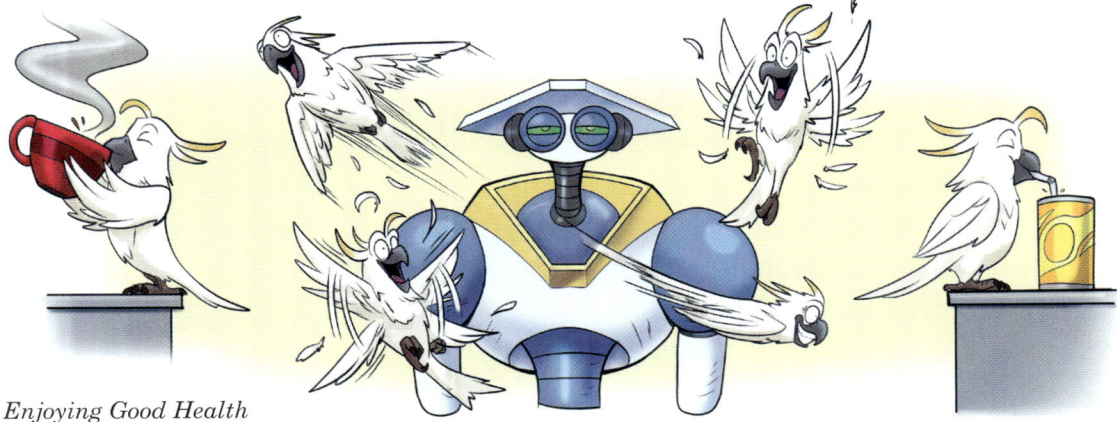

Urologist and Nephrologist

A urologist [yoō·rŏl′ə·jĭst] is a doctor who specializes in disorders of the urinary system. Someone may need to visit a urologist if he wets his bed at night, has difficulty urinating, or has blood in the urine. A urologist can also treat kidney stones and certain types of cancer. The urologist will take urine or blood samples, perform physical examinations, or take pictures of the urinary organs with an ultrasound. He can also perform surgery on the urinary system.

A nephrologist [nə·frŏl′ə·jĭst] is a doctor who specializes in the kidneys. A nephrologist can

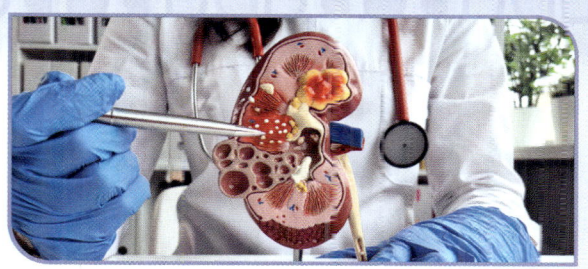

diagnose and treat a wide range of problems with the kidneys. Unlike a urologist, a nephrologist does not perform surgeries. Because of how their specialties differ, urologists and nephrologists often work together to treat diseases that affect several parts of the urinary system.

Comprehension Check 5.3

Identify: *Label the parts of the urinary system.*

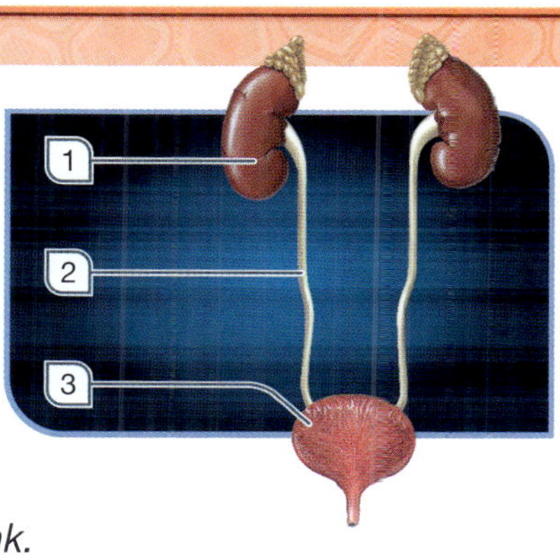

1. _____

2. _____

3. _____

Short Answer: *Write the correct answer in the blank.*

4. What is replacing water that has been lost from the body called? _____

5. What is the removal of unneeded substances from the body? _____

6. What is the job of the urinary system? _____

_____

7. What is the waste-containing fluid remaining in the kidneys after filtration?

_____

8. How does caffeine affect the urinary system? _____

_____

_____

_____

Concepts Review

Chapter 5

1 Digestion Begins (5.1)

A. True/False: *If the statement is true, write* true *in the blank. If the statement is false, replace the underlined word(s) with a word that will make the statement true. Do not write* false *in any blank.*

_____ 1. The breaking down of food into a form that can be used by the body is <u>absorption</u>.

_____ 2. Food travels through the digestive system in a long, muscular tube called the <u>alimentary canal</u>.

_____ 3. The digestive glands in the mouth are the <u>intestinal</u> glands.

_____ 4. Chemical reactions within the body are performed by special chemicals called <u>chyme</u>.

_____ 5. Food is broken down and stored in the <u>stomach</u>.

B. Multiple Choice: *Write the letter of the correct answer in the blank.*

_____ 1. Which teeth bite and cut food?
- a. bicuspids
- b. cuspids
- c. incisors
- d. molars

_____ 2. Which teeth grind food into tiny pieces?
- a. bicuspids
- b. cuspids
- c. incisors
- d. molars

_____ 3. Which digestive juice is produced in the mouth?
- a. bile
- b. gastric juice
- c. pancreatic juice
- d. saliva

_____ 4. What tiny flap of cartilage covers the windpipe when you swallow?
- a. epiglottis
- b. pancreas
- c. pharynx
- d. trachea

_____ 5. What is the thick liquid that the stomach forms from softened food and digestive juices?
- a. bile
- b. chyme
- c. saliva
- d. urine

2 Digestion Continues (5.2)

A. Matching: *Write the letter of the correct answer in the blank.*

> A. gallbladder   B. large intestine   C. liver
>
> D. pancreas   E. small intestine

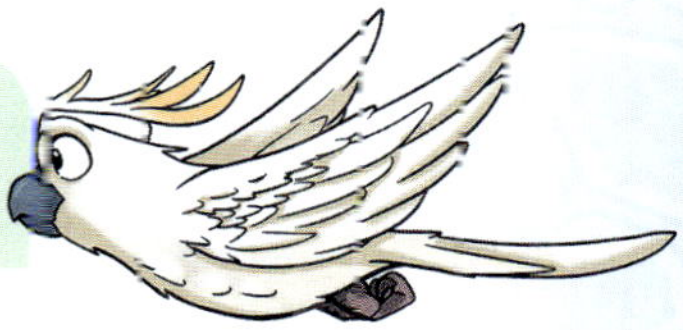

_____ 1. digests most food and absorbs most nutrients

_____ 2. prepares waste to leave the body

_____ 3. recycles blood cells, stores nutrients, and filters blood

_____ 4. produces insulin

B. Short Answer: *Write the correct answer in the blank.*

1. What is absorption? _____

_____

_____

2. How do the villi help with digestion? _____

_____

_____

_____

3. How does bile help with digestion? _____

_____

_____

_____

_____

C. Think!

What would happen if your liver stopped working properly?

_____

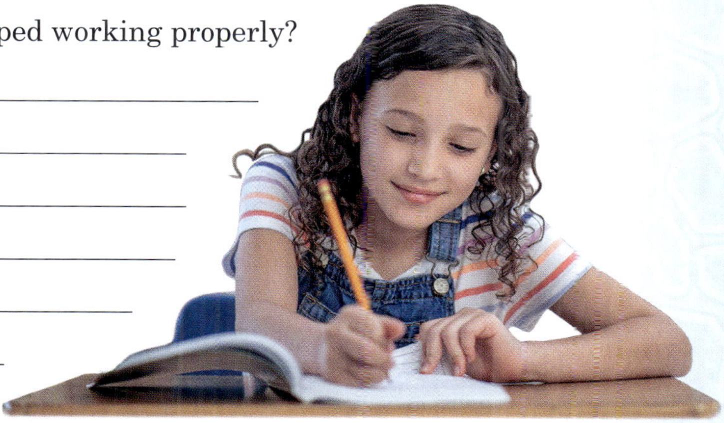

_____

_____

_____

_____

_____

_____

3 Digestive System Review (5.1–5.2)

A. Identify: Label the organs of the digestive system.

1. _____

2. _____

3. _____

4. _____

5. _____

6. _____

7. _____

8. _____

9. _____

10. _____

11. _____

B. Classify: Write A *if the organ is part of the alimentary canal and* N *if it is not part of the alimentary canal.*

_____ 1. esophagus

_____ 2. gallbladder

_____ 3. kidney

_____ 4. large intestine

_____ 5. liver

_____ 6. mouth

_____ 7. pancreas

_____ 8. small intestine

_____ 9. stomach

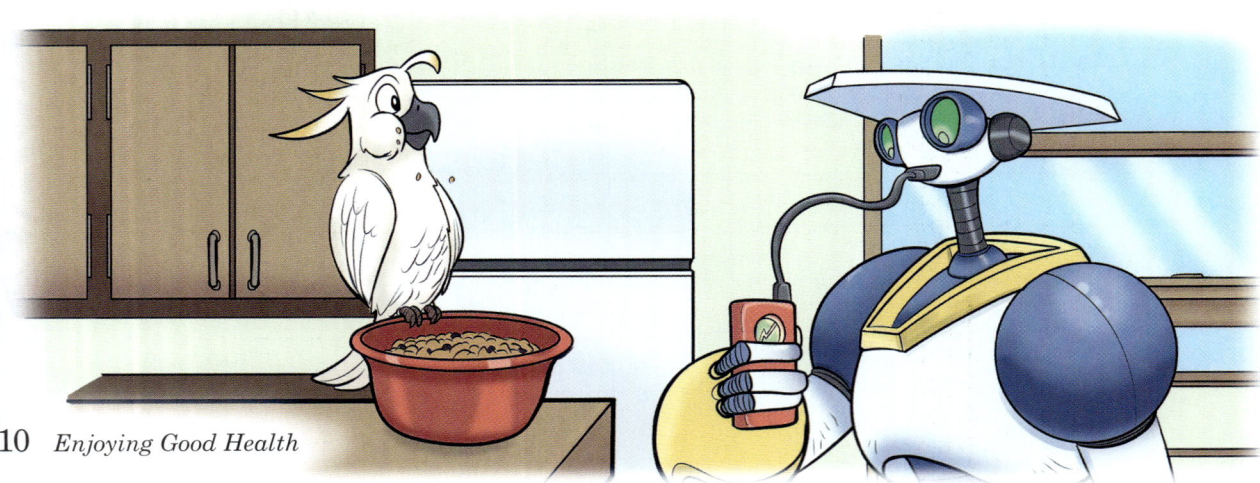

4 Hydration and Excretion (5.3)

A. True/False: *If the statement is true, write* true *in the blank. If the statement is false, replace the underlined word with a word that will make the statement true. Do not write* false *in any blank.*

_____ 1. The replacement of water that has been lost from the body is <u>hydration</u>.

_____ 2. The removal of unneeded substances from the body is <u>digestion</u>.

_____ 3. Liquid waste is removed by the <u>digestive</u> system.

_____ 4. The bean-shaped organs that filter blood are the <u>ureters</u>.

_____ 5. Urine is stored in an expandable pouch called the <u>bladder</u>.

_____ 6. Coffee, tea, soft drinks, and energy drinks usually contain a drug called <u>caffeine</u>.

B. Short Answer: *Write the correct answer in the blank.*

How does caffeine affect the body's water content? _____

_____

_____

_____

_____

C. Think!

Place a check mark ✓ in the box for the healthiest drink. Explain your choice.

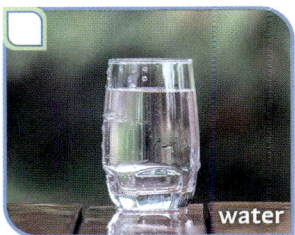 water

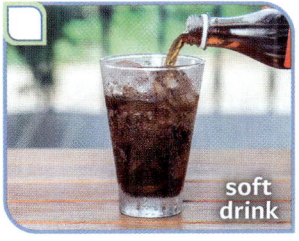 soft drink

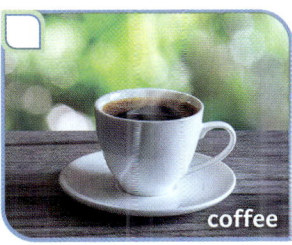 coffee

_____

_____

_____

_____

_____

_____

Chapter 6 — Disease Prevention

Terms

disease: any condition that causes the body to work in an incorrect way

communicable disease: disease that can be spread from person to person

noncommunicable disease: disease that cannot be spread from person to person

microorganism: microscopic organism; also called microbe

pathogen: microorganism that can cause disease; a germ

bacterium: single-celled microorganism that does not have a cell nucleus (bacteria, *plural*)

virus: pathogen much smaller than a bacterium; reproduces by using a host cell of the body

vector: animal that can carry a pathogen and transmit it to humans

cancer: disease caused by the uncontrolled growth of body cells

diabetes mellitus: disease that causes extra sugar to collect in the blood

obesity: the condition of having too much body fat

6.1 Types of Disease

Wherefore, as by one man sin entered into the world, and death by sin; and so death passed upon all men, for that all have sinned. **Romans 5:12**

In the beginning, God created a perfect world. Genesis 1:31 tells that He looked at all He had created and said that it was "very good." There was no pain or suffering because there was no sin. Everything changed when Adam disobeyed God. Because of the Fall, death entered the world. The human body began to break down and stop working properly. Now, our bodies suffer from **disease**, *any condition that causes the body to work in an incorrect way.*

There are several ways that diseases can be classified. One way is by how long they last. An *acute disease occurs suddenly and lasts only a short time.* Other diseases, called *chronic diseases, last for a long time.* The common cold is an acute disease, while diabetes is a chronic disease. Diseases can also be classified by whether they can spread to other people. *A disease that can be spread from one person to another* is a **communicable disease**. A **noncommunicable disease** *cannot be passed from one person to another*. Communicable diseases are usually acute; noncommunicable diseases are usually chronic.

Communicable Diseases

Your body is constantly being attacked by very small invaders. They live by the millions on your skin and in the air you breathe. You cannot get away from them. These *microscopic organisms* are known as **microorganisms**, or *microbes*. Although some microorganisms help the body, many attack the body's cells. If they enter your body and begin to reproduce, they cause an infection. *A microorganism that can cause disease* is called a **pathogen**, or *germ*. *Communicable diseases are caused by pathogens*. A communicable disease spreads as pathogens are transferred from one person to another. *The most common pathogens are bacteria and viruses.*

A **bacterium** is a *single-celled microorganism that does not have a cell nucleus. Bacteria live in water, air, soil, and inside other living creatures.* Many types of bacteria are helpful to the body. For example, good bacteria live in the intestines and help the

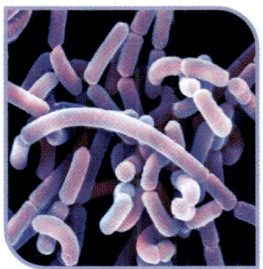
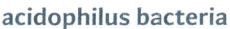
acidophilus bacteria

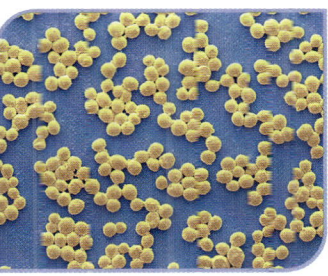
streptococcus bacteria
(cause strep throat)

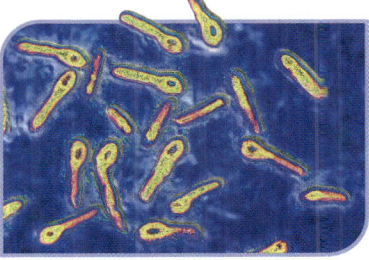
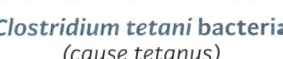
Clostridium tetani bacteria
(cause tetanus)

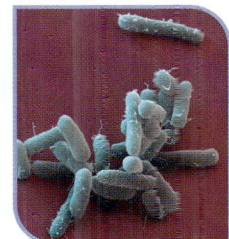
salmonella bacteria

body digest food. Some helpful bacteria even protect the body from diseases.

Harmful bacteria are pathogens that can cause diseases. Bacteria reproduce by dividing repeatedly to make exact copies of themselves. In a matter of hours, just a few bacteria can reproduce to form millions of tiny invaders that can cause the body to be very sick. *Strep throat, tetanus, and food poisoning are common diseases caused by bacteria. Bacterial infections are usually treated with medications called antibiotics, which can stop bacterial growth.*

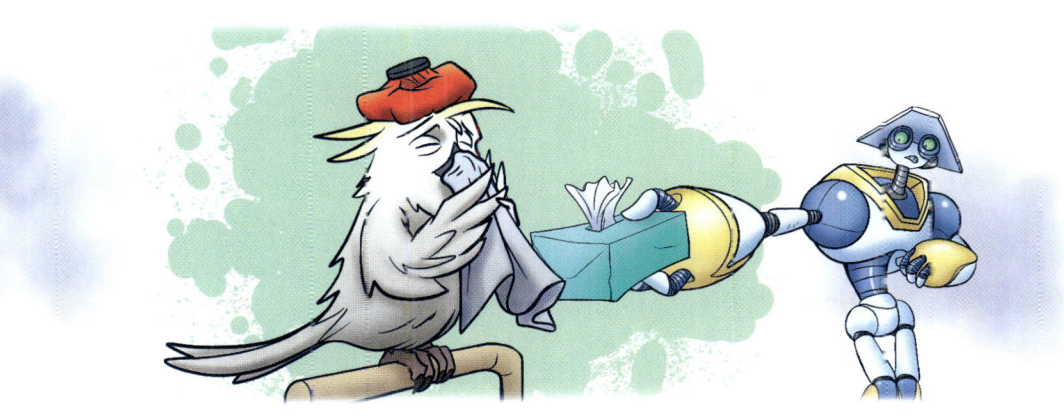

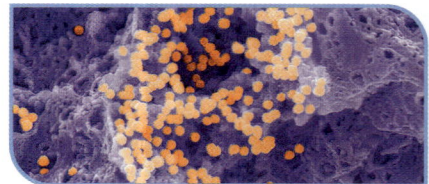
adenovirus
(causes symptoms similar to cold and flu)

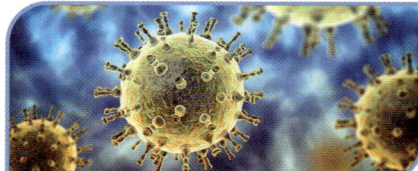
chickenpox virus

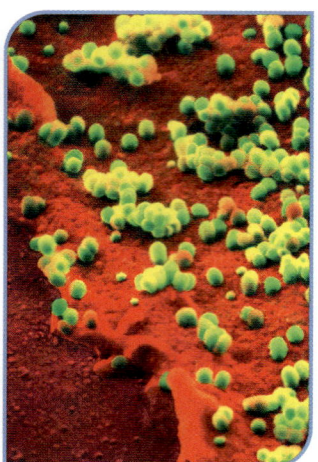
influenza virus

A **virus** is a tiny *pathogen that is much smaller than a bacterium. The common cold, COVID-19, and influenza (the flu) are all caused by viruses.* Although viruses are often classified as microorganisms, scientists do not consider viruses to be living creatures. A virus is made only of genetic material and must invade a host cell to survive. *When a virus enters the cell of a body, it forces the host cell to reproduce viruses exactly like itself.* These new viruses can then enter more cells and cause them to reproduce the virus as well. *An antibiotic cannot treat a disease caused by a virus.* Doctors will prescribe other medicines and treatment plans to manage a viral disease.

Although bacteria and viruses are the most common pathogens, some diseases are caused by other organisms. *Fungi* [fŭn′jī; *fungus, sing.*] *are plant-like organisms that do not make their own food. Athlete's foot* and *ringworm* are caused by fungus pathogens. *Dandruff*, the flaking of skin cells of the scalp, can also be caused by a fungus. *Protozoa* [prō′tə·zō′ə; *protozoan, sing.*] *are singled-celled animal-like organisms.* Protozoan pathogens can cause a variety of serious and often life-threatening diseases, including *malaria* and *African sleeping sickness.*

Communicable diseases spread when pathogens pass from one person to another. Although many communicable diseases are transmitted directly from person to person, some are transmitted by animals. *An animal that can carry a pathogen and transmit it to humans* is called a **vector**. *Common vectors include mosquitoes, fleas, lice, and ticks.* Controlling the population of these pests greatly helps with preventing the spread of diseases. Different vectors carry different types of diseases; the treatment will depend on what specific pathogen the vector transmitted.

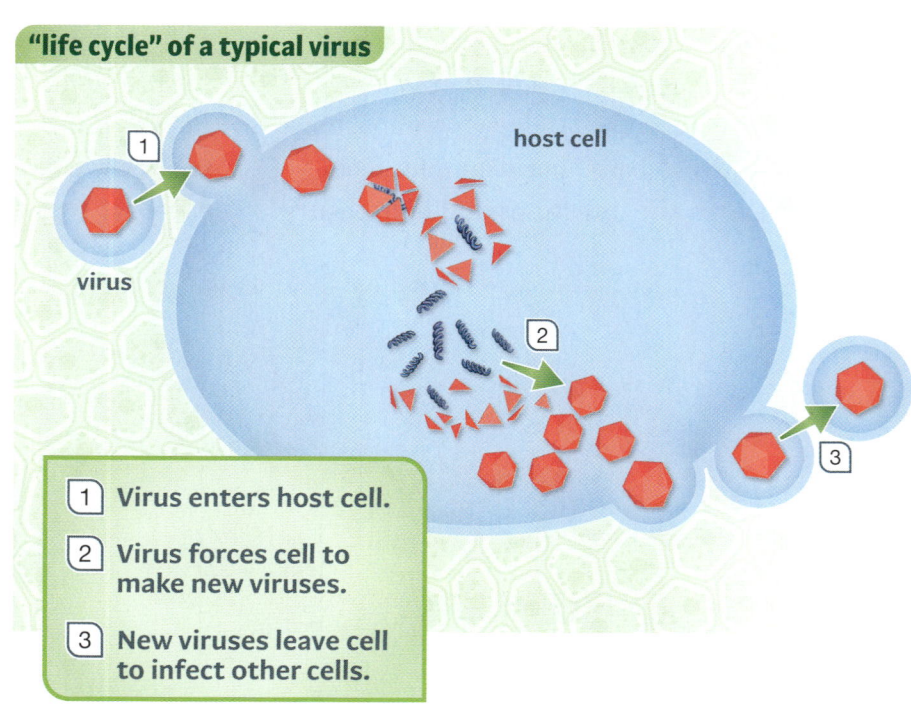
"life cycle" of a typical virus

host cell

virus

1. Virus enters host cell.
2. Virus forces cell to make new viruses.
3. New viruses leave cell to infect other cells.

Effects of Diseases

Every disease affects how your body works. For example, the common cold affects your body by causing symptoms like a runny nose, scratchy throat, cough, sneezing, mild headache, body ache, low-grade fever, shortness of breath, ear pain, and loss of appetite.

Diseases also affect you, your family, and your community in other ways. What are some of the effects of a cold? First, you can spread the disease by passing the pathogen to those around you. Because you feel sick, you may be less able to participate in activities at home, school, and church. If you are very sick, you may have to stay home; this may require your family to adjust schedules with very little notice and make up appointments and responsibilities once you are well.

You may struggle to concentrate on your lessons and schoolwork. This can affect your ability to learn and to do well on tests. You may also have difficulty participating in sports. This difficulty can also affect your team.

You cannot avoid getting sick, and you cannot avoid affecting others when you do get sick. But you can practice health habits that reduce your risk of disease and reduce the effects of your disease on others. If you are feeling very sick, your parents will have to determine if you need to avoid being around others to prevent spreading disease. If you are around others, reduce the risk of spreading disease by washing your hands frequently and covering your mouth when you cough or sneeze. Also limit close contact with young children and older adults, who are often more greatly affected by disease than others are.

Common Childhood Illnesses

Disease	Pathogen	Symptoms	Treatment
athlete's foot	fungus	burning, itchy rash between the toes	antifungal cream
bronchitis	virus	constant coughing, sometimes a fever	antiviral medications, cough medicines
common cold	virus	stuffy or runny nose, sneezing, coughing and sore throat, lasts 1 to 2 weeks	no cure, treated by over-the-counter medicines that reduce symptoms
COVID-19	virus	cough, fever; sometimes sore throat, weak feeling, shortness of breath	antiviral and over-the-counter medications
dandruff	fungus	itchy scalp and skin flakes	medicated shampoo
influenza	virus	stuffy or runny nose, sneezing, fever, weak feeling	antiviral and over-the-counter medications
pneumonia	bacterium, virus, or fungus	high fever, fast breathing, coughing up mucus, chest pain	antibiotics, antiviral and antifungal medications, oxygen treatment, IV fluids
strep throat	bacteria	sore throat, fever, swollen neck glands	antibiotics, over-the-counter medications

Noncommunicable Diseases

Noncommunicable diseases cannot be spread from person to person. A few noncommunicable diseases are caused by pathogens. Most noncommunicable diseases are instead caused by factors such as age; genetics; poor health behaviors, including poor nutrition and lack of physical activity; and environmental factors, including pollution. *Some of the most common noncommunicable diseases are heart disease, cancer, diabetes, and obesity.*

The leading cause of death in the United States is heart disease, which is responsible for about one out of every five deaths. You have already learned that *atherosclerosis* is a buildup of fatty deposits in the arteries. This buildup of fats causes the blood vessels to narrow and restrict blood flow. The heart must then work harder to pump the same amount of blood. *This strain on the heart can cause many different heart diseases, such as coronary artery disease or congestive heart failure.* A *heart attack* occurs when the arteries in the heart become blocked, while a *stroke* is caused by blockage of arteries in the brain. *The best way to reduce the risk of developing heart disease is to maintain a healthy diet and stay physically active.*

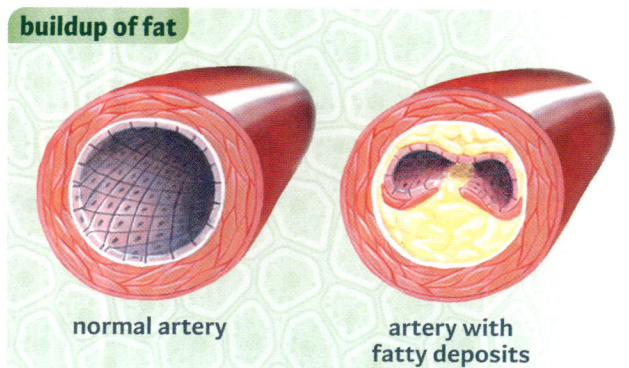

buildup of fat

normal artery

artery with fatty deposits

Mental Workout

Tetanus is caused by bacteria that normally live in the soil. The disease occurs when these bacteria infect a deep cut or wound. Is tetanus a communicable disease or a noncommunicable disease? Explain your answer.

Cancer is a disease caused by the *uncontrolled growth of body cells. It is the second most common cause of death in the United States.* Your cells are designed to reproduce only when new cells are needed. Sometimes, a malfunction causes cells to reproduce rapidly and form a mass of cells called a *tumor.* Not all tumors cause problems, but sometimes cells will leave the tumor and travel to another part of the body. A person has cancer when the tumors begin to spread throughout the body. If the cancer is not stopped, the tumors will damage important organs and eventually cause death. There are many types of cancer, depending on what organs and tissues are affected. Modern medicine has developed many ways to treat cancer, but it is still important to *reduce your risk of developing cancer by maintaining a healthy lifestyle. Some specific ways to limit cancer risk are to avoid tobacco and other drugs, to take steps to prevent sunburn, and to eat a healthy diet.*

Another common noncommunicable disease is **diabetes mellitus** [dī′ə·bē′tĭs mə·lī′təs], a *disease that causes extra sugar to collect in the blood.* Diabetes is caused by an error in how the body produces or responds to the chemical messenger insulin, which is made in the pancreas. There are two forms of diabetes. The less common form is *type 1* diabetes; it is often caused by heredity. The more common form is *type 2 diabetes*. A *healthy diet and sufficient physical activity reduce the risk of developing type 2 diabetes.*

Obesity is the *condition of having too much body fat*. Although a variety of factors, including heredity and medications, affect the likelihood of developing obesity, this disease is often at least partly caused by poor health behaviors. *You can reduce your risk of obesity by maintaining a healthy diet and sufficient exercise, so that you eat only the calories that your body will use.* Obesity increases the risk of developing other diseases, including heart disease and diabetes. A person with obesity should work with his physician to develop a plan to reach a healthy weight.

Comprehension Check 6.1

Classify: *Write* B *for bacterium and* V *for virus.*

_____ 1. uses a host cell to reproduce

_____ 2. smallest pathogen

_____ 3. can be treated with antibiotics

_____ 4. can cause strep throat

_____ 5. can cause the flu

Short Answer: *Write the correct answer in the blank.*

6. What is a condition that causes the body to work in an incorrect way called?

_____

7. What is the difference between an acute disease and a chronic disease? _____

_____

_____

8. What is a vector? _____

9. Give an example of a noncommunicable disease. _____

_____

10. What is the most common cause of death in the United States? _____

_____

11. What disease causes extra sugar to collect in the blood? _____

Think about It.

12. How can obesity cause heart disease? _____

_____

_____

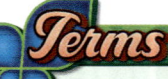
immunity: the body's ability to resist and protect itself against infectious diseases

immune system: the body system that defends against pathogens

mucus: thick, sticky fluid that traps pathogens; produced by mucous membranes

cilia: hair-like projections that keep pathogens from getting into the lungs (cilium, *sing.*)

lysozyme: special enzyme found in tears that can kill bacteria

phagocytes: white blood cells that find, surround, and destroy pathogens

lymphocytes: white blood cells that recognize and attack invading pathogens, produce antibodies, and can become memory cells

antibodies: Y-shaped molecules made by lymphocytes to help protect the body from disease and infection

histamine: chemical messenger that triggers inflammation

inflammation: increased blood flow caused by histamine; makes the tissue become red, swollen, and tender

6.2 The Immune System

Your body is constantly being attacked by invading pathogens. However, the average healthy person usually gets sick only a few times a year. This is because of **immunity**, *the body's ability to resist and protect itself against infectious disease.* Your body is like a fort designed to keep out enemy invaders. A fort has strong walls and gates that act as protective barriers. Soldiers inside the fort defend the walls, and each soldier has a specific job. Their primary goal is to prevent the enemy from getting past them. If enemies do get inside the fort, the soldiers will fight to drive the enemies out. Similarly, your body also has protective barriers and soldiers that work together to keep pathogens out and destroy pathogens that get in. *The body system that defends against pathogens* is the **immune system**.

A Protective Barrier

Your body's first line of defense is your skin. Skin is made of tough, flattened cells, which provide a strong defense against infection and disease. This tough outer layer prevents bacteria and other harmful substances from entering the body. "Helpful" bacteria on

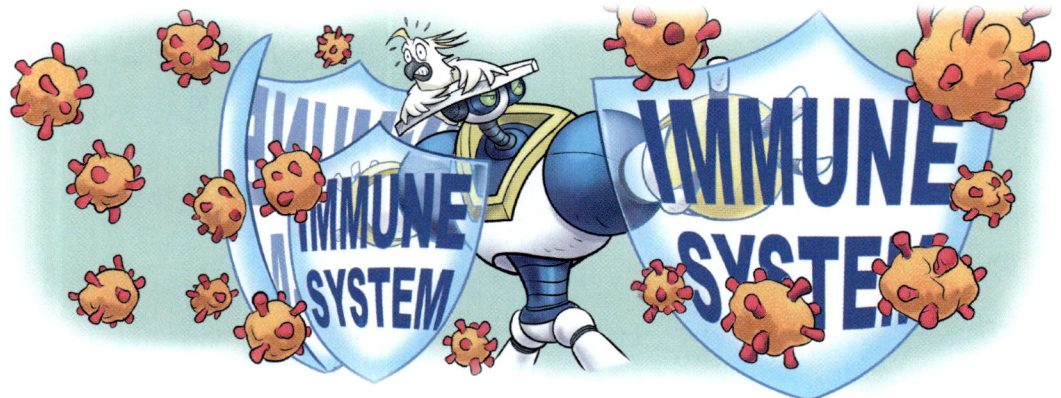

the skin also prevent the growth of harmful pathogens. On clean and dry skin, pathogens do not multiply as quickly as they would otherwise. Pathogens cannot enter through the skin unless there is a cut or other opening in the skin's surface.

Just as a fort has gates, your body has vulnerable areas that are not protected by skin, such as your nose, mouth, and eyes. Your body has special defenses that keep pathogens from invading through body openings, such as your nose and mouth. *Special kinds of cells form a tissue called mucous membrane. Your mouth, nose, throat, and other body openings are lined with mucous membranes that produce a thick, sticky fluid called* **mucus**. The *mucus traps many pathogens* and prevents them from entering farther into your body. The mucous membranes are also lined with *hair-like projections* called **cilia**. Cilia *help keep pathogens from getting into the lungs.* When pathogens and dust enter the body, they irritate the cilia and cause you to sneeze. If pathogens enter the throat, the irritated cilia will cause you to cough. Sneezing and coughing forcefully discharge pathogens from your body.

Your eyes have special defenses that protect them from pathogens. Eyelids and eyelashes prevent dust and other particles from getting on the eye itself. Tears help to keep the eye clean. *Tears contain a special enzyme* called **lysozyme** [lī′sə·zīm′], *which can kill bacteria by destroying their cell walls.* The tears then wash the pathogens and dust from your eyes.

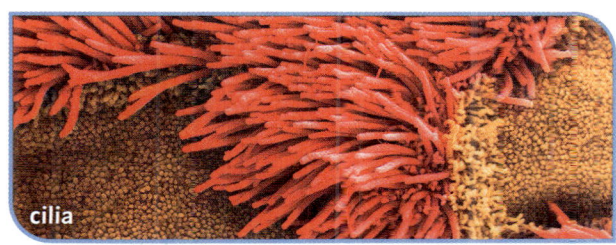
cilia

White Blood Cell Warriors

Sometimes, pathogens can get past the body's protective barriers. These enemy invaders are quickly met by soldiers that fight to defend the body. You have already been introduced to *the most important defenders of the body: white blood cells. White blood cells are made in the bone marrow,* a jelly-like substance found in the center of your bones. When the body is invaded by pathogens, white blood cells travel from the bloodstream to the places that need defense. *The two main types of white blood cells are phagocytes* [făg′ə·sīts′] *and lymphocytes* [lĭm′fə·sīts′]. God gave each of them a design suited to their different purposes.

A **phagocyte** is *designed to find, surround, and destroy pathogens.* The word *phagocyte* means "eater cell" in Greek. *Phago-* means "eater"; *-cyte* means "cell." Some phagocytes patrol the bloodstream and move toward places of infection in the body. Others stay in one area, such as in a particular organ. Some can capture and destroy many pathogens with special chemicals.

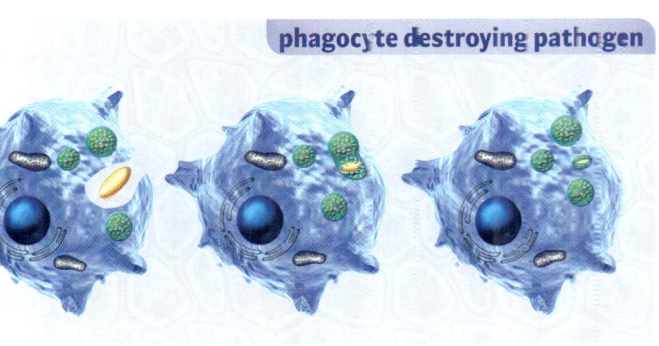
pathogen

phagocyte destroying pathogen

phagocyte

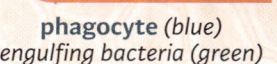
white blood cells destroying pathogens

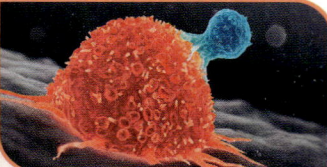
lymphocyte *(blue)* *attacking cancer cell (orange)*

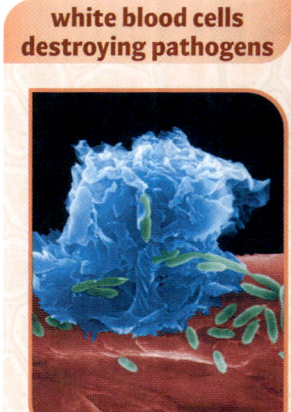
phagocyte *(blue)* *engulfing bacteria (green)*

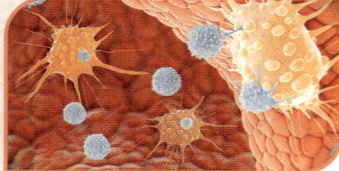
lymphocytes *(gray) attacking cancer cells (orange)*

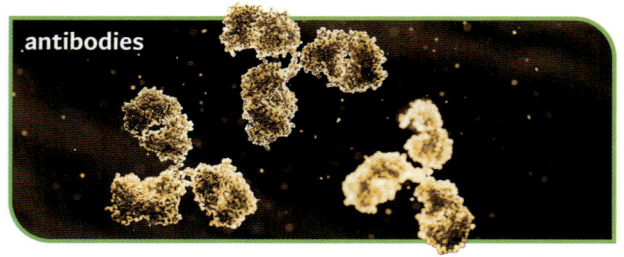
antibodies

Lymphocytes perform a variety of different jobs. Some lymphocytes *recognize and attack invading pathogens*. Other lymphocytes *make antibodies*. **Antibodies** are *Y-shaped molecules that help protect the body from disease and infection*. Antibodies defend against pathogens in two main ways. Some antibodies inactivate pathogens by "gluing" them together. Other antibodies mark the pathogens for destruction by roaming phagocytes. After the immune system has defeated a disease, *some lymphocytes become memory cells*. A memory cell "remembers" how to make antibodies against the specific pathogen, helping the body to develop immunity against the disease.

Your white blood cells can communicate with body cells and with each other. When body cells are injured, they send chemical signals asking for help. White blood cells receive the signal and quickly rush to the site of injury. Some white blood cells produce *a chemical messenger* called **histamine** [hĭs′tə·mēn′]. Histamine *causes the blood vessels to get larger*, allowing more blood to rush into the injured area. This *increased blood flow makes the tissue become red, swollen, and tender*, a condition called **inflammation**. *Inflammation allows other white blood cells and antibodies to get to the injured site more quickly*. Phagocytes, lymphocytes, and antibodies all work together to fight against the invading pathogens. As the battle continues, *dead white blood cells and destroyed pathogens form a whitish-yellowish fluid called pus*. When all the pathogens have been eliminated, the inflammation stops and the wound begins to heal.

Community HEALTH CORNER

Vaccinations

When you go to your regular checkup appointment, your doctor may recommend that you be vaccinated. Vaccinations help your body develop immunity against a particular disease. A vaccine is a substance made from a weakened or dead pathogen. This substance does not cause the disease but tricks the body into thinking that it is infected. The immune system produces memory cells and antibodies that will protect you against future attacks by the actual pathogen.

In the past, many people became sick or died because of infectious diseases such as smallpox, polio, or measles. In modern times, it is rare for people in the United States and other developed nations to get these diseases, since most people receive vaccinations during childhood. Some vaccines provide immunity for your entire life. Other vaccines work for only a certain amount of time and require more than one dose to be effective. Since some viruses can change their structure, new vaccines sometimes must be developed. For example, new flu vaccines are made each year because the flu virus frequently changes. Antibodies from the old flu virus may not recognize the new flu virus.

Although vaccines are generally effective and safe, some people experience side effects from getting vaccinated. They may experience an allergic reaction or get sick from the vaccine. Your parents will consider your doctor's advice and determine which vaccines may be beneficial in your specific situation.

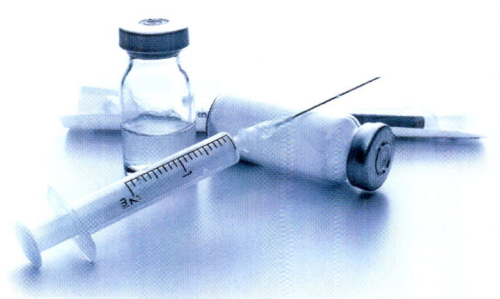

Immune-Boosting Chicken Soup

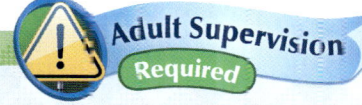
Adult Supervision Required

Homemade chicken soup contains foods that are rich in immune-boosting nutrients; these nutrients can help you fight sickness. You can make a homemade chicken soup with your family!

Be aware of allergies or sensitivities before you handle or eat food.

Ingredients:

- 1 tbsp. olive oil
- 1 c. each onions, carrots, and celery; chopped
- 2 cloves garlic, minced
- ½ tsp. fresh ginger, grated

- ½ tsp. turmeric
- salt and pepper to taste
- 2 tbsp. fresh parsley, chopped
- 3 c. chicken broth*
- 2 c. cooked chicken, chopped

- 2 c. cooked rice or noodles

*Bone broth has the most nutrients and can be made at home or purchased in most supermarkets.

Directions:

1. With an adult's help, prepare the ingredients.
2. Add olive oil, onions, carrots, and celery to a large saucepan. Heat over medium heat, while stirring, to sauté for five minutes.
3. Add garlic, ginger, turmeric, salt, pepper, and half the parsley; sauté for one more minute.
4. Add chicken broth and stir. Bring to a low boil; simmer until vegetables are tender. Add chicken.
5. Add rice or noodles and garnish with parsley, if you would like. Share with your family and enjoy!

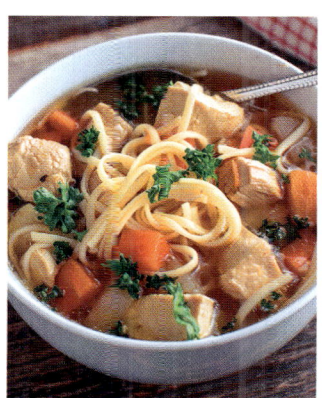

Matching: *Write the letter of the correct answer in the blank.*

_____ 1. the body's first line of defense against pathogens

_____ 2. thick, sticky fluid that traps pathogens

_____ 3. hair-like projection that keeps pathogens from getting into the lungs

_____ 4. special enzyme found in tears that can kill bacteria

_____ 5. Y-shaped molecule made by white blood cells

_____ 6. chemical messenger that triggers inflammation

A. antibody

B. cilium

C. histamine

D. lymphocyte

E. lysozyme

F. mucus

G. skin

Short Answer: *Write the correct answer in the blank.*

7. What is the body's ability to resist and protect itself against infection? _____

_____

8. What is the immune system? _____

9. Where are white blood cells made? _____

10. What type of white blood cells surround and destroy pathogens? _____

_____

11. What is the condition in which increased blood flow makes tissue red, swollen, and tender? _____

Think about It.

12. Why does a cut in the skin make you more vulnerable to infection?

_____

_____

_____

_____

_____

_____

_____

_____

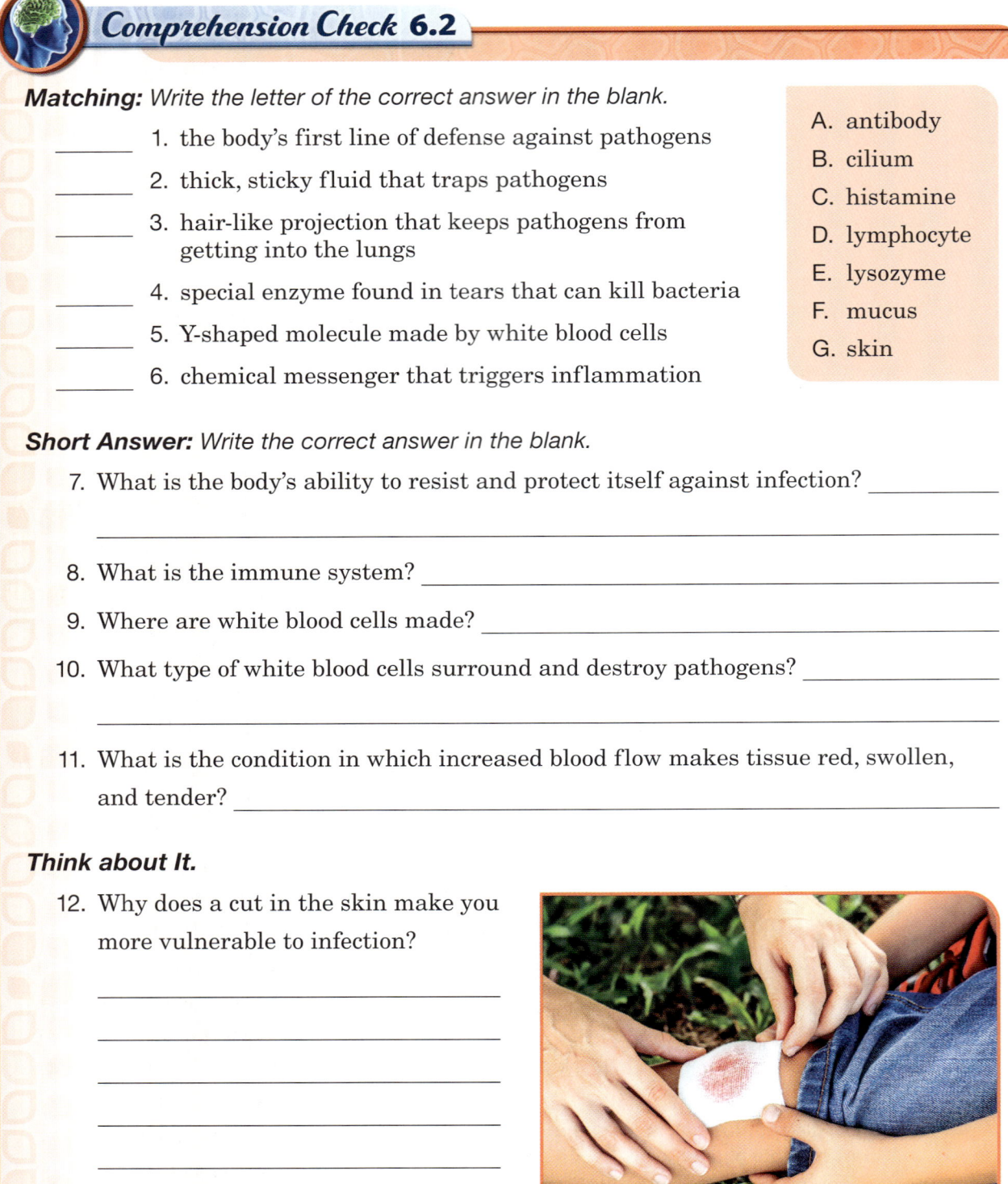

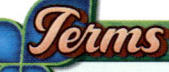
lymphatic system: part of the immune system that collects tissue fluid and cleans the body of pathogens

tissue fluid: fluid that surrounds cells; keeps cells clean and balanced with liquid

lymph capillaries: the smallest vessels of the lymphatic system

lymph: tissue fluid that has been forced into lymph vessels

lymph vessel: a transportation vessel for lymph

lymph nodes: large bunches of lymphatic tissue located throughout the body

tonsils: a group of lymph nodes at the back of the throat

adenoids: a group of lymph nodes at the back of the nose

Peyer's patches: groups of lymph nodes in the walls of the small intestine

spleen: largest organ of the lymphatic system; cleanses the blood

thymus: lymphatic organ that prepares lymphocytes to fight pathogens

6.3 The Lymphatic System

White blood cells are assisted by the body's **lymphatic system**. *Your lymphatic system is the part of the immune system that collects fluid from tissues of the body and cleans the body of pathogens.* Fluid-filled vessels of the lymphatic system also help transport the white blood cells throughout the body.

Tissue Fluid

All the cells in your body are surrounded by a liquid called **tissue fluid**. This liquid comes from the blood plasma. Tissue fluid *helps keep the cells clean and balanced with liquid*. Without the right water balance, the cells could either collapse from too little water or burst from too much water. Once the tissue fluid

has cleaned the cells of pathogens, it is forced into **lymph capillaries**, *the smallest vessels of the lymphatic system. The tissue fluid is called* **lymph** *after it has been forced into the lymph vessels.* The tiny lymph capillaries then empty the lymph into larger *transportation vessels* called **lymph vessels**.

The lymphatic system carries lymph in a way similar to how blood vessels transport blood. However, the heart does not pump lymph through lymph vessels. Instead, lymph is forced through the lymph vessels by a squeezing action of the muscles. Lymph is transported only one direction. Special valves inside lymph vessels prevent the lymph from flowing in the wrong direction. Lymph vessels join with other vessels and empty into two large *lymph ducts*. Each lymph duct returns lymph to the bloodstream.

As lymph travels through the lymph vessels, it passes through **lymph nodes**. Lymph nodes are *large bunches of lymphatic tissue along the lymph vessels throughout the body*. Lymph nodes are most numerous in your armpits and neck. The lymph nodes contain white blood cells, which clean the lymph of debris and pathogens. Your lymph nodes may become swollen and painful when your body is fighting an infection or disease. This is because the white blood cells start attacking the pathogens carried by the lymph, and the lymph nodes become a battle zone.

Lymphatic Organs

In addition to your lymph vessels and lymph nodes, the lymphatic system contains several other organs. These lymphatic organs work together to fight invading pathogens. *The organs of your lymphatic system include the tonsils, adenoids, Peyer's* [pī′ərz] *patches, spleen, and thymus.*

Your **tonsils** are a *group of lymph nodes at the back of your throat*. The **adenoids** are a *group of lymph nodes at the back of the nose*. Tonsils and adenoids protect these entrances into the body by trapping pathogens before you inhale or swallow them. If your tonsils or adenoids become frequently infected, they may have to be surgically removed. *Your small intestine also contains groups of lymph nodes* called **Peyer's patches**. Any pathogen that makes its way into the intestine is destroyed by white blood cells in the Peyer's patches.

Your **spleen**, the *largest lymphatic organ*, is about the size of your fist and is located behind the stomach and beneath the diaphragm. *The main job of the spleen is to cleanse the blood* that passes through it. When you breathe, your diaphragm provides

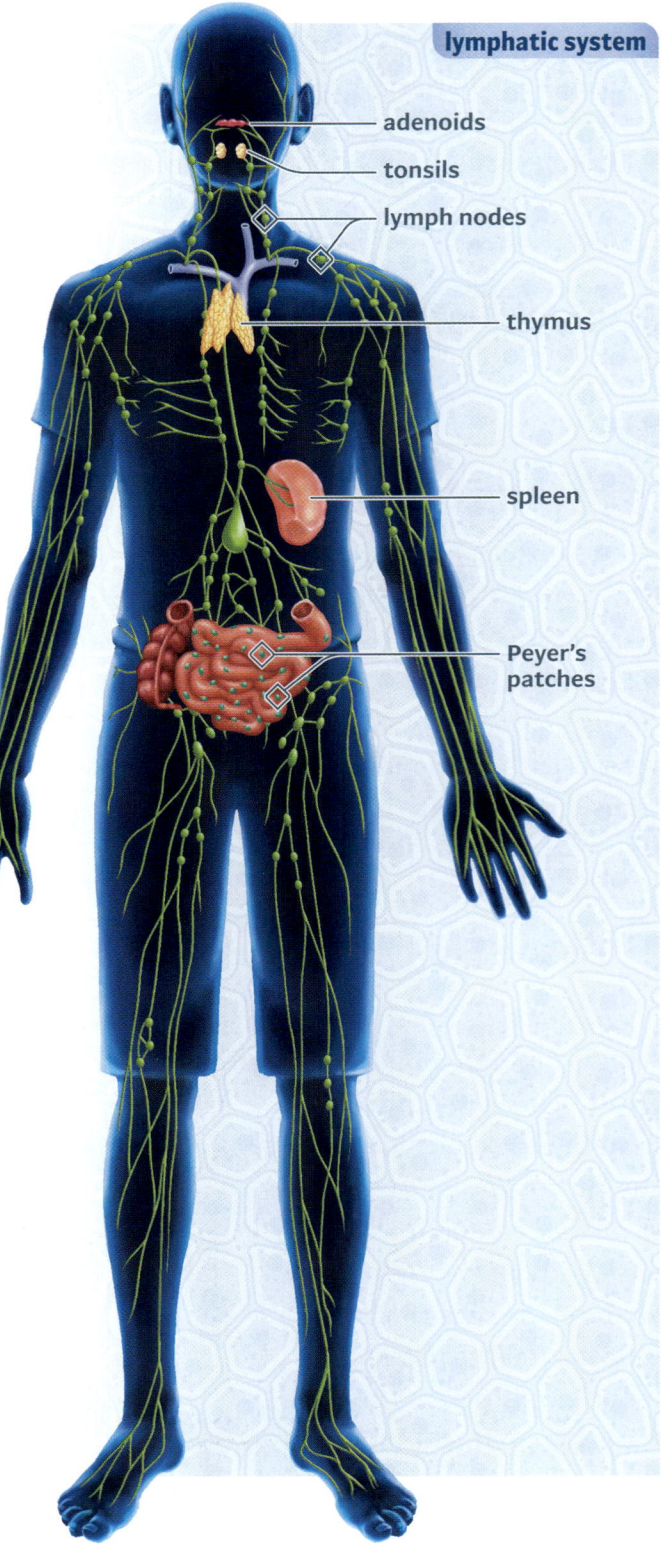

lymphatic system

adenoids

tonsils

lymph nodes

thymus

spleen

Peyer's patches

a squeezing action to transport blood to your spleen. Dead cells and pathogens are quickly filtered out and disposed of through this amazing organ. *The spleen also stores extra blood that can be used in an emergency.*

The **thymus** is located between the lungs and above the heart. The thymus *prepares lymphocytes for their battle against pathogens.* Undeveloped lymphocytes travel from the bone marrow through the bloodstream to the thymus. The thymus "trains" lymphocytes as they develop and grow. *By the time you become an adult, your thymus will have done most of its job and will eventually shrink.*

Preventing the Spread of Pathogens

Proper hygiene habits can help prevent the spread of disease-causing pathogens. *Keeping your skin clean will help prevent the spread of disease.* Millions of pathogens live on your skin, especially on your hands. You should avoid touching your face or putting your fingers in your nose or mouth. *Hand washing is one of the best ways to prevent the spread of pathogens and avoid getting sick.* To wash

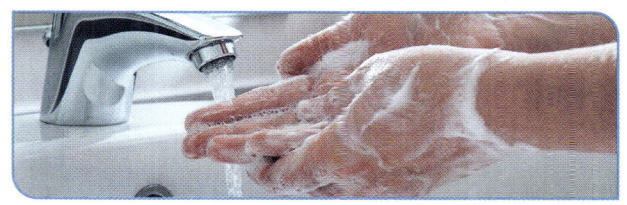

correctly, you should first wet your hands then apply soap and *scrub for at least 20 seconds.* Be sure to wash every surface of your hands, including your fingertips, thumbs, and under your fingernails. Singing or humming the song "Happy Birthday to You" twice is a good way to make sure that you have scrubbed for long enough. After scrubbing, rinse your hands until all the soap is gone. Dry your hands with a clean paper towel or hand towel.

Pathogens can also be transferred through body fluids, such as saliva, sweat, and blood. A cough or sneeze propels droplets into the air; these droplets can be inhaled by someone else. *Instead of coughing or sneezing into your hands, use a tissue or the inside of your elbow to cover your nose and mouth.* This will keep pathogen-containing droplets from spreading. After using a tissue, throw it away and wash your hands. If you cannot wash your hands right away, use an alcohol-based hand sanitizer and wash your hands later.

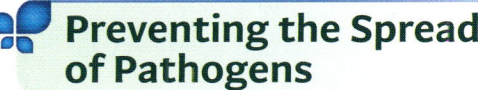

Hands-On Health

See the effects of soap.

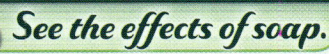

Materials needed:
- clear bowl or dish
- water
- ground black pepper
- liquid soap (hand soap or dish detergent)

You can demonstrate how soap helps to wash away pathogens.

1. Fill the clear bowl or dish with water.

2. Sprinkle pepper into the water.

3. Place your finger in the water. Observe what happens to the pepper.

4. Put some soap on your finger. Place your finger in the water again. Observe what happens to the pepper this time.

The CDC

The *Centers for Disease Control and Prevention*, or *CDC*, is a national public-health agency of the United States. The main goal of the CDC is to protect public health and safety. The CDC also seeks to provide reliable sources of health information. Scientists perform research and develop technology to prevent and treat diseases. This research is presented to the public through educational materials that promote healthy and safe behaviors in individuals

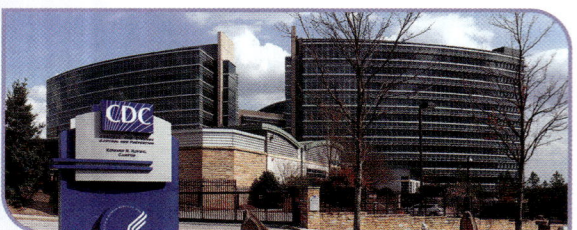

and communities. The CDC also provides doctors and other medical professionals with information that helps them diagnose and treat disease. Whenever there is a health or safety threat, the CDC will quickly respond with guidelines that should save lives and protect people.

State and local organizations work with the CDC to develop public-health policies. These public-health policies are intended to improve the overall health of individuals, communities, and the nation. Your local community is greatly impacted by the work of public-health organizations. You can learn more about disease prevention by reading material published by the CDC and other public-health organizations. You can also encourage your friends and family to promote health and safety in your community.

Family Health History

When you visit the doctor for a general checkup or sick appointment, you may be asked to provide a record of your family health history.

Many chronic diseases, including diabetes, heart disease, and cancer, run in families. If one of your relatives has a particular disease, you have a higher risk of developing that same disease. Some diseases are genetic and are passed from parent to child. Other diseases are caused by unhealthy behaviors such as poor nutrition, lack of exercise, or drug use. If you share similar health behaviors as your relatives, you are more likely to get the same diseases.

You can learn about your family history by talking to your family members. Make a list of your parents, siblings, grandparents, aunts, uncles, and cousins. Ask each person about any medical conditions they might have. How old

were they when they first developed the disease? Was the disease caused by poor health decisions, or was it caused by genetics? What are they doing to treat or manage the condition? If some of your relatives are no longer living, you can ask a parent or other family member for their causes and ages of death. The information that you discover may help you know if you are at risk of developing a specific disease. If your doctor knows your family history, he can help you take necessary steps to prevent or manage high-risk diseases.

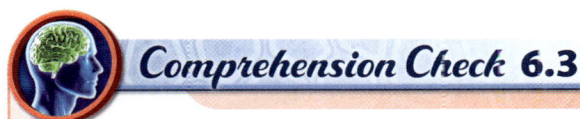

Short Answer: *Write the correct answer in the blank.*

1. What is the lymphatic system? _____

_____

_____

2. What is the purpose of tissue fluid? _____

_____

3. What are the smallest vessels of the lymphatic system? _____

4. What are lymph nodes? _____

_____

5. How should you cover your mouth when you cough? _____

_____

_____

Matching: *Write the letter of the correct answer in the blank.*

_____ 6. lymph nodes at the back of the throat

_____ 7. lymph nodes at the back of the nose

_____ 8. lymph nodes in the small intestine

_____ 9. lymphatic organ that stores extra blood

_____ 10. lymphatic organ that prepares lymphocytes to fight pathogens

A. adenoids
B. liver
C. Peyer's patches
D. spleen
E. thymus
F. tonsils

Think about It.

11. Explain the relationship between blood plasma, tissue fluid, and lymph. _____

_____

_____

_____

_____

_____

_____

_____

Concepts Review

1 Types of Diseases (6.1)

A. Pathogens: *Complete this information table. Name each pathogen and give an example of a disease it causes.*

Pathogen	Description	Disease
	single-celled microorganism that does not have a cell nucleus	
	forces a host cell to produce more of the pathogen	
	plant-like organism that can cause disease	
	single-celled animal-like organism	

B. True/False: *If the statement is true, write* true *in the blank. If the statement is false, replace the underlined word with a word that will make the statement true. Do not write* false *in any blank.*

1. A disease that lasts for a short time is <u>chronic</u>.
2. A disease that cannot be spread from one person to another is a <u>communicable</u> disease.
3. A microorganism that causes disease is a <u>pathogen</u>.
4. Because it is caused by a bacterium, strep throat is probably a <u>communicable</u> disease.
5. The second most common cause of death in the United States is <u>diabetes</u>.

C. Think!

1. Can a vector cause coronary heart disease? Explain why or why not. _____

_____

_____

_____

_____

2. How might an unhealthy diet affect someone with diabetes? _____

_____

_____

_____

_____

_____

2 The Immune System (6.2)

A. Multiple Choice

_____ 1. The body's first barrier against pathogens is __?__ .

a. blood

b. mucus

c. sebum

d. skin

_____ 2. A hair-like projection that helps prevent pathogens from getting to the lungs is a __?__ .

a. cilium

b. mucus

c. sebum

d. skin

_____ 3. The blood cells that surround and destroy pathogens are __?__ .

a. lymphocytes

b. phagocytes

c. platelets

d. red blood cells

_____ 4. The Y-shaped molecules that help protect against disease and infection are __?__ .

a. antibodies

b. enzymes

c. histamines

d. phagocytes

_____ 5. The chemical messenger that causes the blood vessels to get larger is __?__ .

a. antibody

b. histamine

c. inflammation

d. phagocyte

B. Short Answer: Write the correct answer in the blank.

1. Where are white blood cells made? _____

2. How does inflammation help with fighting pathogens? _____

_____

_____

_____

_____

3 The Lymphatic System (6.3)

A. Identify: *Label the parts of the lymphatic system.*

1. _____

2. _____

3. _____

4. _____

5. _____

6. _____

B. True/False: *If the statement is true, write* true *in the blank. If the statement is false, replace the underlined word with a word or phrase that will make the statement true. Do not write* false *in any blank.*

_____ 1. The liquid that surrounds cells and keeps them clean and balanced with liquid is <u>lymph</u>.

_____ 2. Lymph is first forced into lymph <u>ducts</u>.

_____ 3. White blood cells in your <u>spleen</u> clean the lymph of debris and pathogens.

_____ 4. Pathogens that enter your throat are trapped by your <u>tonsils</u>.

_____ 5. When washing your hands, scrub for at least <u>30</u> seconds.

C. Think!

1. What will happen to your body cells if there is not enough tissue fluid? _____

_____

_____

2. At what point in your life is your thymus the largest? Why does the thymus change in size? _____

_____

_____

_____

4 Your Body's Defenses (6.1–6.3)

A. Crossword: *Fill in the answer to complete the crossword puzzle.*

Down

1. an animal that can carry a pathogen and transmit it to humans

2. any condition that causes the body to work in an incorrect way

3. "trains" lymphocytes to fight pathogens

4. lasts for a long time

5. fluid that has been forced into lymph vessels

6. special protein in tears that can destroy bacteria

Across

7. the body's ability to resist or protect itself against infectious diseases

8. the condition of having too much body fat

9. organ that cleans and stores blood

10. thick, sticky fluid that traps pathogens

B. Think!

How do the immune and lymphatic systems work together to protect your body from disease? _____

_____

_____

_____

_____

_____

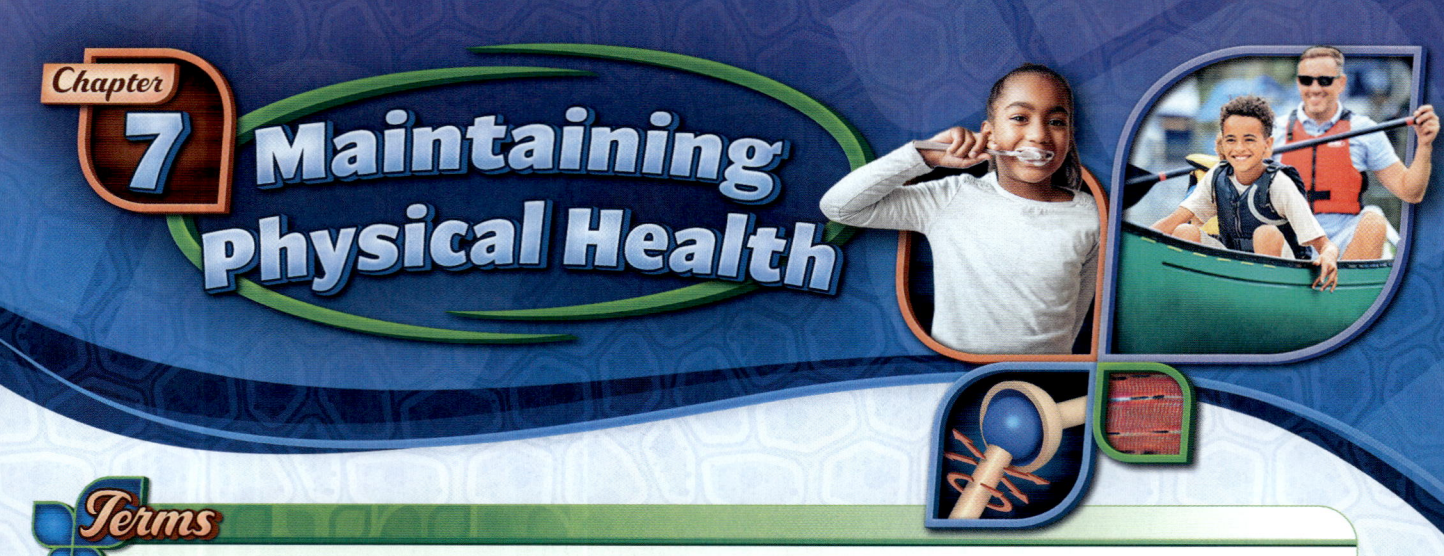

Chapter 7 Maintaining Physical Health

Terms

adolescence: transitional time of growth and development between childhood and adulthood

puberty: process of physical changes during adolescence

hormone: chemical messenger that regulates how the body works

hygiene: cleanliness habits that prevent disease and promote health

integumentary system: the body system that covers and protects the body; includes the skin, hair, and nails

epidermis: outer layer of skin

dermis: inner layer of skin beneath the epidermis

hypodermis: layer of fat cells below the dermis; deepest layer of the integumentary system

hair follicle: small tube in the dermis that makes hair

sebum: oily substance produced by sebaceous glands

acne: skin condition in which clogged pores cause blemishes, or pimples

enamel: protective outer covering of a tooth's crown; hardest substance in the body

dentin: hard, bone-like tissue that gives a tooth its shape

pulp: soft tissue within the dentin that contains nerves and blood vessels

plaque: film of harmful bacteria that forms on teeth

dental caries: disease caused by bacteria inside the mouth; also called cavities

7.1 Caring for Yourself

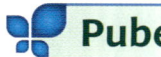 Puberty

When God created you, He designed your body to automatically grow. As you grow, your body goes through many changes. The body you have now is very different from the body you had as a baby because of the many ways you have developed physically. The way you are growing now is quite special. You are in *a transitional time of growth and development between childhood and adulthood* called **adolescence** [ăd′l·ĕs′əns]. Your body will continue to grow and develop until you reach adulthood.

During adolescence, your body goes through a process of physical changes called **puberty**. You will go through many physical

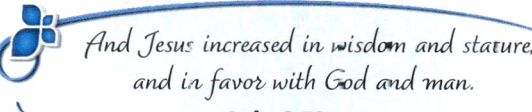

Build on TRUTH

Jesus' human body went through the stages of growth, just like every other person's body. Have you wondered how Jesus acted when He was going through adolescence? Luke 2:41–52 describes a situation that occurred when Jesus was twelve years old. What kinds of things was Jesus interested in doing? As you go through the changes of adolescence, remember that the God Who created you understands what you are going through.

And Jesus increased in wisdom and stature, and in favor with God and man.
Luke 2:52

and emotional changes during puberty. Your body will grow rapidly in sudden spurts, and you may notice many emotional changes in a short period of time. As you mature, you will learn to manage these emotions. Some people experience puberty quickly at an early age. Other people may take longer to go through this process. *Physical characteristics that distinguish men and women develop during puberty.* For example, boys will develop facial hair, and their voices will get lower pitched. If you have questions about the changes you experience, ask your parents or other trusted adults to help you.

The changes that happen during puberty are controlled by hormones. A **hormone** is a *chemical messenger in the body that regulates, or controls, the way the body works.*

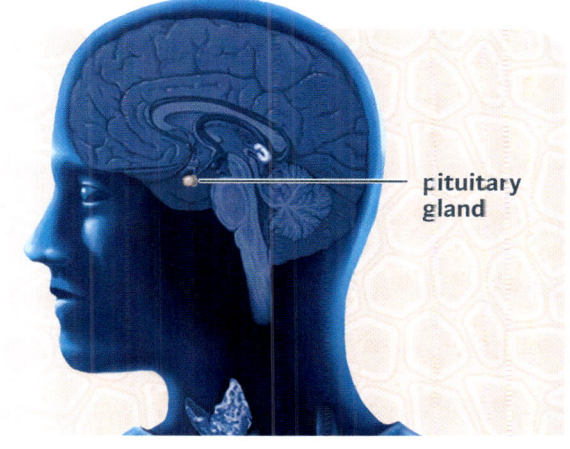

pituitary gland

Hormones are produced by glands that are part of the endocrine system. Puberty is coordinated by the *pituitary* [pĭ·too′ĭ·tĕr′ē] *gland*, located inside the brain. The pituitary gland directs other glands to produce hormones that cause the body to grow and develop.

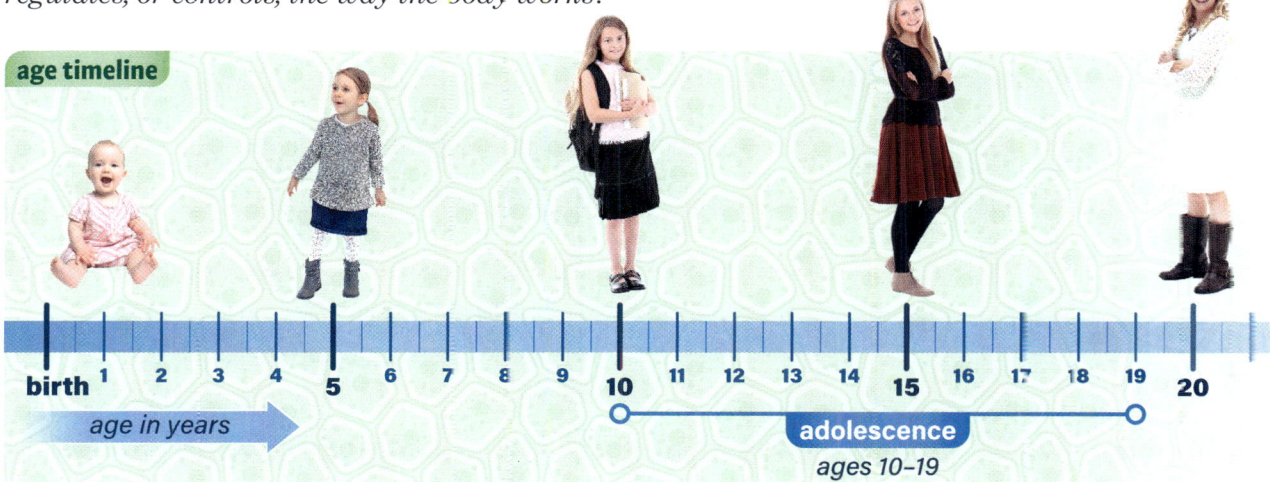

age timeline

birth 1 2 3 4 5 6 7 8 9 10 11 12 13 14 15 16 17 18 19 20

age in years

adolescence
ages 10–19

Maintaining Physical Health **133**

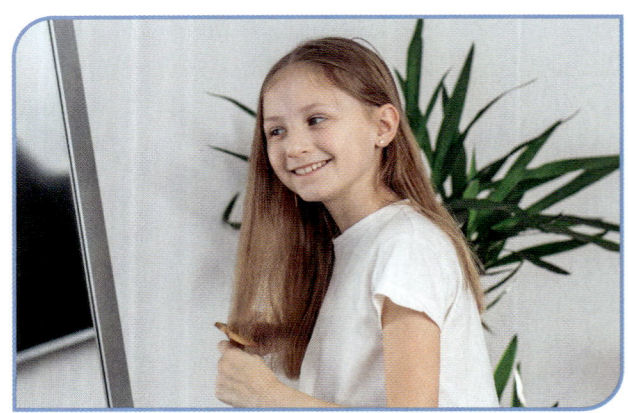

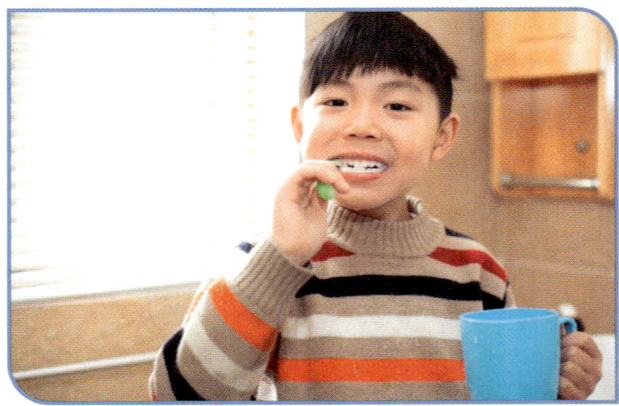

Integumentary Hygiene

When you were younger, your parents helped you take care of your body. As you mature, you have the responsibility to start developing your own habits. **Hygiene** is *cleanliness habits that prevent disease and promote health*. Your body needs daily maintenance to keep it neat looking and to prevent disease. Proper cleaning makes it more difficult for pathogens to invade and infect your body. Developing hygiene habits is especially important as you begin adolescence. If you develop good hygiene habits now, you will enjoy better health throughout your life.

The Integumentary System

One essential part of hygiene is caring for your *skin*, the largest organ of your body. Your skin is part of the **integumentary** [ĭn·tĕg′yo͝o·mĕn′tə·rē] **system**, *the body system that covers and protects your body*. *Your skin, hair, and nails are all part of the integumentary system.* The integumentary system is your body's first line of defense against invading pathogens; proper care of your integumentary system will help to reduce the number of pathogens that enter your body.

The *outer layer of the skin* is the **epidermis**. The epidermis is made of tough, flattened cells that prevent pathogens from entering the body. *Beneath the epidermis is an inner layer* called the **dermis**. The dermis has a complex structure, with many parts. *The deepest layer of the integumentary system is the* **hypodermis**, *a layer of fat cells below the dermis*. This tissue connects the skin to the muscles below it.

Each part of the dermis has an important job. Connective tissue gives the skin elasticity and attaches it to muscles. *Hair is made by small tubes in the dermis* called **hair follicles**. *Attached to each hair follicle is a*

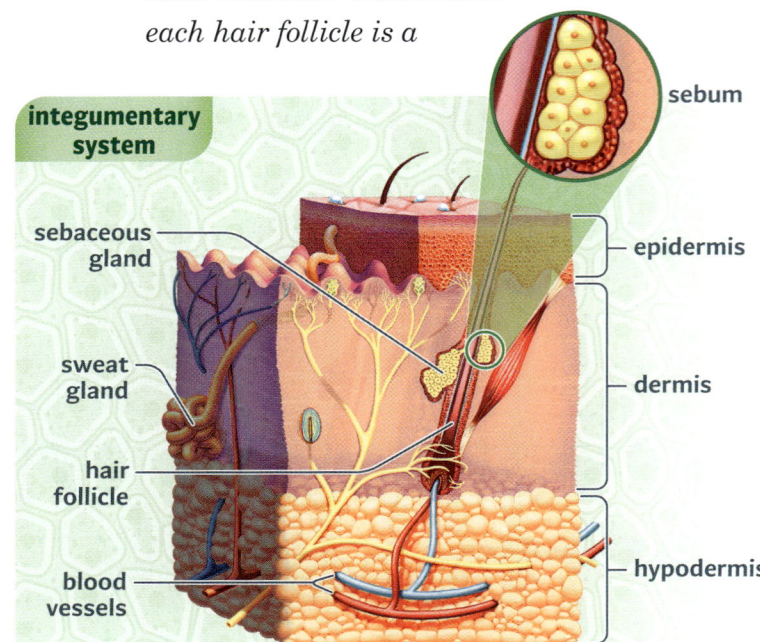

sebaceous [sĭ·bā′shəs] *gland, or oil gland. Se-baceous glands produce* **sebum**, *an oily substance that keeps the skin soft and prevents it from cracking open.* Sebum is released through hair follicles. Sweat glands help your body maintain a normal temperature and release *sweat, or perspiration*, when your body gets hot. Blood vessels bring nutrients and oxygen to the skin cells. Nerve endings allow your skin to sense touch, temperature, and pain.

Skin Care

When puberty begins, hormones cause sebaceous glands to produce more sebum. This extra sebum can combine with bacteria and dead skin cells, clogging the pores of the skin. A condition called **acne** occurs when *the clogged pores cause blemishes, or pimples.* Many people develop acne during puberty. To prevent and manage acne, gently wash your face with a mild cleanser twice a day.

Hormones during puberty also make the sweat glands produce more perspiration. Bacteria on the skin mix with this perspiration and produce an unpleasant odor. *Frequent bathing with soap and water, as well as wearing deodorant or antiperspirant, can* help to eliminate unpleasant body odor. If you have been physically active or in a hot environment, then it is especially important to wash the perspiration from your body.

The clothes next to your skin become soiled from perspiration, oil, and bacteria on the epidermis; to protect your body from diseases, your clothes should be changed daily and cleaned between wearings Your outer clothing can sometimes be worn more than one time between cleanings. Wear clean socks and dry shoes to help prevent common foot problems such as *athlete's foot*. Since the fungus that causes athlete's foot grows in damp areas, wear sandals in areas such as locker rooms and pool decks. If your shoes become wet, do not wear them again until they are dry.

Hair Care

Your integumentary system includes your hair. Sebum from your sebaceous glands keeps your hair soft and shiny. Gentle brushing or combing helps remove tangles and spreads the sebum evenly throughout your hair. *Regular shampooing will keep your hair clean and remove excess sebum.* Since different types of hair have different needs, find a shampoo and hair-washing frequency that work for your hair type. Some hair types may also need conditioner to keep them moisturized.

Never share anything that touches your hair, including combs, hats, headphones, or pillows. If a person

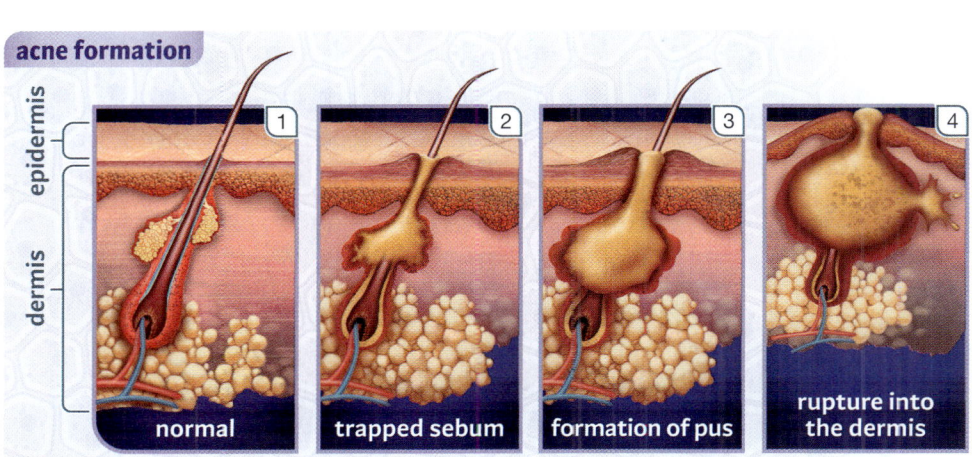

acne formation

epidermis

dermis

1 | 2 | 3 | 4

normal | trapped sebum | formation of pus | rupture into the dermis

is infected with head lice, sharing such objects can spread the lice to others. Chlorine in swimming pools can damage your hair; you may need to wear a swim cap or to wash your hair after swimming. Since excess heat can damage your hair, limit your use of heat products such as blow dryers, curling irons, or flatirons. Find a hairstyle that flatters your appearance and is easy to maintain; such a hairstyle can encourage self-confidence.

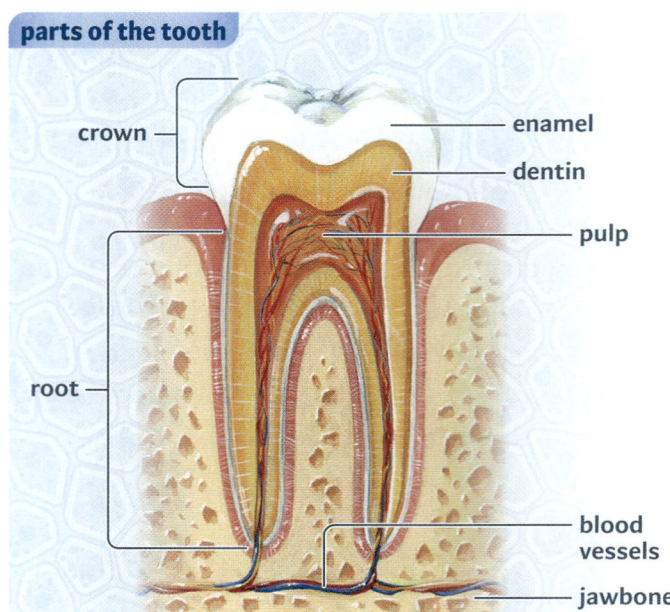

parts of the tooth

crown — enamel — dentin — pulp — root — blood vessels — jawbone

 ## Dental Care

Another aspect of hygiene is caring for your teeth. Teeth are important because they prepare food for digestion and help you speak clearly. Each tooth has two parts: the *crown*, which is the part you can see, and the *root*, which holds the tooth in the jawbone. Like the skin, the tooth has three layers. The outer layer is **enamel**, which forms a *protective outer covering of the tooth's crown*. Enamel is the *hardest substance in the body*. *Underneath the enamel is a hard, bone-like tissue* called **dentin**. Dentin *forms and shapes the tooth*. Inside the dentin is a *soft tissue* called **pulp**. Pulp *contains nerves and blood vessels that provide nutrients to the dentin*. These nerves and blood vessels come up through an opening at the tip of the root. The *gums* are tissues that surround each tooth to hold it firmly in place.

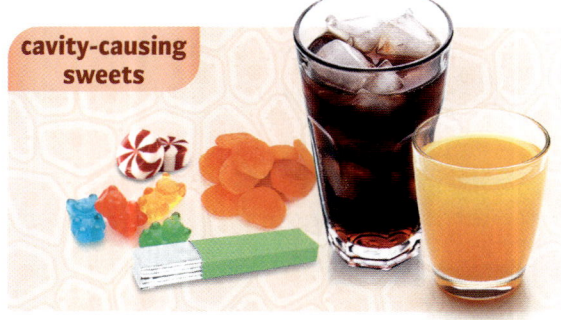

cavity-causing sweets

Teeth are durable but are under continual attack. *Harmful bacteria in the mouth form a sticky, colorless film called* **plaque** *on your teeth*. The bacteria use sugar from the food you eat to create acid, which attacks the enamel. Over time, *continual acid attacks can make holes in the enamel* called **dental caries**, or *cavities*. A *toothache* will occur when the decay reaches the nerves in the pulp. Plaque can also cause *gum disease*. Gum disease infects the bones supporting the teeth. As gum disease progresses, the bones supporting the teeth break down, and the teeth loosen enough to fall out.

You can protect your teeth from acid attacks by practicing good oral hygiene. If you take care of your teeth, they will remain healthy throughout your life. Brushing and flossing remove plaque and excess food from your teeth. *Brush your teeth for at least two minutes twice a day with a soft-bristled toothbrush*. Use a toothpaste that contains fluoride, a substance that helps teeth resist the destructive acids caused by plaque. Daily flossing between your teeth also helps prevent cavities and keeps your teeth clean. If you cannot brush your teeth after eating, rinse your mouth with water to wash away some of the sugar. You can also rinse your mouth with a mouthwash that contains fluoride or an antiseptic that kills bacteria.

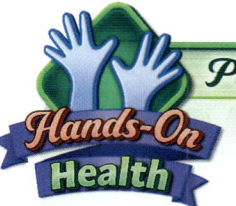

Plaque Attack

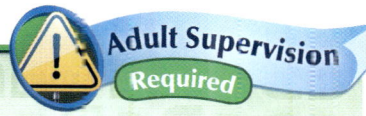

Adult Supervision
Required

Materials needed:
- two clear plastic cups
- fine-point permanent marker
- two packets of yeast
- 1 tablespoon of sugar
- warm (not hot) water

1. Label one cup "sugar" and the other cup "no sugar."

2. Empty one packet of yeast into each cup.

3. Add 1 tablespoon of sugar into the cup marked "sugar."

4. Fill each cup with warm water. Observe how the sugar causes the yeast to activate faster. Record your observations.

Sugar reacts with plaque in your mouth in a similar way to cause tooth decay.

Developing Good Hygiene Habits

LIVE IT OUT!

Think about your current habits for caring for your skin and teeth. For each of these body parts, make a goal to develop healthier habits, identify at least one strength that will help you reach the goal, and identify one challenge that you must overcome to reach your goal. After two weeks, evaluate how well you were able to reach your goals.

	Skin Care	Dental Care
Goals		
Strengths		
Challenges		
Evaluation		

Dentist

Not only does a healthy smile help you look better, but oral health also affects your overall health. Poor oral hygiene can lead to toothaches, cavities, or gum disease; the resulting infections can spread throughout your body. Besides brushing and flossing your teeth, you should visit a dentist every six months. A dentist is a medical professional who treats oral health conditions. Some dentists specialize in a certain area of oral health. If you have crooked teeth, an orthodontist [ôr′thə·dŏn′tĭst] can straighten your teeth by applying braces. A periodontist [pĕr′ē·ə·dŏn′tĭst] treats gum diseases, while an oral surgeon conducts surgeries on the mouth. A dental assistant or hygienist helps the dentist. All these professionals work together to keep your teeth healthy.

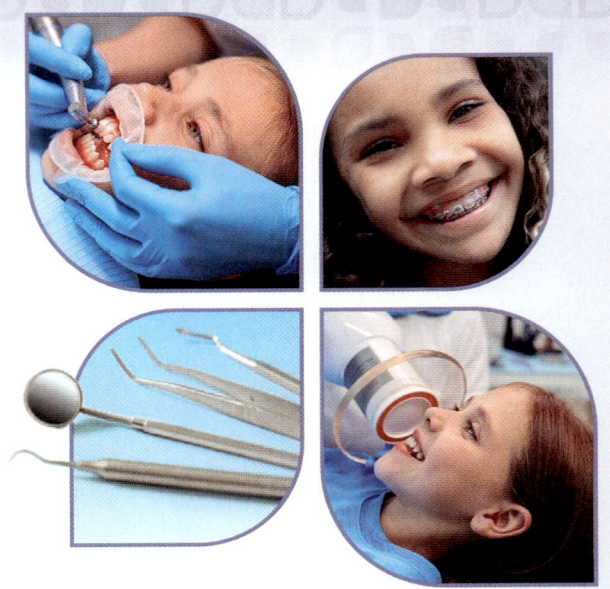

Although some people get nervous about seeing a dentist, most dental offices provide excellent care. When you go for a general checkup, the dentist will inspect and x-ray your teeth. The dental assistant or hygienist will then clean your teeth and apply fluoride to strengthen the enamel. If there is a cavity, the dentist will need to stop the damage by filling it or by placing a crown, or cap, over the tooth. If the infection goes down into the root, then you may need to get a root canal or have the tooth removed. Missing teeth can be replaced by a dental implant.

Dentists will sometimes come to schools, churches, or other community events to teach children and adults about the importance of brushing and flossing. They will also explain how diet can impact oral health. By practicing good dental habits yourself, you can encourage your friends and family to avoid sugary foods and take care of their teeth.

Many dentists are passionate about teaching the community good oral health. In the United States, dentists work with the American Dental Association, or ADA, to provide resources for the public.

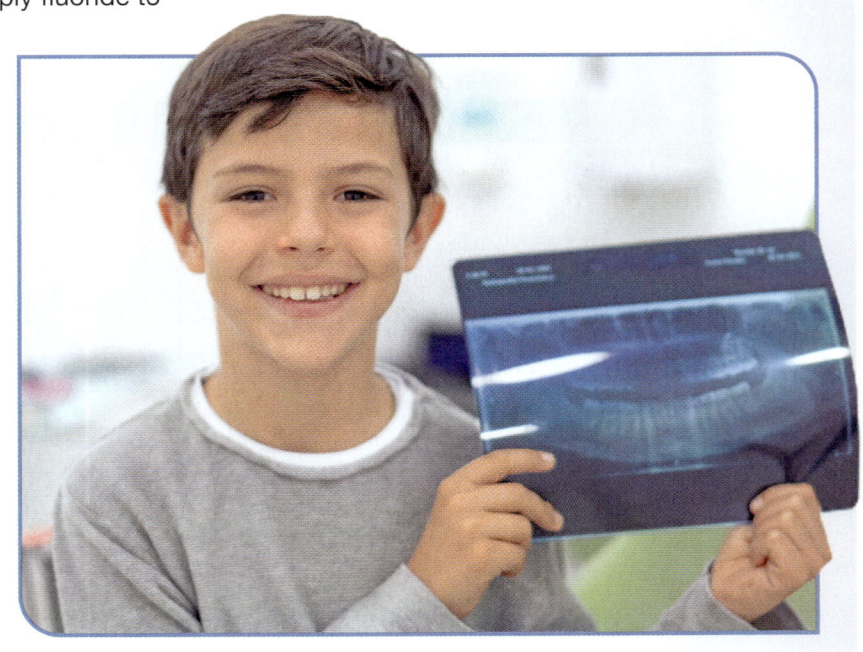

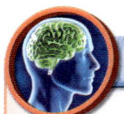

Comprehension Check 7.1

Short Answer: *Write the correct answer in the blank.*

1. What is adolescence? _____

   _____

2. What is puberty? _____

   _____

3. What are chemical messengers that regulate how the body works?

   _____

Identify: *Label the parts of the skin.*

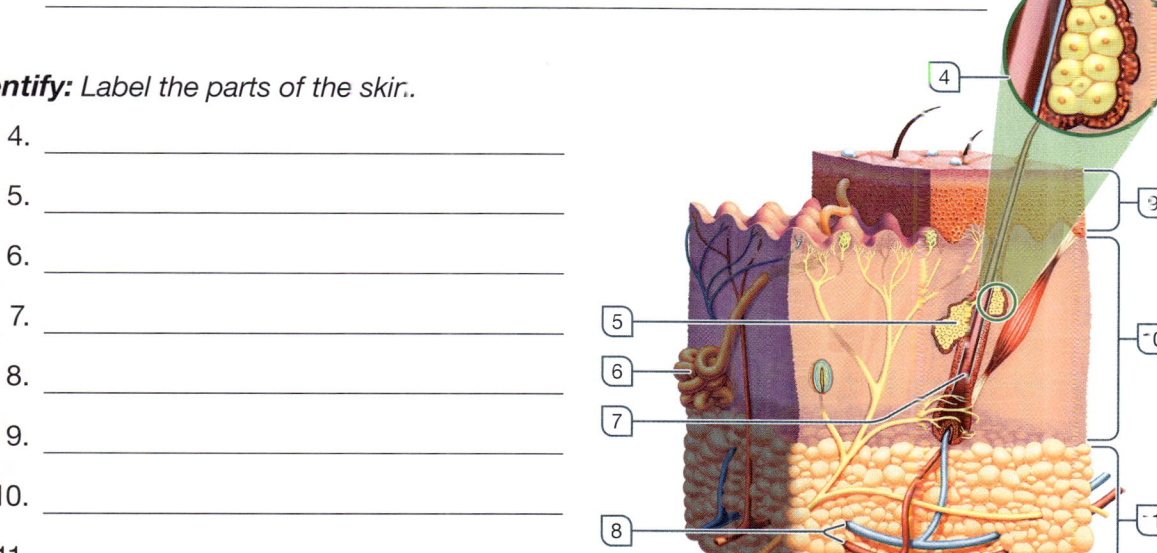

4. _____

5. _____

6. _____

7. _____

8. _____

9. _____

10. _____

11. _____

Matching: *Write the letter of the correct answer in the blank.*

A. acne	B. dental caries	C. hygiene
D. plaque	E. sebum	F. sweat

_____ 12. cleanliness habits that can prevent disease

_____ 13. released from sebaceous glands

_____ 14. skin condition in which clogged pores cause pimples

_____ 15. film of bacteria that forms on teeth

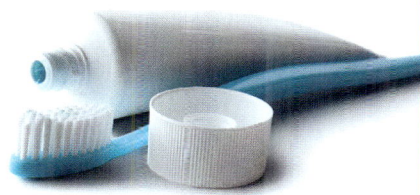

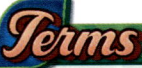

Terms

physical fitness: body's ability to function at its best during daily physical activities without tiring easily

muscular system: body system that provides movement

involuntary muscles: muscles that work automatically without your thinking about them

voluntary muscles: skeletal muscles that can be moved when you want them to move

tendon: cord of white fibers that connects muscle to bone

trapezius: back muscle that moves the shoulder and turns the head

deltoid: muscle that forms the curve of the shoulder and lifts the arm

biceps: upper-arm muscle that bends the arm

triceps: upper-arm muscle that straightens the arm

abdominal muscles: muscles that cover the abdomen; help balance and posture

quadriceps: group of muscles in the front of the upper leg; straighten the knee

hamstrings: group of muscles in the back of the upper leg; bend the knee

muscle tone: the steady contraction of muscles against each other

aerobic exercise: exercise that causes muscles to use more oxygen; endurance exercise

anaerobic exercise: exercise in which muscles do not use more oxygen; requires strength, speed, and agility rather than endurance

lactic acid: waste product formed during strenuous exercise

7.2 Physical Fitness

God designed your body for physical activity. A truly healthy body needs to engage in regular physical activity. Think of all the ways that you are active, such as the sports you participate in and the hobbies you enjoy. Staying active helps your body function at its best. *When your body can function at its best during daily physical activities without tiring easily, you have developed* **physical fitness**.

Being physically fit has many advantages, from helping you control your weight to giving you a restful night's sleep. It helps you look and feel well. Even more importantly, research shows that those who exercise regularly are less likely to get chronic diseases such as heart disease. If you are physically fit, you will have the energy you need to complete your daily activities. *Your muscular and skeletal systems work together so that you can be active and develop physical fitness.*

The Muscular System

Your **muscular system** is *responsible for producing the movements of your body.* All your movements are made by over 600 muscles in your body. Muscles allow you to eat and digest your food. Without muscles, you cannot breathe, and your heart cannot beat. You use muscles when you work or play. *About half of your body weight is muscle.* **Involuntary muscles** *work automatically without your thinking about them.* The two types of involuntary muscles are cardiac muscle tissue, which the heart uses to pump blood, and smooth muscle tissue, which moves food, liquids, and blood through your body. **Voluntary muscles** *can be moved when you want them to move. Voluntary muscles, or skeletal muscles, are connected to the bones of the skeleton by strong white fibers, or cords,* called **tendons**.

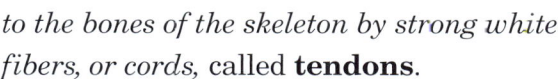
tendons

Skeletal muscles help you to move in many ways. Most of the skeletal muscles work in pairs; *each movement involves two partner muscles.* One muscle relaxes while its partner muscle tightens, or contracts. When a muscle contracts, it gets shorter and thicker; when it relaxes, it gets longer and thinner. Each muscle does its work by pulling—*muscles never push.*

Your *facial muscles* control the movements of your face, allowing you to talk, eat, and make facial expressions. *You can turn your head and shrug your shoulders by using your* **trapezius** [trə·pē′zē·əs], *a large, triangular muscle in your back.* The **deltoid** *forms the curve of your shoulder and lifts your arm.*

Your **biceps** is a *muscle in your upper arm that bends the arm.* Its partner, the **triceps**, *pulls to straighten the arm.* You have many muscles in your forearm and hand that help to move your wrist and fingers.

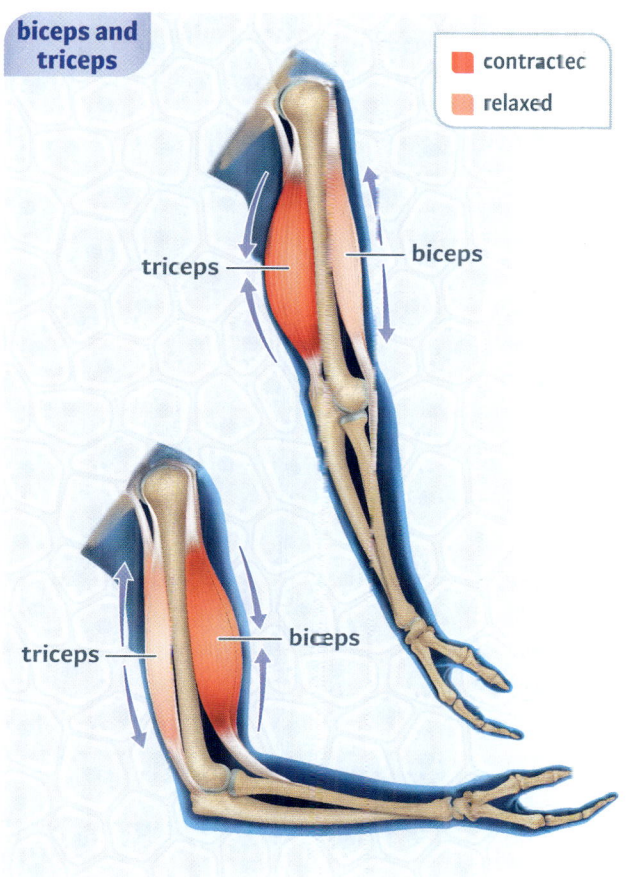

biceps and triceps

contracted
relaxed

triceps — — biceps

triceps — — biceps

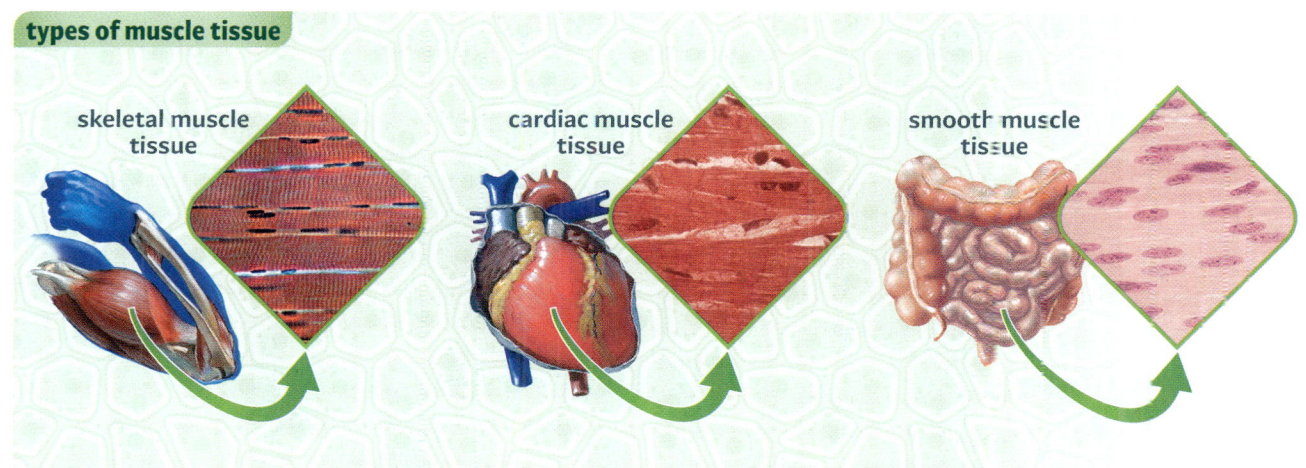

types of muscle tissue

skeletal muscle tissue

cardiac muscle tissue

smooth muscle tissue

Maintaining Physical Health **141**

The **abdominal muscles** *cover your abdomen*. Abdominal muscles, back muscles, and hip muscles are part of your *core muscles*. Your core muscles *help you have better balance and posture when you are doing physical activities* because they give you strong support.

Your legs have strong muscles that work together to walk, kick, and climb. The **quadriceps** [kwŏd′rĭ·sĕps′] are a *group of muscles on the front of your upper leg that straightens your knee*. The *muscles at the back of your upper leg* are called **hamstrings**. The hamstrings *allow you to bend your knee*. A variety of other muscles allow you to move your leg in all directions and rotate your ankle.

muscular system

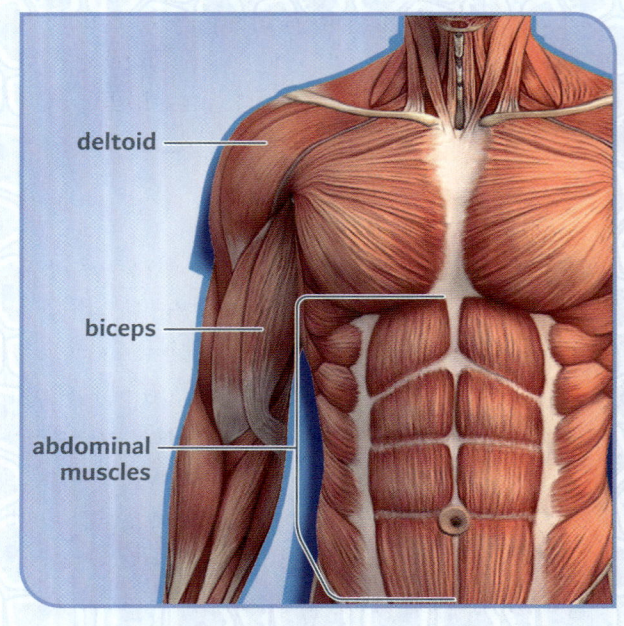

deltoid

biceps

abdominal muscles

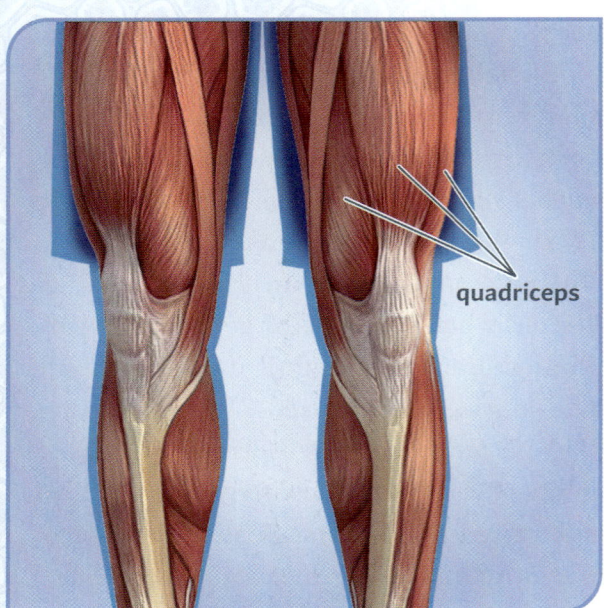

quadriceps

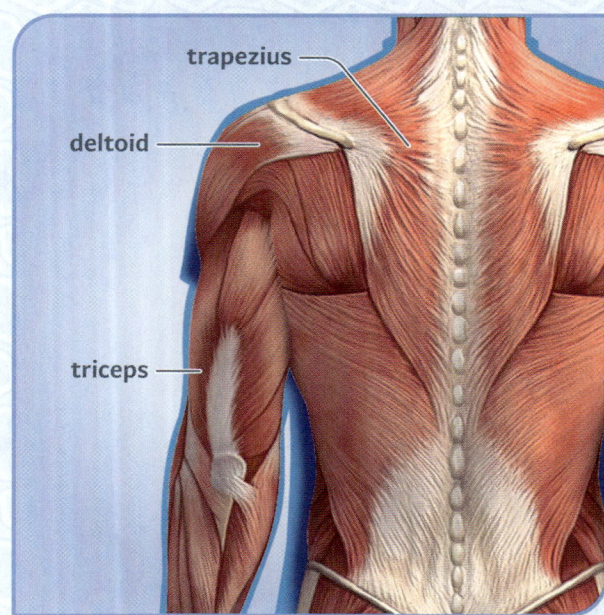

trapezius

deltoid

triceps

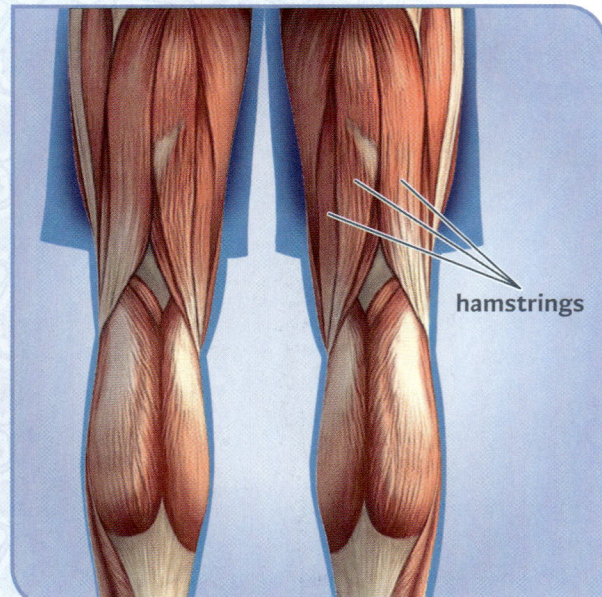

hamstrings

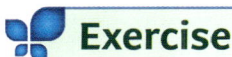

Exercise

Regular exercise gives your body the endurance, strength, and flexibility it needs to be physically fit. You are exercising when you move your body. When your muscles are exercised regularly, your heart supplies them with more blood and nutrients to make the *muscle fibers*, or muscle cells, thicker. Thus, the more muscles are used, the larger and stronger they become.

Exercise also improves muscle tone. **Muscle tone** is *the steady contraction, or gentle pulling, of muscles against each other*. Muscles with good muscle tone are firm and elastic; they respond quickly and easily when the brain tells them to do something. To keep all your muscles strong and toned, you need a variety of activities during work and play.

The Physical Activity Guidelines for Americans recommends that young people get at least 60 minutes of physical activity daily. *There are two types of exercise: aerobic and anaerobic* [ăn′ə·rō′bĭk] *exercises*. Aerobic exercise especially benefits the heart and lungs, while anaerobic exercise benefits bones and muscles. Both types of exercises are important for physical fitness.

Aerobic Exercise

Aerobic exercise *helps your muscles use large amounts of oxygen and builds your endurance by strengthening your heart and lungs*. Aerobic exercise causes muscles to use more oxygen. Your heart must beat faster, and you must breathe more quickly to supply your muscles with oxygen. Most of your daily 60 minutes of activity should be aerobic exercise. Any activity that increases your heart rate for an extended period of time is an aerobic exercise. Aerobic activities include jogging, brisk walking, jumping rope, and swimming.

Anaerobic Exercise

In **anaerobic exercise**, *muscles do not use more oxygen* the way they do during aerobic exercise. Anaerobic activities *require strength, speed, and agility but do not maintain a raised heart rate*. Your body needs anaerobic exercise at least three times a week. Stop-and-go activities, such as baseball, football, bowling, and weightlifting, are anaerobic sports. Using your body strength to hold a certain position is also anaerobic. Gymnasts are anaerobic athletes because of their acrobatic and tumbling skills.

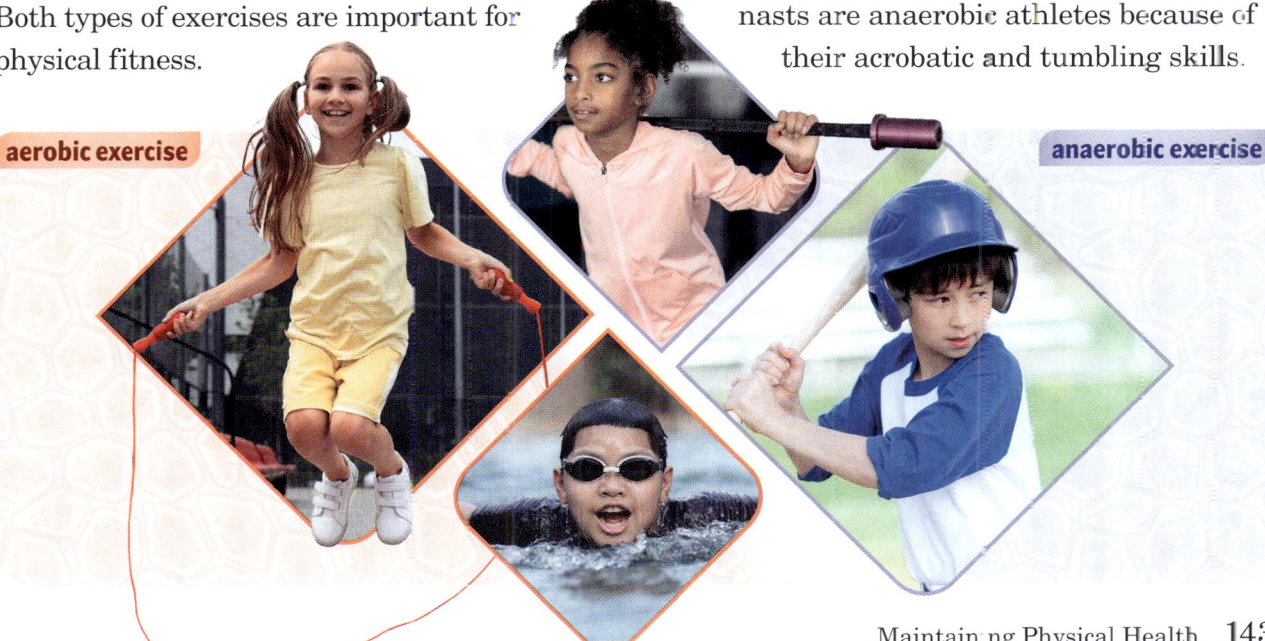

aerobic exercise

anaerobic exercise

Warming Up

Before you begin any strenuous game or activity, your body needs to warm up. Warmups are light exercises that send warm blood flowing to your muscles, raising the muscles' temperature. Warmth from the increased circulation makes your muscles looser and more elastic, reducing the chance of injury. If you begin vigorous exercise before your muscles are warmed up, you may suffer from sore or injured muscles. Light exercises also speed up the work of your heart and lungs and prepare them for more strenuous exercises. You should warm up by doing the strenuous exercise at a lower speed and intensity.

Stretching

After warming up, you can stretch. Stretching lengthens your muscles, tendons, and connective tissue. You should always stretch slowly, just to the point of tightness. Stretching to the point of pain can cause injury and loss of flexibility. Hold the stretch for 15–30 seconds. Never bounce or jerk while stretching; doing so can cause you to overstretch and injure a muscle or tendon.

Cooling Down

Properly caring for your muscles also means allowing them to cool down and return to normal once you have finished any strenuous exercise. You should gradually decrease the intensity of your activity until both your heart rate and breathing have slowed down. Stretch again after energetic exercise to help reduce stiffness and soreness.

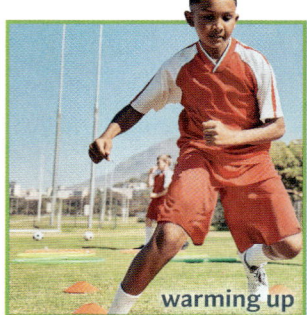
warming up

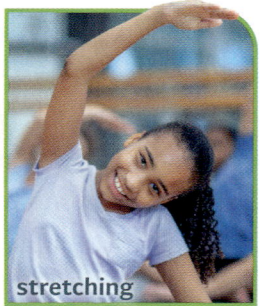
stretching

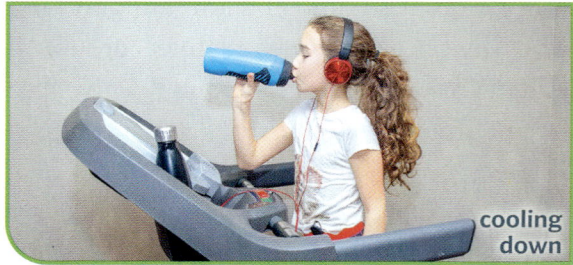
cooling down

Rest and Sleep

To maintain physical fitness, your body needs periods of rest. When your muscles work, food and oxygen are used up and waste materials are formed. **Lactic acid** is *a waste product formed during strenuous exercise.* When lactic acid is formed faster than it can be removed by the blood, it accumulates in the muscles. This makes your muscles feel sore. *Rest gives your body a chance to remove waste materials.* It allows your muscles to rebuild worn parts and to restore some of the energy that has been used up. Rest when you begin to feel tired, because tiredness is a sign that your body is becoming fatigued. When you are fatigued, you cannot work or play as well as when you are rested; it is easy to make mistakes because your body and brain are not alert.

The best rest comes from quiet and peaceful sleep. When you are sleeping, your heart rate slows down and less blood is pumped to your voluntary muscles. Your breathing also slows down, because your body has less carbon dioxide to rid itself of than when you are active. Your body does most of its resting, growing, and fighting of infections while you sleep. *A long period of uninterrupted sleep is better than the same length of interrupted sleep.*

The amount of rest and sleep you need depends on your age, how active you are, and how fast you are growing. *Children between the ages of five and twelve years old need between 9 and 11 hours of sleep each night.* Whenever your body is growing rapidly, you need extra sleep. When you are sick, you need more sleep and rest than when you are well. After strenuous work or activity, it is a good idea to go to bed earlier than usual.

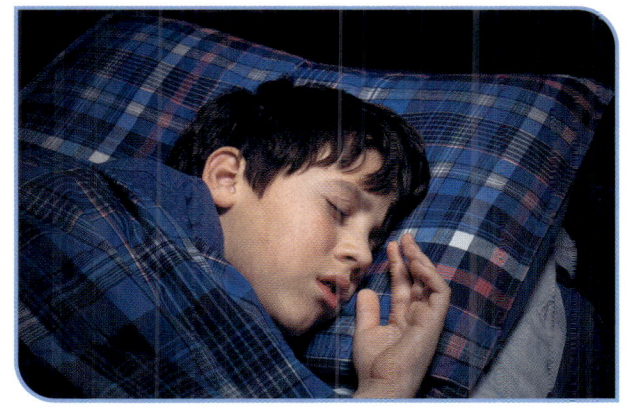

Because activity helps eliminate waste products, strenuous activity relaxes your body and helps you to get restful sleep. When your body is rested, it is able to function at its best throughout the day.

Managing Screen Time

What are some recreational activities that you enjoy? Perhaps you enjoy reading, writing, or doing crafts. You may enjoy gardening or building things. Many people enjoy team sports or other outdoor activities. Other people enjoy watching TV or playing video games. All of these activities can be enjoyable hobbies, but some promote physical fitness more than others. Recreational activities that allow you to get fresh air and exercise help develop your physical fitness.

Activities like watching TV and playing video games can be enjoyable, but it is important to manage screen time. Screen time is the amount of time you spend looking at the screens of televisions, computers, electronic tablets, and cellphones. Screens are often needed for education and work, but too much time looking at screens for recreation can harm your overall health. Looking at screens right before bedtime makes it harder for you to fall asleep. Your relationships with family and friends will also suffer if you are too distracted by a screen. Limit the amount of your screen time each day; your parents may also set a limit on your screen time. Instead of looking at a screen, participate in enjoyable physical activities. Getting plenty of fresh air and exercise are healthy habits to develop for a lifetime.

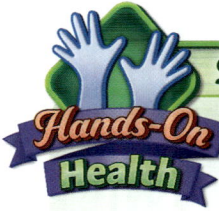

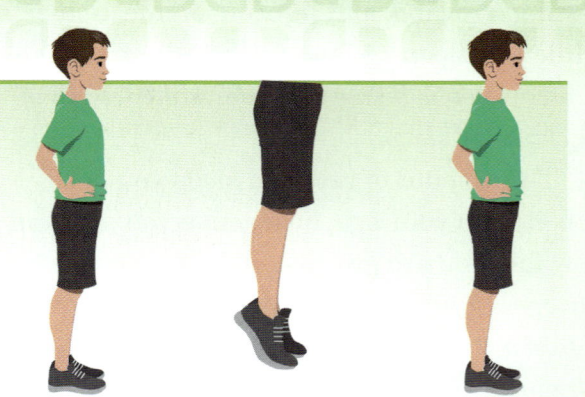

Exercise to build strength.

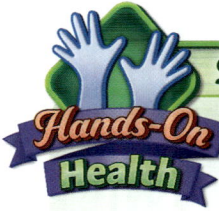
Hands-On Health

Lower-Body Exercises

Calf Raises

Begin by standing with your feet hip-width apart with your toes pointing forward. Place your hands on your hips and keep your back straight. Lift your heels up so that your body weight is on the balls of your feet. After a few seconds, lower your heels back to the ground.

Crab Walk

Sit on the floor with your hands behind your body. Keeping your hands and feet flat on the floor with your knees bent, lift your hips up. Step forward with your left hand and right leg. Then take another step with your right hand and left leg. Continue to use your opposite hand and leg to walk backward and forward.

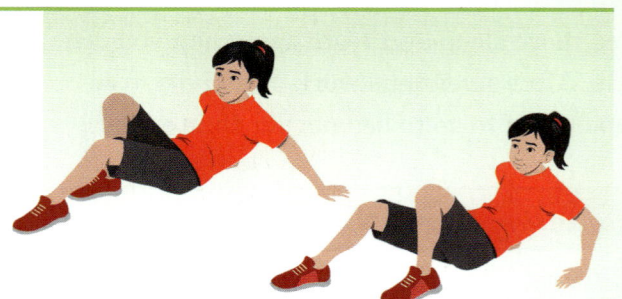

Lunges

Begin by standing with your feet hip-width apart with your toes pointing forward. Keeping your back straight, take a giant step forward with your right foot. Keep your knees bent, and don't push your knee too far forward. Return to your starting position, pushing away from the floor with your heel as you stand up. Repeat with your left leg.

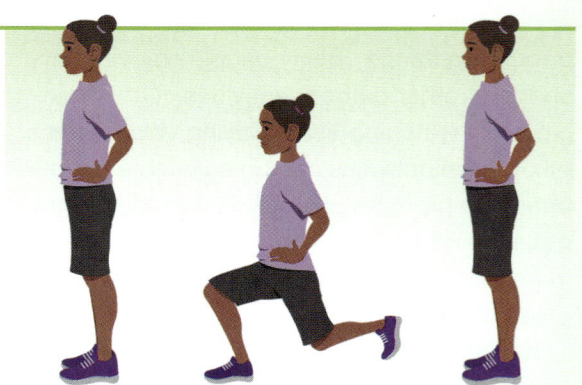

Squats

Begin by standing with your feet slightly wider than hip-width apart with your toes turned out. Keeping your back straight, bend your knees and lower your body as if you were going to sit in a chair. Exhale as you squat down; inhale as you stand up.

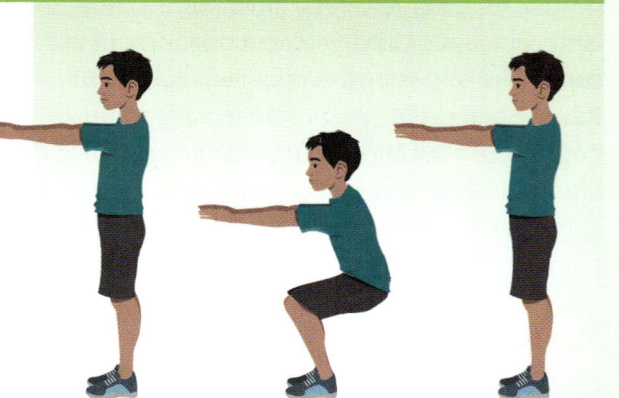

146   *Enjoying Good Health*

Biceps Curls

Begin by standing with good posture. Place a small, squeezable ball in the joint between your biceps and forearm. Make a fist and bring it toward your shoulder. Count ten biceps curls, exhaling each time you curl. Switch to the other arm and repeat.

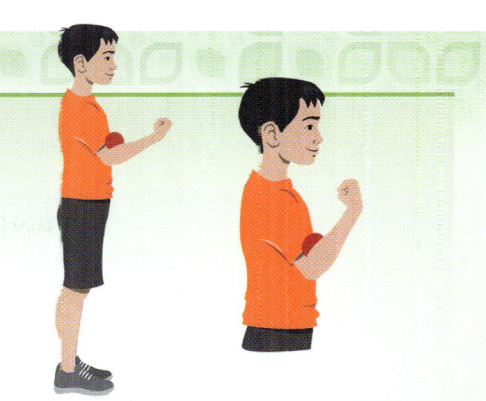

Pushups

Get down on the floor. Place your hands palm down, slightly wider than your shoulders, and bend your elbows. Extend your legs back so that you are balanced on your toes; keep your back straight. Lower yourself so that your chest almost touches the floor, and then raise yourself back to the starting position. You can also modify the pushup by keeping your knees on the ground. Be sure to keep your back straight throughout the whole exercise.

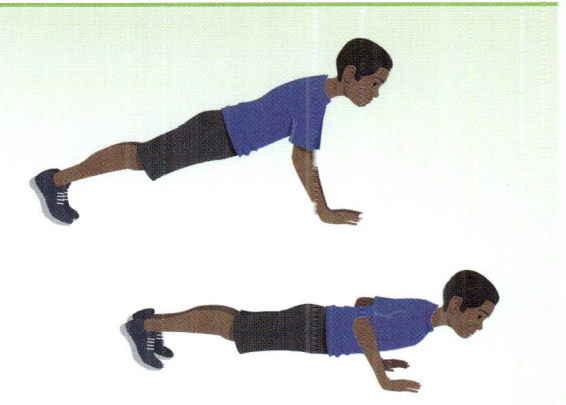

Overhead Press

Begin by standing with good posture. Hold your arms out and keep your elbows bent across from your shoulders. Make two fists and push your arms up overhead as you exhale; inhale as you bring your fists back down again.

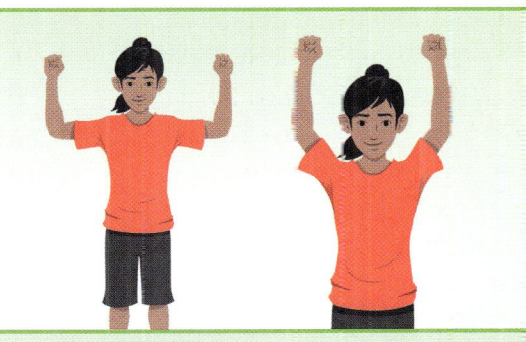

Wall Pushups

Stand about an arm's length away from a wall. Place both palms on the wall at shoulder height. Slowly bend your elbows and lean your body toward the wall; be sure to keep your heels down. Return to the starting position.

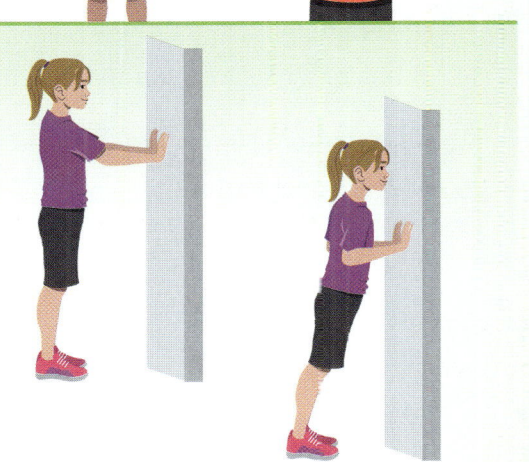

Matching: *Write the letter of the correct answer in the blank.*

_____ 1. shrugs the shoulder and turns the head

_____ 2. forms the curve of the shoulder and lifts the arm

_____ 3. bends the arm

_____ 4. straightens the arm

_____ 5. found in the front of the upper leg

_____ 6. found in the back of the upper leg

A. abdominal muscles
B. biceps
C. deltoid
D. hamstrings
E. quadriceps
F. trapezius
G. triceps

True/False: *If the statement is true, write* true *in the blank. If the statement is false, replace the underlined word(s) with a word or phrase that will make the statement true. Do not write* false *in any blank.*

_____ 7. The body's ability to function at its best is <u>physical fitness</u>.

_____ 8. Your heart and stomach are made of <u>voluntary</u> muscles.

_____ 9. Muscles are connected to bones by <u>ligaments</u>.

_____ 10. The muscles use more oxygen in <u>anaerobic</u> exercise.

_____ 11. Weightlifting is an <u>aerobic</u> exercise.

_____ 12. Your muscles become sore when <u>lactic acid</u> is formed faster than it can be removed.

_____ 13. Each night, a child between the ages of five and twelve years old needs <u>9 to 11</u> hours of sleep.

Think about It.

14. What muscles are you using when you throw a baseball? _____

_____

15. Name an exercise that engages your core muscles. Which muscles are involved?

_____

_____

_____

_____

7.3 The Skeletal System

Your muscles could not move your body without the help of the **skeletal system**, the *framework of bones that support and protect your body*. The skeletal system of an adult has 206 bones. The skeleton has two main divisions. The **axial** [ăk′sē·əl] **skeleton** is *the division of the skeleton that includes the head, spine, and ribs*. The 80 bones of the axial skeleton *protect important organs* such as your brain, eyes, heart, lungs, and spinal cord. The **appendicular** [ăp′ən·dĭk′yə·lər]

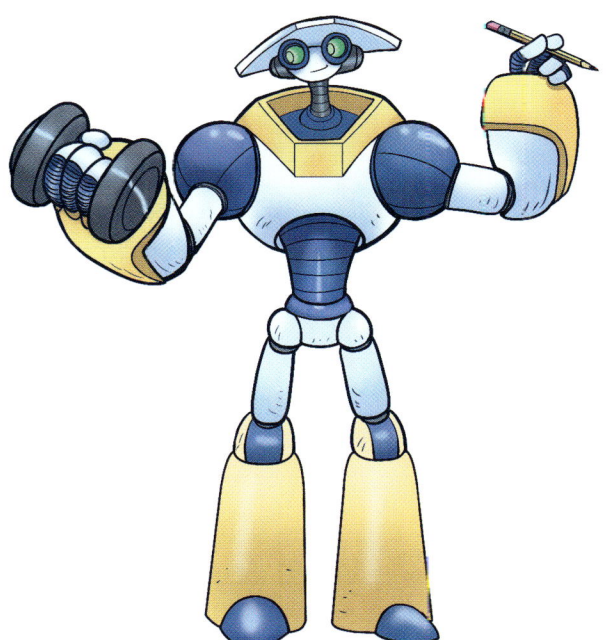

skeleton is *the division of the skeleton that includes the shoulders, hips, arms, and legs*. The 126 bones of the appendicular skeleton *work with your muscles to move your body*.

Structure of a Bone

Your bones were engineered to be strong. Consider the structure of a typical arm or leg bone; these bones are classified as **long bones** because they are *longer than they are wide and have enlarged ends*. A long bone is not completely solid; instead, it has an outer shell of hard bone that surrounds a hollow interior. This design enables it to bear weight. *The outer shell of compact bone gives the bone strength and rigidity*. The bone's interior is made of a *lightweight, porous tissue* called **spongy bone**. Although the spongy bone resembles a porous sponge, *it is actually strong and rigid*. This scaffold-like inner structure *reduces the bone's weight*. The tiny open spaces in spongy bone are filled by **bone marrow**, the *soft tissue in the open spaces of a bone*.

Bones not only provide structure and protection to your body but also make blood cells and store minerals. *Red bone marrow* makes both red and white blood cells. These cells are used by the circulatory and immune systems. In adults, some of the red marrow is replaced by *yellow bone marrow*, which stores fats. *Your bones store minerals such as calcium, magnesium, and phosphorus*, all of which help make the bones strong. If your blood does not have enough of these minerals, your bones will release them into the bloodstream.

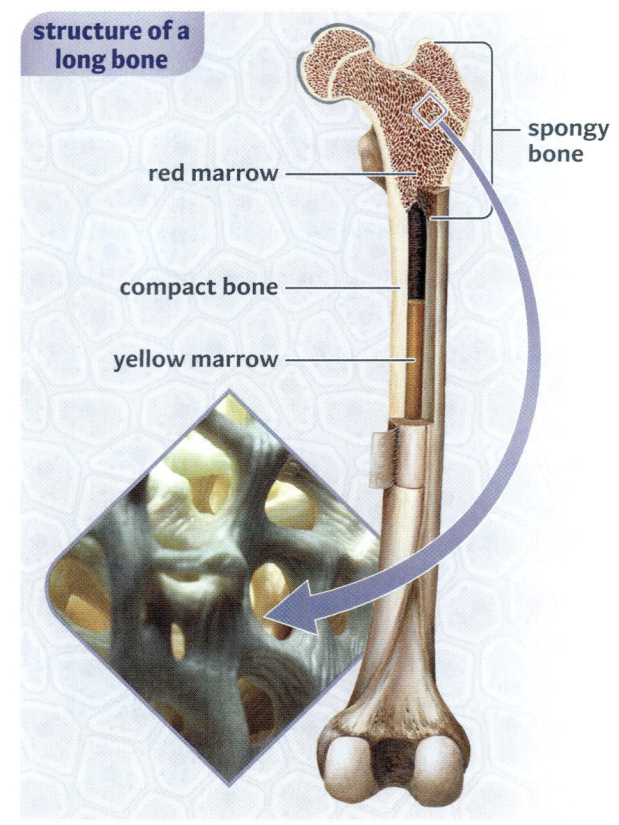

structure of a long bone

red marrow

compact bone

yellow marrow

spongy bone

Mental Workout

What types of food are good sources of calcium, magnesium, and phosphorus? (Refer back to Chapter 4.) What would happen to your bones if you do not eat enough of these foods?

Types of Bones

Bones are classified into four types based on their shape. Remember, long bones are longer than they are wide and have enlarged ends. They support your body's weight and work with your muscles to provide movement. Long bones are found in your arms and legs.

Short bones are roughly cube-shaped; they are as long as they are wide. Short bones are found in your wrists and ankles.

Flat bones are thin, flattened bones that protect vital organs. Flat bones include your ribs, shoulder blades, and cranium.

Irregular bones have odd shapes and cannot be easily classified into any other category. Irregular bones include the bones of the spinal column and the hammer, anvil, and stirrup bones in your middle ear.

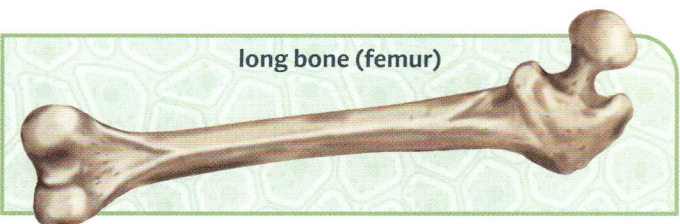

long bone (femur)

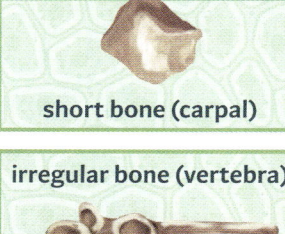

short bone (carpal)

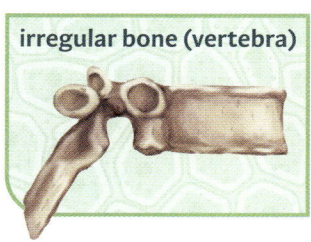

irregular bone (vertebra)

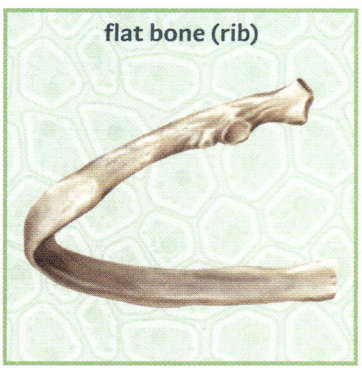

flat bone (rib)

Joints

Like puzzle pieces that fit together, your bones are joined to make your skeleton. *A place where two or more bones join is called a* **joint**. At a joint, *bones are connected by strong, elastic bands of fibrous tissue called* **ligaments** [lĭg′ə·mənts]. The elasticity of ligaments *helps keep bones and joints stable in their movements.*

There are many types of joints in your body. Some joints are *immovable*. They hold the bones tightly together and do not allow any movement. Your skull has immovable joints. Other joints are *slightly movable*. They allow the bones to bend or twist only a little. Your backbone has slightly movable joints. Most

joints of the body are *freely movable*, which allow for a wide range of motion. Freely movable joints are found in your arms and legs.

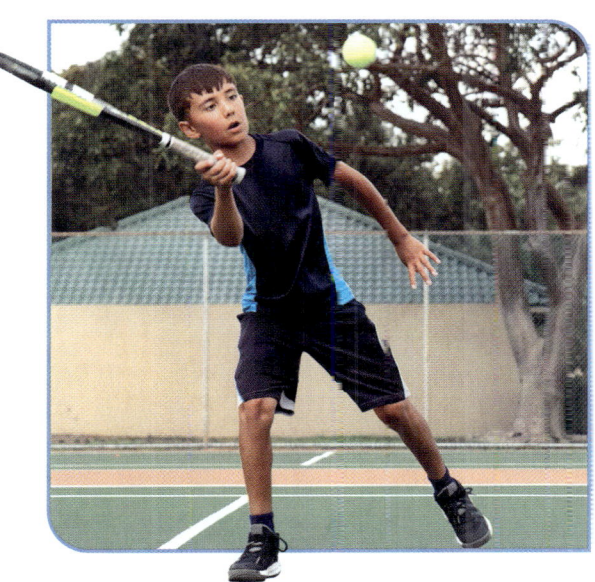

Types of Freely Movable Joints

Most of your freely movable joints are found in the appendicular skeleton. These joints allow your arms, legs, hands, and feet to bend and help your skeletal muscles make many types of movements.

Ball-and-socket joints allow the widest range of motion. They allow your arms and legs to move in many directions. Your shoulder joints and hip joints are the only ball-and-socket joints in the body.

Hinge joints allow back-and-forth movement, like the hinges of a door. Hinge joints are found in your elbows, knees, and fingers.

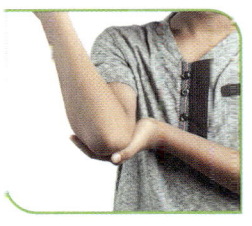

Pivot joints allow turning movements. Pivot joints in your neck allow you to turn your head. Your elbow has pivot joints that let you turn your hands over.

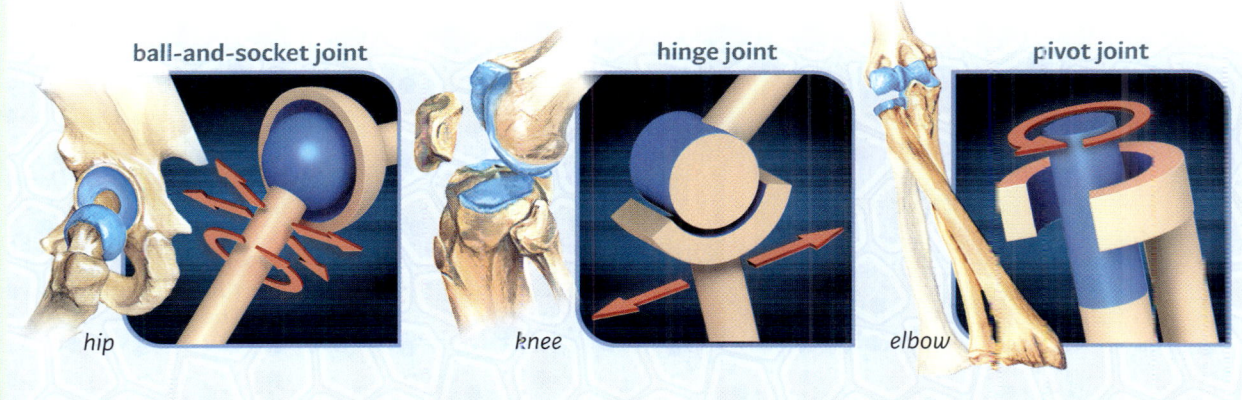

ball-and-socket joint   hinge joint   pivot joint

hip   *knee*   *elbow*

skeletal system

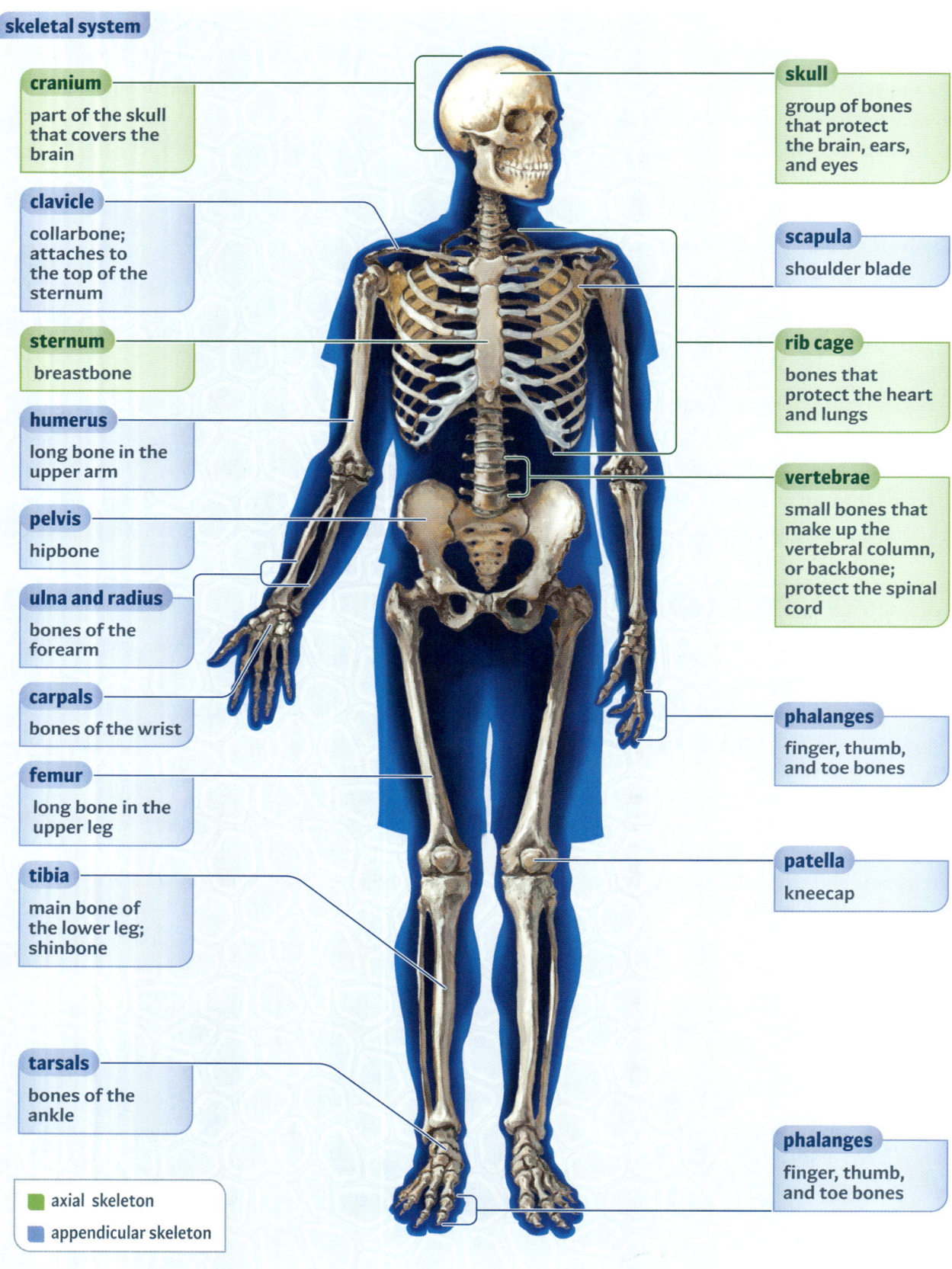

cranium
part of the skull that covers the brain

clavicle
collarbone; attaches to the top of the sternum

sternum
breastbone

humerus
long bone in the upper arm

pelvis
hipbone

ulna and radius
bones of the forearm

carpals
bones of the wrist

femur
long bone in the upper leg

tibia
main bone of the lower leg; shinbone

tarsals
bones of the ankle

skull
group of bones that protect the brain, ears, and eyes

scapula
shoulder blade

rib cage
bones that protect the heart and lungs

vertebrae
small bones that make up the vertebral column, or backbone; protect the spinal cord

phalanges
finger, thumb, and toe bones

patella
kneecap

phalanges
finger, thumb, and toe bones

■ axial skeleton
■ appendicular skeleton

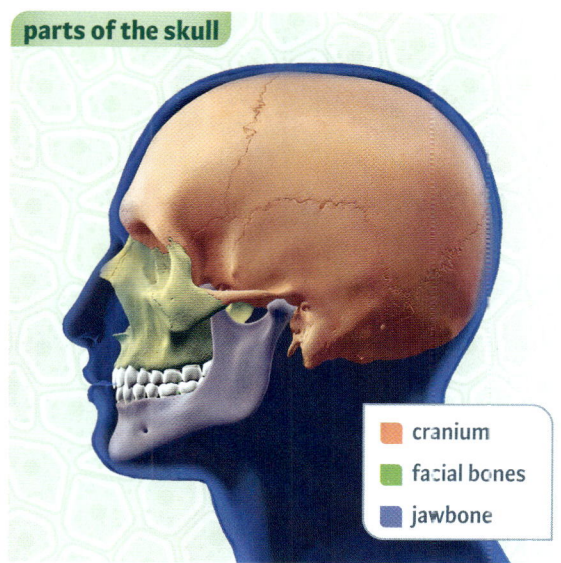

cranium
facial bones
jawbone

The Axial Skeleton

Your **skull** is made of twenty-two bones that *protect your brain, ears, and eyes from injuries*. The eight flat *skull bones that cover your brain* form the **cranium**. The fourteen *facial bones* form the shape of your face. Your lower jawbone, while part of your skull, is different from the other skull bones. It holds the lower teeth and is the only movable bone of the skull.

Your vertebral [vûr′tə·brəl] *column, or backbone, is your body's main support.* Without it, you cannot sit up or stand. *The adult vertebral*

vertebrae

column is made up of thirty-three small bones called **vertebrae** [vûr′tə·brā′; *sing.* vertebra: vûr′tə·brə]. The vertebrae are joined by slightly movable joints so that you can bend and twist your spine. *The spinal cord is protected in a hollow tube formed by your vertebral column.*

Attached to the vertebrae are twelve pairs of *long, thin bones called ribs*. The ribs wrap around to the front of your body, where the upper ten pairs attach to the **sternum**, or *breastbone*. The lowest two rib pairs also wrap around the body but attach only to the vertebral column. *Together, the ribs and sternum form the* **rib cage**, *which protects your heart and lungs*. The tissue that attaches the ribs to the sternum is flexible, letting the rib cage expand during breathing.

The Appendicular Skeleton

Bones of the Shoulders and Arms

Your arms are attached to the axial skeleton at the **scapulas** [skăp′yə·ləz], or *shoulder blades*. Muscles allow you to raise and lower your scapulas. Each scapula is braced by a **clavicle**, or *collarbone*, that *attaches to the top of the sternum*. Your two clavicles hold your arms in proper position at the sides of your body. They also give your upper body structural support so that it moves correctly.

Your arm is made of three long bones called the *humerus, ulna, and radius*. The **humerus** is *the long bone in the upper arm that attaches to the scapula at the shoulder joint. The forearm has two bones*, the **ulna** and **radius**. These bones work together to *let you rotate your forearm and wrist.*

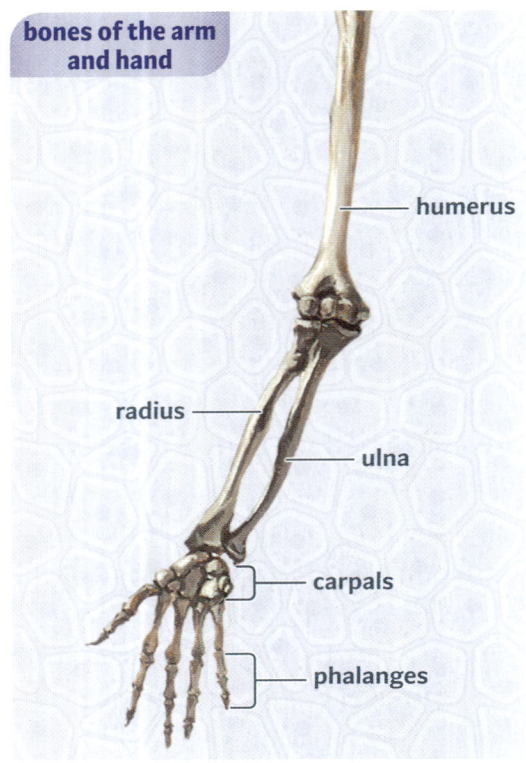

bones of the arm and hand

humerus

radius

ulna

carpals

phalanges

Your hand is attached to the ulna and radius by the **carpal** bones in your wrist. The carpals *allow the wrist to bend in various directions. Each of your fingers has three slender bones* called **phalanges** [fə·lăn′jēz]. Your thumb has only two phalanges. Your hand bones perform a variety of complex movements. Over the next week, observe them as you work and play. You will be amazed at the abilities God gave the human hands.

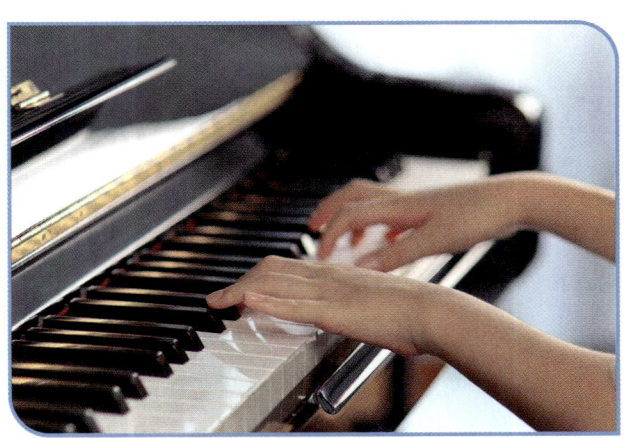

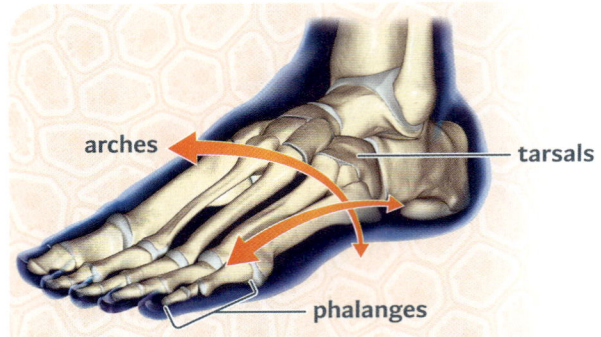

arches

tarsals

phalanges

Bones of the Hips and Legs

Your legs are attached to the axial skeleton by the bones of the **pelvis**, or *hipbone*. The pelvis forms a rigid ring of thick bone that supports most of the body's weight. *The longest bone of the body is the thighbone*, or **femur**. Your femur is attached to the lower leg at the *knee joint. Your* **patella**, *or kneecap, protects your knee joint.* The **tibia**, or *shinbone*, is *the main bone of the lower leg.* Your tibia must be very strong because it has to carry the weight of the body with each step.

One-fourth of the bones in your body are found in your feet and ankles. The tibia attaches to the **tarsals**, or *ankle bones.* The bones that make up the main part of your foot are arched so that they can support the weight of the body. Like the finger bones, *the toe bones are called phalanges*. The phalanges in your toes are shorter and wider than the phalanges in your fingers. This wise design helps keep your body balanced when you stand or walk.

Growing Pains

Have you ever woken up in the middle of the night because your legs hurt? You may have been experiencing growing pains. Many young people feel pain in the front of the thighs, in the muscles of the lower legs, or behind the knees. Some also have abdominal pain or headaches. The symptoms usually happen at night and go away in the morning. Although it was once thought that growing pains result from rapid growth spurts, research has shown that the leg pain results from overuse of muscles. Children who spend a lot of time running, climbing, and jumping are more likely to experience growing pains.

If you experience growing pains, you can ask a parent or trusted adult to rub or massage your legs to help ease the pain. Heat from a heating pad or a warm bath can help soothe sore muscles. You can also take an over-the-counter pain medicine or do stretching exercises. You may need to see a physician if the pain continues during the day or if you get a fever. Growing pains usually stop once you become a teenager.

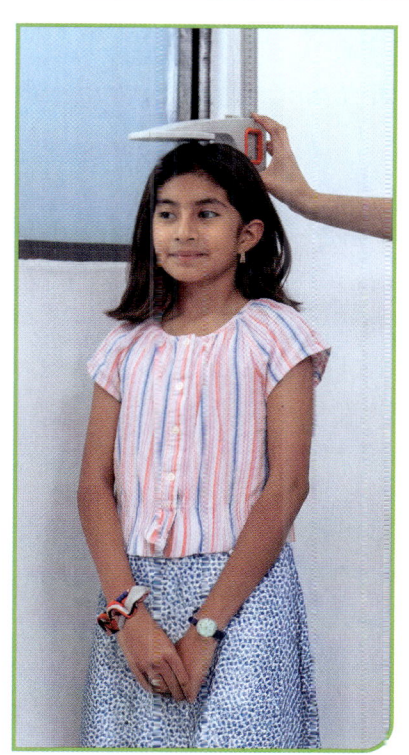

Protein-Packed Yogurt Bowl

Greek yogurt is helpful for your muscular and skeletal systems because it has plenty of protein and calcium and other important nutrients. Here is a delicious Greek yogurt bowl that you can make with your family!

Be aware of allergies or sensitivities before you handle or eat food.

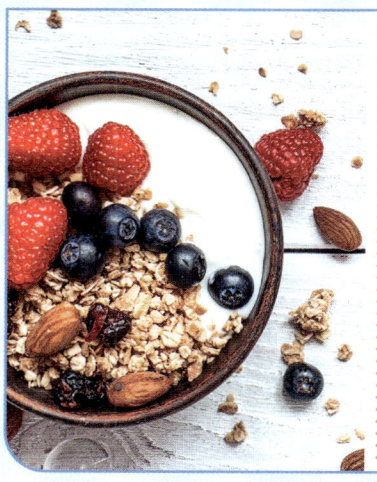

Ingredients:

- plain Greek yogurt
- granola
- fresh or dried fruit, whole, sliced or chopped (for example, bananas, strawberries, blueberries, pineapple, or mango)
- nuts, whole or chopped (for example, walnuts, almonds, or pecans)

Directions:

1. Place the Greek yogurt in a bowl.
2. Top with granola, fruit, and nuts of your choice.
3. Share with your family and enjoy!

Matching: *Write the letter of the correct answer in the blank.*

> A. clavicle   B. cranium   C. rib cage   D. tibia   E. vertebra

_____ 1. covers the brain

_____ 2. protects the spinal cord

_____ 3. protects the heart and lungs

_____ 4. collarbone

Short Answer: *Write the correct answer in the blank.*

5. Which division of the skeleton includes the head, spine, and ribs? _____

_____

6. How does spongy bone help the bone? _____

_____

7. What elastic bands of fibrous tissue connect bones? _____

8. What long bone is found in the upper arm? _____

Think about It.

9. Why does your body need several different types of joints? _____

_____

_____

_____

10. What two parts of the body contain bones called phalanges? _____

_____

Identify: *Label the bones.*

11. _____

12. _____

13. _____

14. _____

15. _____

16. _____

1 Caring for Yourself (7.1)

A. Matching: *Write the letter of the correct answer in the blank.*

A. dentin
B. dermis
C. enamel
D. epidermis
E. hair follicle
F. hypodermis
G. pulp
H. sebum

_____ 1. the outer layer of the skin

_____ 2. small tube that makes new hair

_____ 3. oily substance that keeps the skin soft

_____ 4. the hardest substance of the body

_____ 5. bone-like tissue that shapes a tooth

_____ 6. soft tissue inside a tooth

B. True/False: *If the statement is true, write* true *in the blank. If the statement is false, replace the underlined word with a word or phrase that will make the statement true. Do not write* false *in any blank.*

_____ 1. The process of physical changes during adolescence is called <u>hygiene</u>.

_____ 2. Puberty is coordinated by the <u>pituitary</u> gland.

_____ 3. Your body is covered and protected by the <u>endocrine</u> system.

_____ 4. The condition in which clogged pores cause pimples is <u>acne</u>.

_____ 5. Combs and hats <u>should</u> be shared with other people.

_____ 6. Harmful bacteria in the mouth form a sticky, colorless film called <u>plaque</u>.

C. Fill in the Blank: *Write the correct word in the blank.*

1. The transitional time of growth and development between childhood and adulthood is called _____.

2. Chemical messengers called _____ regulate how the body works.

3. Acid attacks create holes in the tooth enamel called cavities, or _____.

continued

D. Short Answer: *Write the correct answer in the blank.*

1. Why is it important to develop good hygiene habits during adolescence? _____

   _____

   _____

2. What can you do to eliminate unpleasant body odor? _____

   _____

3. What can you do to keep your hair clean? _____

2 Physical Fitness (7.2)

A. Short Answer: *Write the correct answer in the blank.*

1. What is physical fitness? _____

   _____

   _____

2. What type of muscles can be moved when you want them to move? _____

   _____

3. What is muscle tone? _____

   _____

4. What waste product is formed during strenuous exercise? _____

   _____

5. Why is rest important for your body? _____

   _____

B. Multiple Choice: *Write the letter of the correct answer in the blank.*

_____ 1. What muscle forms the curve of your shoulder and helps lift your arm?
   - a. biceps
   - b. deltoid
   - c. quadriceps
   - d. trapezius

_____ 2. What muscles allow you to bend your knee?
   - a. deltoid
   - b. hamstrings
   - c. quadriceps
   - d. triceps

_____ 3. Which of the following is an anaerobic exercise?
   - a. jumping rope
   - b. running
   - c. swimming
   - d. weightlifting

C. Identify: *Label the muscles.*

_____ 1.
_____ 2.
_____ 3.
_____ 4.
_____ 5.
_____ 6.
_____ 7.

A. abdominal muscles
B. biceps
C. deltoid
D. hamstrings
E. quadriceps
F. trapezius
G. triceps

D. Think!

Why do almost all muscles work in pairs? _____

_____

_____

3 **The Skeletal System (7.3)**

A. True/False: *If the statement is true, write* true *in the blank. If the statement is false, replace the underlined word with a word that will make the statement true. Do not write* false *in any blank.*

_____ 1. The bones in the arms and legs are part of the <u>axial</u> skeleton.

_____ 2. The interior of a bone is made of lightweight, porous tissue called <u>spongy</u> bone.

_____ 3. The soft tissue inside a bone that makes blood cells is the bone <u>joint</u>.

_____ 4. Bones are connected by fibrous tissue called <u>tendons</u>.

_____ 5. The vertebral column is made of <u>33</u> vertebrae.

continued

B. Identify: *Label the bones of the body. Circle the numbers for bones of the appendicular skeleton.*

_____ 1.

_____ 2.

_____ 3.

_____ 4.

_____ 5.

_____ 6.

_____ 7.

_____ 8.

_____ 9.

_____ 10.

_____ 11.

_____ 12.

_____ 13.

_____ 14.

_____ 15.

_____ 16.

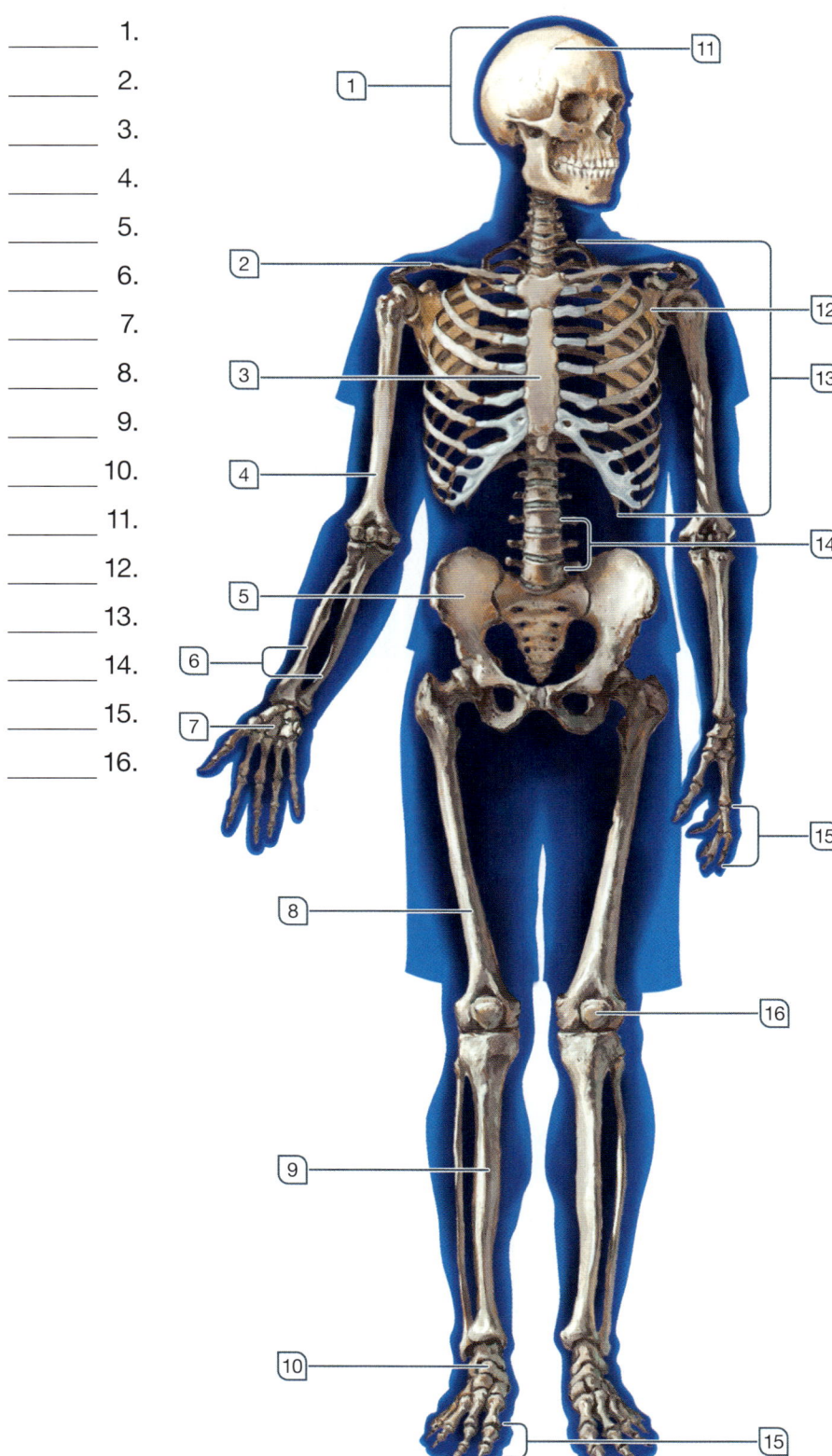

A. carpals

B. clavicle

C. cranium

D. femur

E. humerus

F. patella

G. pelvis

H. phalanges

I. rib cage

J. scapula

K. skull

L. sternum

M. tarsals

N. tibia

O. ulna and radius

P. vertebrae

C. Multiple Choice: *Write the letter of the correct answer in the blank.*

_____ 1. Your brain is covered by your __?__ .
   a. clavicle
   b. cranium
   c. pelvis
   d. vertebrae

_____ 2. Your heart and lungs are protected by your __?__ .
   a. cranium
   b. patella
   c. pelvis
   d. rib cage

_____ 3. The longest bone in the body is the __?__ .
   a. femur
   b. humerus
   c. tibia
   d. ulna

_____ 4. The main bone of the lower leg is the __?__ .
   a. femur
   b. radius
   c. scapula
   d. tibia

_____ 5. The ankle bones are called __?__ .
   a. craniums
   b. patellas
   c. tarsals
   d. vertebrae

D. Think!

How are the bones in your fingers and toes similar? _____

_____

_____

_____

How are they different? _____

_____

_____

_____

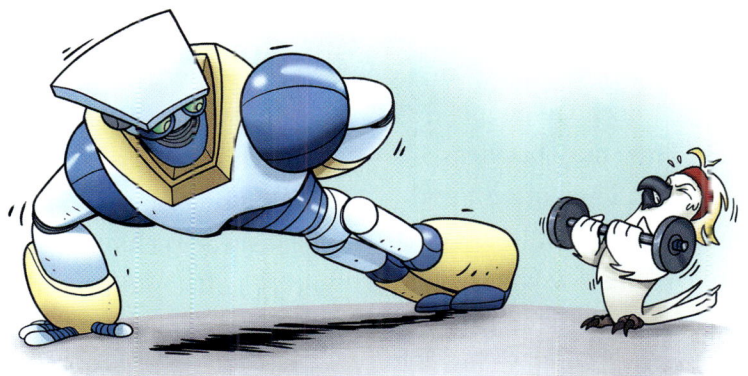

Chapter 8 Safety and First Aid

8.1 Staying Safe

You have learned about many behaviors that are part of a healthy lifestyle, such as a healthy diet, physical activity, and personal hygiene. However, these behaviors cannot prevent accidents that could harm or injure your body. You can lower health risks that could harm you or others by developing safety habits, knowing basic first aid, and avoiding harmful substances.

Accidents often happen because people take unnecessary risks. They may be careless, rushing, or showing off. They often have not learned the procedures that would keep them safe. *A person who is prudent, or wise and careful, takes precautions to avoid injuring himself or others.* You can help prevent accidents by learning and following safety rules and procedures.

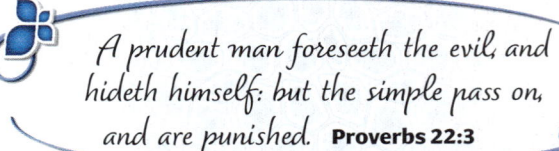

A prudent man foreseeth the evil, and hideth himself: but the simple pass on, and are punished. **Proverbs 22:3**

Sports Safety

Recreational sports are a fun way to stay physically active. Accidents and injuries can occur while playing sports, often because of careless or reckless behavior. Every sport has safety rules and procedures that help prevent injuries. *Each participant should learn and follow the safety rules of the sport.*

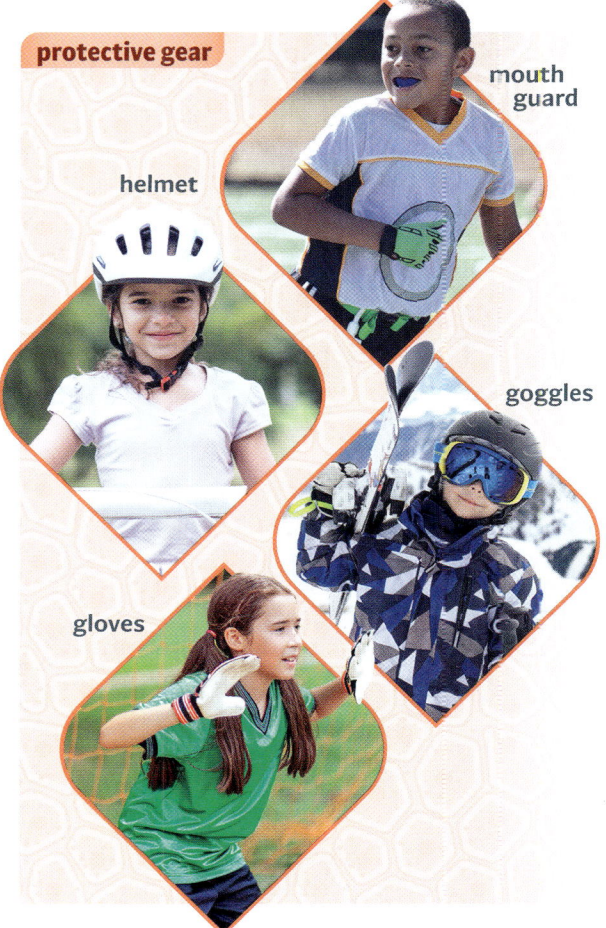

protective gear

mouth guard

helmet

goggles

gloves

Many serious sports injuries can be prevented or reduced by using protective gear. A *helmet* lowers the chance of a head injury. *Protective pads* shield joints, the rib cage, and the back. A *mouth guard* protects the teeth, mouth, and jaw from serious injuries. *When you participate in any sport, make sure that you have proper protective gear that fits well and is in good condition.*

Physical activity such as yard work also requires proper safety habits and protective gear. Wearing *gloves* can protect your hands from blisters, thorns, and insect bites. When using loud lawn equipment, wear *earplugs or other hearing protection* to prevent hearing loss. To protect your eyes, you should wear *safety glasses or safety goggles* while using lawn equipment.

 ## Weather Safety

Being outside is good for your health. Fresh air, exercise, and sunshine all benefit your body. However, weather conditions can harm your body if you do not take proper precautions. Before participating in outdoor activities, check the weather forecast and prepare to protect yourself from any extreme weather.

Cold-Weather Safety

During winter, snow and ice can change the landscape. Many people enjoy winter sports such as ice skating, skiing, snowmobiling, or sledding. Dress warmly when you go outside in cold weather; without adequate clothing, your body parts could be frozen by the cold temperature. **Frostbite**, *the freezing of body tissue*, occurs when body parts are exposed to freezing temperatures for too long. Your hands, feet, cheeks, ears, and nose are most likely to get frostbite.

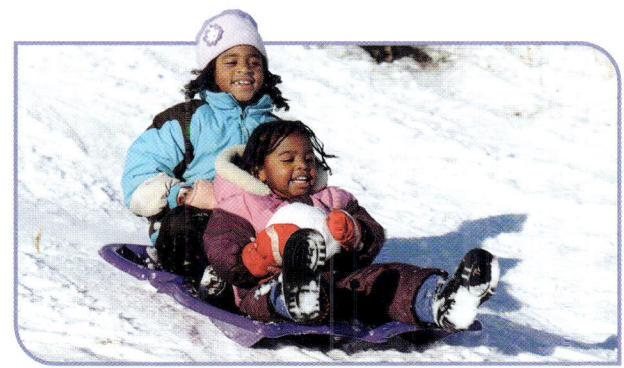

Warm-Weather Safety

Warm weather in spring and summer provides many opportunities for fun outdoor activities. These warmer temperatures can cause your body to sweat. When you sweat, your body loses water and **electrolytes**, *minerals that help regulate the body's water balance.*

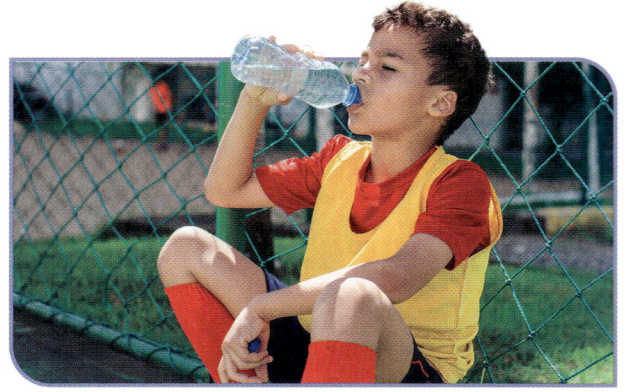

Dehydration occurs when the *body tissues lose too much water. Excessive or prolonged heat and dehydration limit your body's ability to control its internal temperature*, a condition called **heat exhaustion**. On a hot summer day, you may be suffering from heat exhaustion if you start feeling cold; your skin becomes clammy, or cool and moist; and you feel sick to your stomach.

Follow safety precautions to avoid heat exhaustion. Wear loose-fitting clothes that are both lightweight and light in color to keep your body cooler and to reduce sweating. You can also avoid excessive sweating by limiting outdoor activities in hot weather. If you must be outside, drink plenty of water or sports drinks. Sports drinks contain electrolytes that help your body absorb water quickly. If you show symptoms of heat exhaustion, you should rest, take steps to cool yourself, and seek medical attention.

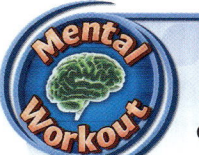

How are sports drinks different from energy drinks?

Sun Safety

Sunlight benefits you in many ways. It helps your body produce vitamin D, which you need for strong bones. Sunlight also helps improve your immune system and sleep quality and boosts your mood. However, sunlight can also be harmful to your skin. The sun produces **ultraviolet radiation**, or *UV rays, invisible rays beyond the violet end of the light spectrum*. The atmosphere protects us from most UV rays, but some of them reach Earth. Although you cannot see or feel their energy, too much exposure to them can cause sunburn or even skin cancer.

If you must be outside when the sun's rays are strong, you can block some UV rays by applying sunscreen. *Sunscreen is rated by its* **SPF***, or sun protection factor*. The higher the SPF, the more UV rays are filtered. Apply sunscreen 30 minutes before going outside, and reapply it every few hours. If you go swimming, reapply sunscreen

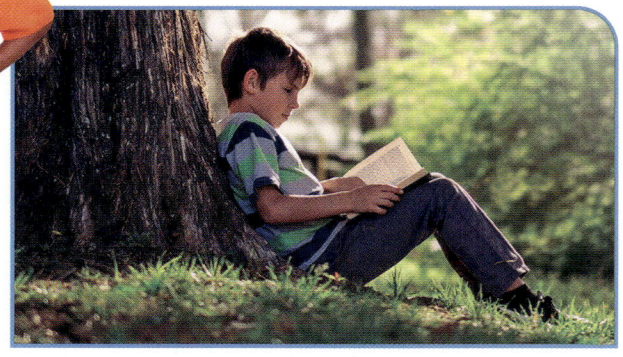

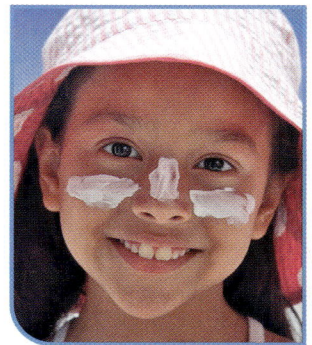

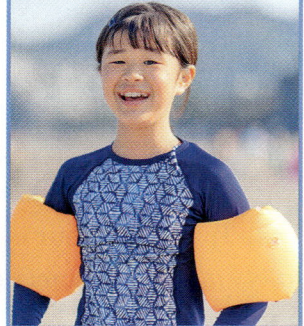

after you get out of the water. You should also wear clothes that cover and protect your body. Long sleeves and pants protect your arms and legs. Sun shirts, swim shirts, and rash guards are made of light materials that keep you cool while providing UV protection. Wear a wide-brimmed hat to protect your ears, neck, and face. Sunglasses that block UV rays protect your eyes and the skin around them.

Water Safety

Some of the most popular warm-weather activities are watersports, such as swimming, surfing, boating, and tubing. These sports have special precautions because of the danger of *drowning*. Drowning results from *suffocation*, or blocked breathing, underwater and is one of the leading causes of accidental deaths. *Many drowning accidents have occurred because a person did not know how to swim or did not follow safety procedures.* Even strong swimmers can drown if they ignore safety procedures.

You can reduce your risk of drowning by learning how to swim. Two important water-safety skills are treading water and floating. To tread water, or swim in place, slowly move your legs as if you were pedaling a bicycle and sweep your arms back and forth. To float, turn over onto your back and relax. Staying calm and relaxed instead of panicking will help you survive in water.

If someone in the water calls for help, find help immediately. If you cannot find someone to help, hold out a towel, fishing pole, branch, or other long object to the person and then pull him in to safety. If you do not have anything long enough to reach him, push or throw something that floats toward him. Encourage him to stay calm and not panic. *Do not swim out to rescue someone.* Attempting a water rescue without proper training puts you in danger of drowning.

Water-Safety Habits

- Never swim alone.
- Listen to adults and lifeguards.
- Be aware of how deep the water is.
- Get out of the water if you get chilled or tired.
- Wear a life jacket when needed.
- Stay away from water during an electrical storm.

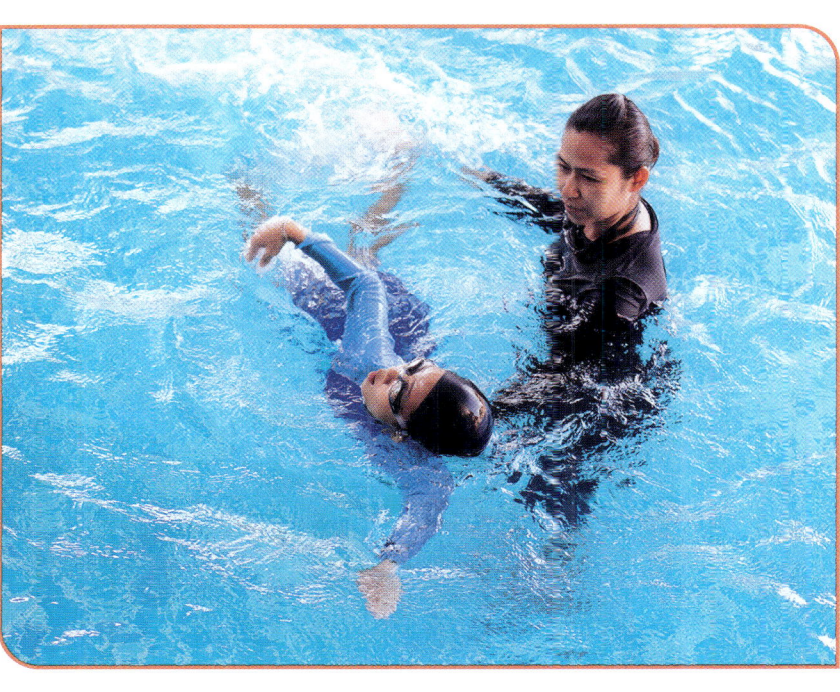

🦋 Fire Safety

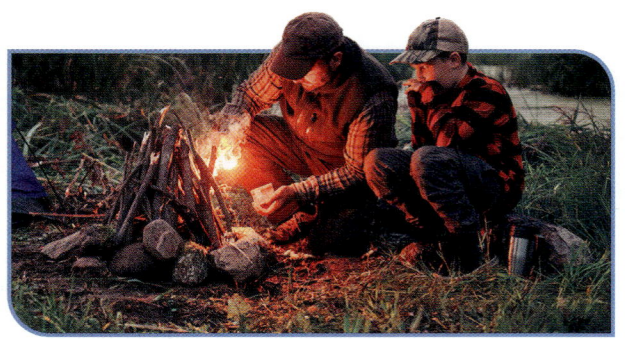

After a day of fun outdoor activities, it is relaxing to sit by a campfire at night. You should always watch a campfire carefully and put it out completely before you leave the area. *An unattended campfire can cause a wildfire*, which can quickly spread and cause much destruction. Although fire can be helpful, it also can be very dangerous if it gets out of control.

House fires can break out suddenly, without warning. Most house fires occur at night, when people are sleeping; therefore, it is important to have smoke detectors that will wake you if a fire starts. If you have a fireplace or gas- or wood-burning appliances, such as a furnace or water heater, you also need carbon-monoxide detectors. Your family can prepare for a possible fire by making an escape plan. Determine how you could get outside from each room. Choose a specific place outside your home where everyone will meet. Practice your escape plan regularly so that you know what to do.

Once you are out of the building, wait at the arranged meeting place. As soon as a cellphone is available, call 911. Remain calm so that you can clearly and accurately give information to the operator. *Never go back into a burning building*. Firefighters are trained to save people from fires and should be the only ones to conduct a rescue.

If your clothes catch fire, do not run; running will make the fire spread faster. Instead *stop, drop, and roll*. **Stop** moving. **Drop** to the floor and protect your face with your hands. **Roll** back and forth, smothering the area where the fire is. Fire needs oxygen from the air to survive; by rolling, you cut off the supply of oxygen. If there is a heavy blanket or rug nearby, wrap yourself in it and roll on the floor to put out the fire.

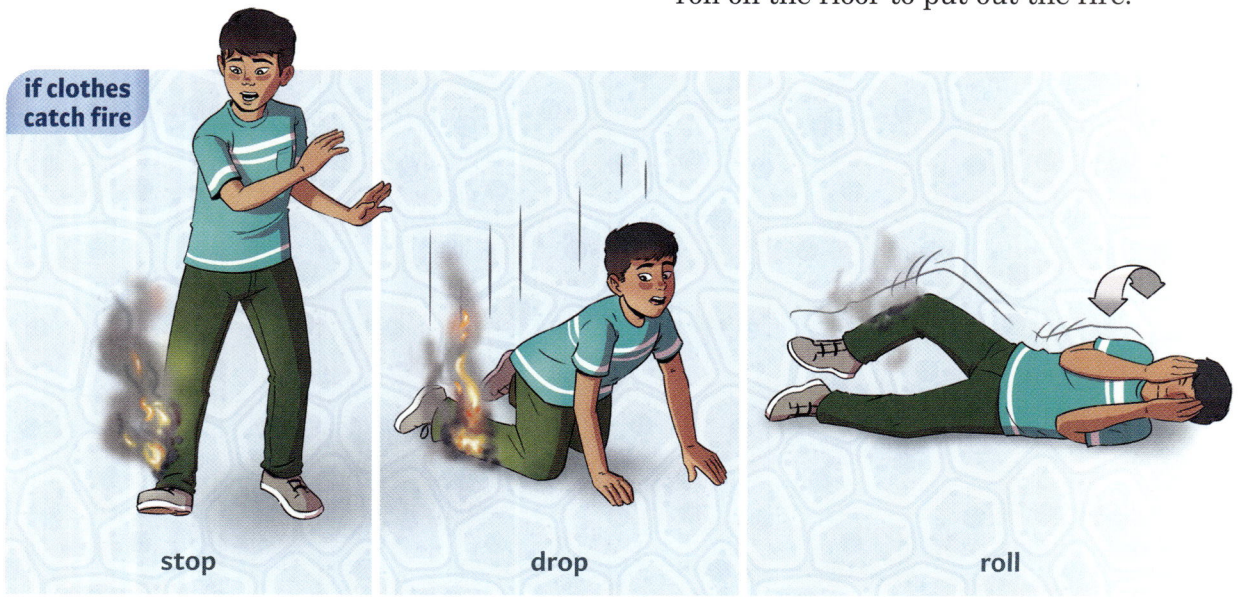

if clothes catch fire

stop   drop   roll

Preparing for Disasters

LIVE IT OUT!

One aspect of safety is being prepared for unexpected events. Natural disasters include lightning, tornadoes, hurricanes, floods, blizzards, and earthquakes. It is not always possible to know when a natural disaster might occur, although some areas are more likely to suffer specific disasters. Warm tropical areas may be hit by hurricanes, while northern areas may have blizzards during the winter. Although you cannot control the damage done by a disaster, you can help protect yourself and members of your family by preparing for disasters. Think about how you can stay safe during a natural disaster.

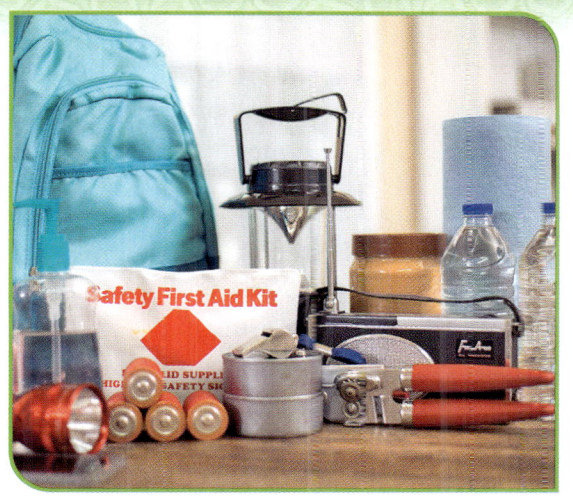

1. What types of natural disasters are most likely to occur in your area?

_____

_____

_____

_____

2. What can you do to prepare for a possible disaster? _____

_____

_____

_____

_____

3. What safety procedures should you follow? _____

_____

_____

_____

4. How can you work with your family to take the necessary steps to be properly prepared?

_____

_____

_____

_____

Comprehension Check 8.1

Multiple Choice: *Write the letter of the correct answer in the blank.*

_____ 1. What type of protective gear lowers the chance of a head injury?

a. helmet
b. mouth guard
c. protective pads
d. safety goggles

_____ 2. Which of the following types of clothing would not protect against frostbite?

a. earmuffs
b. gloves
c. sandals
d. scarves

_____ 3. What condition can occur if you are exposed to excessive heat and dehydration?

a. concussion
b. drowning
c. frostbite
d. heat exhaustion

Short Answer: *Write the correct answer in the blank.*

4. Why is it important to follow safety rules and procedures? ____________________

____

____

5. What protective gear should you use while mowing the lawn? ________________

____

____

6. What are electrolytes? ____

____

____

7. What should you do if your clothes catch on fire? ________________________

____

Think about It.

8. What are two things that you can do to reduce your risk of drowning? __________

____

____

____

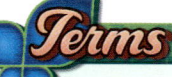

Terms

boundaries: rules or guidelines for appropriate behavior from yourself and others

abuse: situation in which someone deliberately ignores another person's boundaries for the purpose of causing harm

bullying: trying to gain control over someone by taunting him or by making him feel unsafe

gang: group of people who use violence or crime to gain power and who identify themselves with a group name or symbol

cyberbullying: use of electronic devices to bully by sending, posting, or sharing harmful or embarrassing content

8.2 Being Aware, Alert, and Careful

Following safety rules prepares you for dangers in sports and similar activities. Some other dangers are more difficult to prepare for because they are not part of your normal routine. Although these dangers rarely happen, you should be prepared to protect yourself in any situation. Being aware, alert, and careful helps you to stay calm and know what to do in difficult situations.

Fear thou not; for I am with thee: be not dismayed; for I am thy God: I will strengthen thee; yea, I will help thee; yea, I will uphold thee with the right hand of My righteousness. **Isaiah 41:10**

Being Aware and Alert in Public Places

Whenever you go into a public place, be aware of your surroundings. A prudent person is always alert for anything that does not seem right; he uses common sense to evaluate places and situations. Most people that you will encounter in public places are harmless to you, but there are some people who seek to harm others. It is important for your safety that you be cautious of strangers. *Look around as you enter any new environment and stay close to a parent or*

trusted adult. If someone near you is acting in a way that is strange or makes you uncomfortable, let the trusted adult know and leave that area.

If you get lost, stay calm and seek help from a safe adult, like a store employee, security guard, or police officer. You should memorize the phone numbers of at least two trusted adults whom you could call in an emergency. Even if you have these numbers stored in your own cellphone, you should remember them in case you lose your phone.

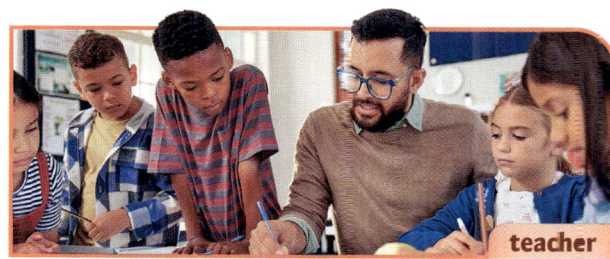

teacher

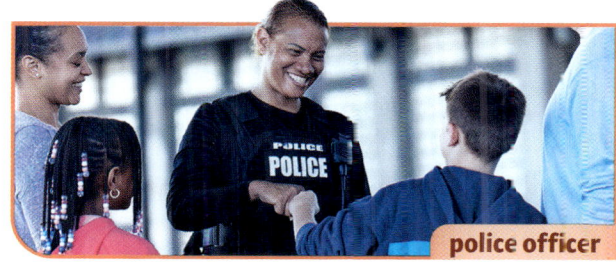

police officer

For God hath not given us the spirit of fear; but of power, and of love, and of a sound mind. **2 Timothy 1:7**

Being Alert to Danger

If you find a gun or other weapon, leave it alone and tell an adult immediately. *Never play with a gun or other weapon.* If you ever find yourself in a dangerous or violent situation, you should remember to *Run—Hide—Fight*:

Run—*Move away from the dangerous situation as quickly as possible.* Find a safe adult and report what you heard and saw. Follow the directions of *first responders, such as policemen, firemen, or security guards.*

Hide—You may not always be able to remove yourself from a dangerous situation, or you may be instructed to hide. Find a place where you are out of sight. *Once you are safely hidden, stay put and remain calm.* Remain completely silent; pray or mentally recite Scripture or sing a song. Stay in your hiding place until a first responder tells you that the area is safe.

Fight—If you cannot run or hide, *you must be ready to defend yourself.* Scream, kick, throw objects, and do anything you can to harm an attacker. This will alert people of the danger and may scare the attacker so that he stops the attack. Once help arrives, you should follow the instructions of first responders until there is no longer a threat.

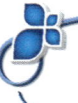 *God is our refuge and strength, a very present help in trouble.* **Psalm 46:1**

Being Careful about Boundaries

An important part of staying safe is setting and respecting boundaries. **Boundaries** are *rules or guidelines for appropriate behavior from yourself and others.* Physical boundaries protect your body, while emotional or mental boundaries protect your mind. Healthy personal boundaries respect the needs of yourself and others and help you stay safe. You can set boundaries in your relationships with others by clearly stating your needs. *Do not be afraid to say no if someone tries to do something that makes you feel unsafe.*

Abuse occurs when *someone deliberately ignores another person's boundaries for the purpose of causing harm.* If anyone tries to harm you or touch you in a way that makes you feel uncomfortable, no matter who the person is or what they say to you, yell for help and run away. *You should always tell a safe adult if you experience abuse or witness someone else suffering from abuse.*

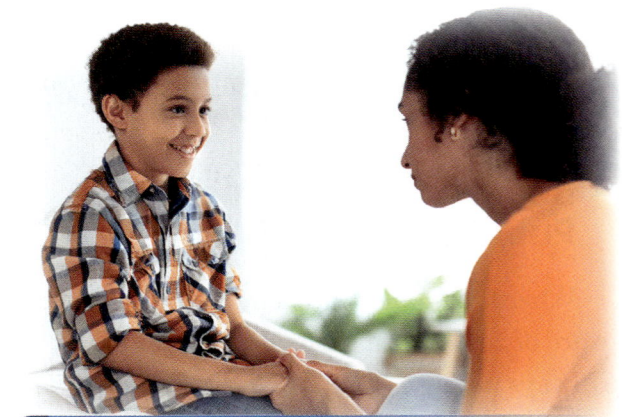

Being Careful around Others

You can also set boundaries about how to interact with people you do not know well or who make you feel uncomfortable. Most people will not hurt you, but some people may have harmful intentions. *It is important to tell* the difference between a safe person and some-one who wants to cause harm. Safe adults do not ask children to keep secrets from their parents, try to be alone with children away from their parents, or try to make children feel uncomfortable or unsafe. If someone makes you feel unsafe, get away as quickly as possible and tell a safe adult. *It is not rude to get away from a person who makes you feel unsafe.*

A child or teenager should never go anywhere with someone without a parent's permission. Be careful if an adult asks you personal questions or offers to give you candy, money, or a ride. *If someone tries to force you to leave with him, make as much noise as possible.* Try to get away and run to a safe place, such as a school, store, or police station. If you cannot get away, continue screaming, kicking, and fighting until help arrives.

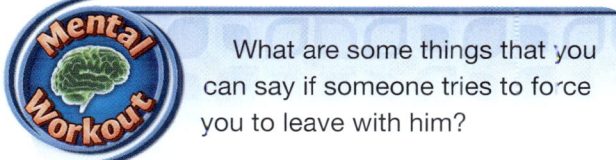

What are some things that you can say if someone tries to force you to leave with him?

You can also practice personal safety habits at home. *Keep doors locked so that an intruder cannot get into your home.* If you are outside in your yard when a stranger approaches, get inside as quickly as possible and tell a trusted adult. If someone knocks on your door, leave the door locked unless a parent or trusted adult gives you permission to open it. *Never answer the door if you are at home alone.* If the person decides to wander around the property or tries to come in, call 911 and ask for the police to check on the person.

Be careful about what information you share over the phone. Most phones have caller ID; answer only if you recognize the phone number.

Let your parents know if you receive a call or text from an unknown number. A caller may ask for personal information, such as your name, age or address, or may try to sell you something. If that happens, quickly end the call and tell your parents. *Never tell a caller that you are home alone.*

Being Careful around Bullies

You should set boundaries about how you interact with your peers, those people who are your age or who are in your group of friends. One of your peers may have a habit of unkind behavior called bullying. **Bullying** involves *trying to gain control by taunting someone else or by making him feel unsafe.* Bullies hurt people by using physical strength, popularity, or embarrassing information.

If you are being bullied, use an assertive tone of voice and calmly tell the person to stop, instead of responding in anger or fear. If speaking up for yourself seems unsafe, turn around and walk away. Find a safe adult to help you if the bullying continues. An adult can protect you from harm and may help the person behaving unkindly. Since bullies often struggle with insecurity or issues in their personal lives, they may need help learning how to be a better friend.

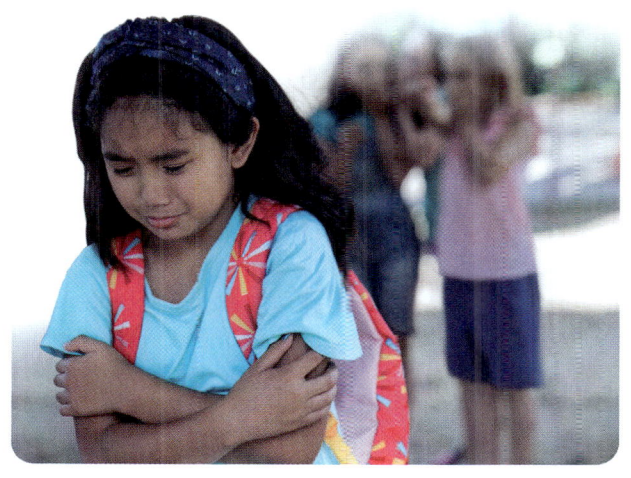

If you see someone else being bullied, you should *be an active bystander by standing up for the person.* Ask the bully to stop; comfort the person who has been hurt by bullying. If the bully refuses to stop, find a safe adult who can help with the situation.

Do not feel pressured to join a peer group that is involved in bullying or violence. A **gang** is a *group of people who use violence or crime to gain power and who identify themselves with a group name or symbol.* Choose friends who value you for who you are and encourage you to make good choices.

Being Careful Online

As you enter adolescence, your parents may give you more access to electronic devices and the internet. Electronic devices can be fun and useful tools, but they can also be dangerous when used carelessly or incorrectly. *Setting boundaries about your online use can help you stay safe.* You should always respect the boundaries that your parents have set for you, even if your peers have different boundaries. For accountability and safety, it is best to stay near an adult while using these devices.

When using the internet, it is not safe to give out personal information such as your phone number, address, age, or passwords. Do not talk about private information or personal issues online. Be careful about clicking on links from strangers or downloading unknown apps or software. If you see something that makes you feel uncomfortable, turn away from the screen immediately and tell a trusted adult.

Smartphones, social media, and online games can give opportunities for **cyberbullying**, the *use of electronic devices to bully by sending, posting, or sharing harmful or embarrassing content.* Since the internet enables cyberbullies to remain anonymous, their harmful actions can affect many people. *Tell a trusted adult if you or someone you know experiences cyberbullying.*

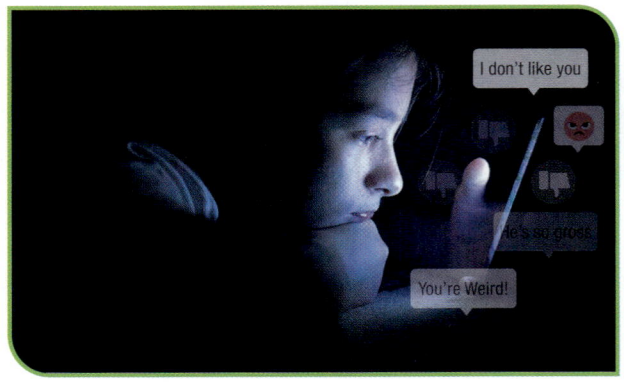

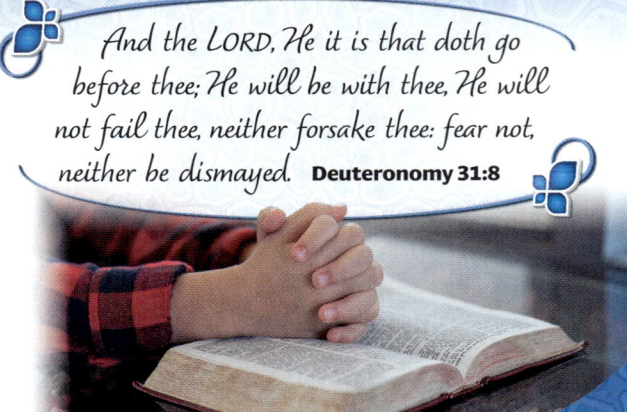

Build on TRUTH

If you find yourself in a scary or dangerous situation, remember that God is always with you. You may not understand why bad things happen, but God has promised that He will never leave you. He will help you when you are in trouble. Praying to God and memorizing Scripture will help you stay calm in difficult situations.

And the LORD, He it is that doth go before thee; He will be with thee, He will not fail thee, neither forsake thee: fear not, neither be dismayed. **Deuteronomy 31:8**

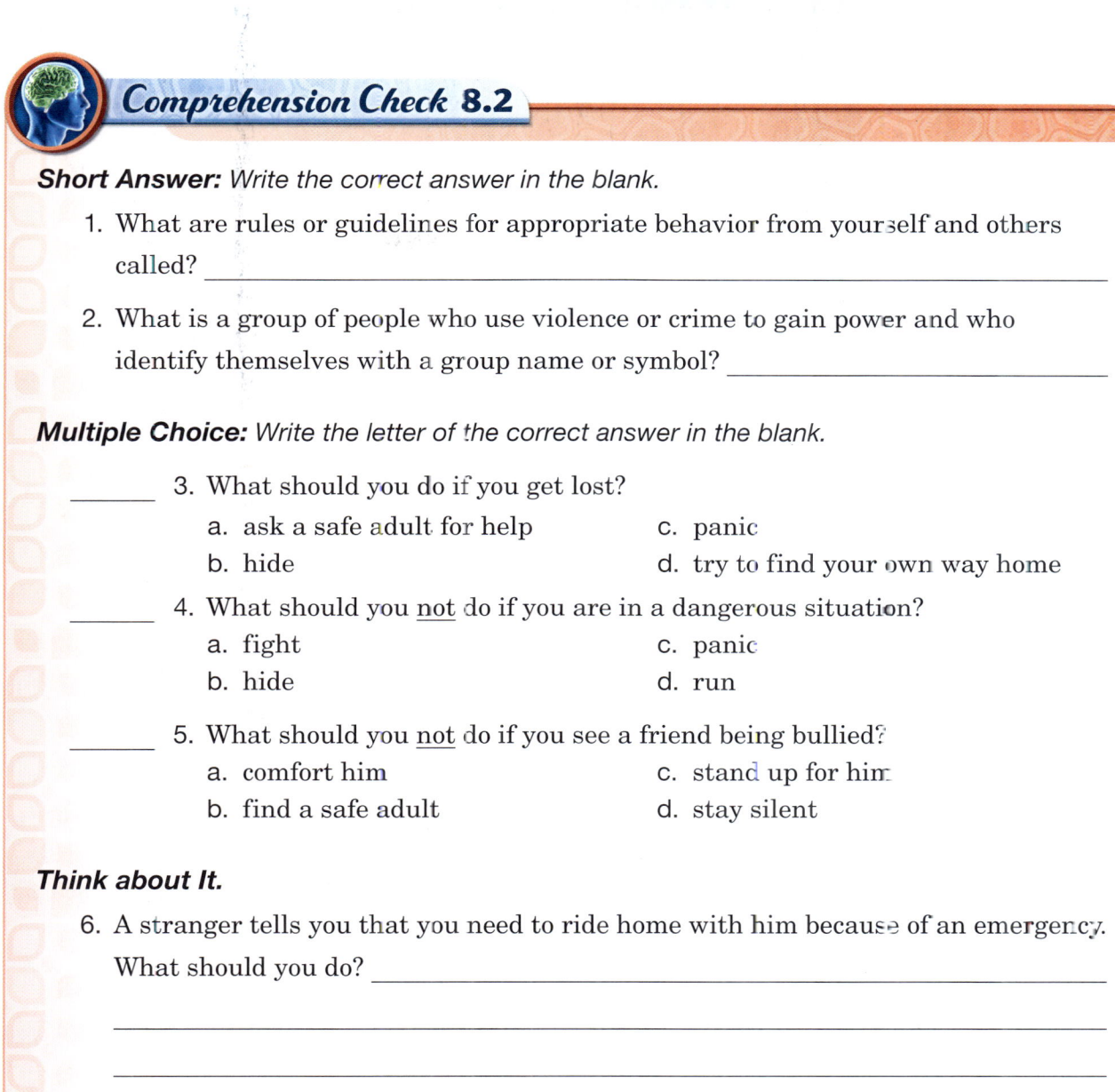

Short Answer: *Write the correct answer in the blank.*

1. What are rules or guidelines for appropriate behavior from yourself and others called? _____

2. What is a group of people who use violence or crime to gain power and who identify themselves with a group name or symbol? _____

Multiple Choice: *Write the letter of the correct answer in the blank.*

_____ 3. What should you do if you get lost?
   a. ask a safe adult for help   c. panic
   b. hide   d. try to find your own way home

_____ 4. What should you <u>not</u> do if you are in a dangerous situation?
   a. fight   c. panic
   b. hide   d. run

_____ 5. What should you <u>not</u> do if you see a friend being bullied?
   a. comfort him   c. stand up for him
   b. find a safe adult   d. stay silent

Think about It.

6. A stranger tells you that you need to ride home with him because of an emergency. What should you do? _____

   _____

   _____

   _____

7. You are playing in your backyard when a stranger approaches you. What should you do? _____

   _____

   _____

8. What should you do if a person that you met online starts asking you personal questions? _____

   _____

   _____

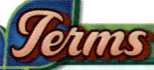

Terms

first aid: emergency care or treatment given to a person who is injured or suddenly becomes ill until professional medical help arrives

medical emergency: any illness or injury requiring immediate care

shock: sudden loss of blood flow that causes blood pressure to drop

cardiac arrest: serious medical emergency in which a person's heart stops beating

cardiopulmonary resuscitation (CPR): life-saving procedure that can be used when the heart stops beating

poison: substance that causes harm, illness, or death when it is consumed or absorbed into the body

strain: pulled muscle or tendon resulting from a tear

sprain: stretched or torn ligament

concussion: brain injury in which the brain is shaken inside the skull

8.3 First Aid

Many injuries can be prevented by following safety procedures, but unexpected accidents can cause severe injuries. Accidents can happen at home, at school, during sports, and on the road. Be prepared for emergencies no matter where you are.

First aid is *emergency care or treatment given to a person who is injured or suddenly becomes ill until professional medical help arrives*. First aid can be given for minor injuries like cuts or scrapes or for more serious injuries like severe bleeding or choking. Learning first aid is important because a minor injury can sometimes become major if either no care or improper care is given. Proper first aid can save someone's life.

Medical Emergencies

A **medical emergency** is *any illness or injury requiring immediate care*. Examples of medical emergencies are severe bleeding, breathing problems, and head injuries. A medical emergency that is not treated immediately could cause permanent disability or death. In a medical emergency, first aid is given until professional help arrives. Paramedics and emergency medical technicians, or EMTs, are first responders trained in rescue and life-saving skills.

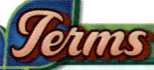

They will give emergency care to the victim and transport him to the hospital, where doctors and nurses will provide medical care.

Medical emergencies can be frightening. It is important to stay calm so that you can think clearly. Follow the procedure *Check—Call—Care*. **Check** that you and the injured person are in a safe place, and quickly examine him for life-threatening conditions. If it is a medical emergency, **call** 911 immediately. Explain your emergency to the operator; be prepared to give your name and location. Follow the operator's directions and remain on the phone until help arrives.

After calling 911, begin administering first-aid **care**. *If the person is conscious, you must receive his consent, or permission, before beginning care.* Check to see if a first-aid kit or medical supplies are available; if possible, wear gloves to protect yourself from blood and other body fluids. Let the injured person know that help is on the way and try to make him as comfortable as possible. Your care and concern for someone in pain can give him hope during unfortunate circumstances.

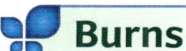

Peace I leave with you, My peace I give unto you: not as the world giveth, give I unto you. Let not your heart be troubled, neither let it be afraid. **John 14:27**

Emergency Procedures

- Check your surroundings.
- Call 911.
- Care for victim.

CHECK **CALL** **CARE**

Burns

Burns, a leading cause of accidental death, can produce extreme pain and may require months of care. Not all burns are alike. A *thermal burn* is caused by flames, hot gases, or hot objects. Burns can also be caused by electricity or chemicals. Knowing the cause of the burn helps first responders and doctors decide how to care for a burn.

A first-degree burn damages only the epidermis. These burns cause redness, swelling, and mild pain but heal rather quickly. Treat a first-degree burn by holding it under cool running water until the pain lessens.

A second-degree burn damages both the epidermis and the dermis. These burns are more painful and can cause blisters. Treat a second-degree burn in the same way you would treat a first-degree burn; then blot the area dry and cover it loosely with a dry, sterile (germ-free) bandage. Second-degree burns sometimes require medical attention.

Third-degree burns damage all the way down to the hypodermis. These burns require emergency medical attention. While waiting for help to arrive, do not remove clothing from the burn or apply cold water. Loosely cover the damaged area with a dry, sterile bandage.

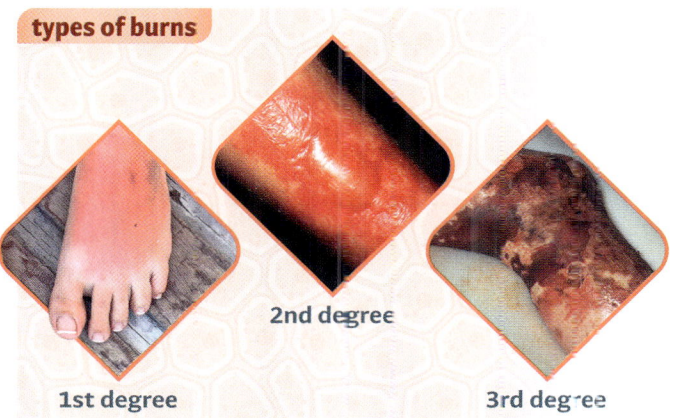

types of burns

1st degree **2nd degree** **3rd degree**

Bleeding

When a blood vessel is damaged, severe bleeding can occur. Severe bleeding is life threatening. *Use direct pressure to stop the bleeding until help comes.* Wear disposable gloves, if available, while placing a sterile gauze pad or clean cloth over the wound and applying firm pressure. Even if you cannot stop the bleeding, slowing it down could save someone's life. If the first cloth gets saturated, do not remove it but cover it with a second clean cloth and continue to apply pressure. Take deep breaths to keep yourself calm.

After a severe injury, a person's body can go into *shock*. **Shock** occurs when there is *a sudden loss of blood flow that causes blood pressure to drop*. This causes the heart to pump harder and may lead to heart 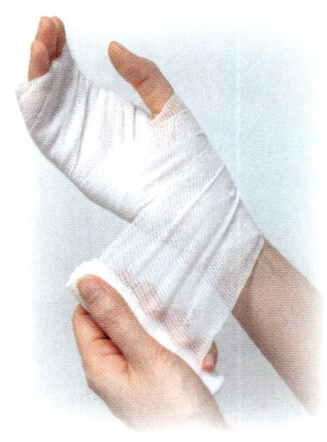 failure. The person's skin will feel cold or lose color. Shock is a serious emergency that needs immediate medical attention. Call 911 and stop any bleeding. *While you wait for help, place a blanket or coat over someone who may be in shock.*

Choking

Choking occurs when an object gets stuck in the trachea, blocking the airway so that the person cannot breathe. A choking person could die if he does not receive immediate medical attention. If he is coughing, his airway is only partially blocked; he should continue to cough until his airway is free. If he cannot talk or breathe, he should place both hands at his neck. This gesture is the universal sign for choking.

If the choking person is conscious, begin care by giving five back blows. Support him by placing one arm in front of his chest; then lean him over so that his chest is parallel to the ground. Use your fist to pound five times between his shoulder blades. If he is still choking, perform five abdominal thrusts. Stand behind him with your arms around his waist. Place one fist with the thumb against his midsection, slightly above the navel, or bellybutton. Hold your other hand over your fist and pull both hands upward and inward toward yourself. *Alternate between five back blows and five abdominal thrusts until the object is dislodged from the trachea and the person can cough or breathe again.* After the person recovers, he should see a doctor to make sure he has not been injured.

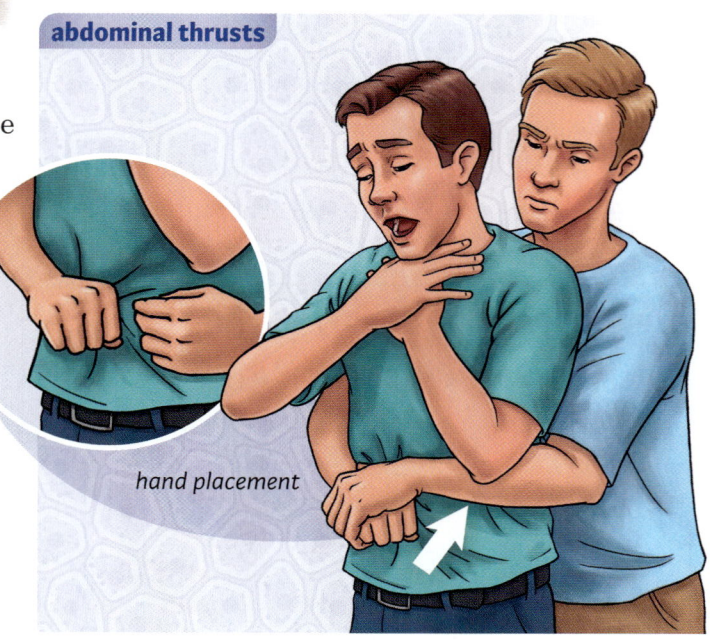

abdominal thrusts

hand placement

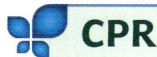

CPR

Cardiac arrest is a *serious medical emergency in which a person's heart stops beating*. Without blood flowing to the brain, the person can die within minutes. Signs of cardiac arrest are that the person appears to be unconscious, does not respond when you tap his shoulder or yell at him, and is not breathing. After calling 911, perform **cardiopulmonary resuscitation** [kär′dē·ō·pool′mə·nĕr′ē rĭ·sŭs′ĭ·tā′shən], or **CPR**, *a life-saving procedure that can be used when the heart stops beating*. *To perform hands-only CPR, use both hands to push hard on the person's chest; give 100 to 120 compressions per minute*. CPR will force blood to flow from the heart and throughout the body, which may keep the person alive until first responders arrive.

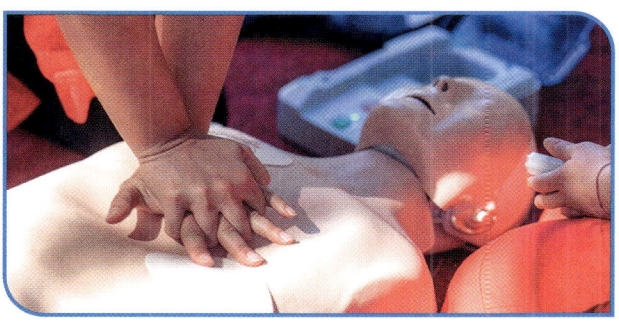

Poisoning

Certain household cleaners contain poisonous substances. A **poison** is a *substance that causes harm, illness, or death when it is consumed or absorbed into the body*. Even medications can be poisonous if taken incorrectly. Poisons can cause body systems to malfunction or shut down. Because a poison victim could stop breathing or even die within minutes, he must have immediate care.

If someone has swallowed something poisonous, call 911 or the local poison control center. If possible, give the name of the poison. Save the container, if there is one, to show first responders. Most products have a warning label that tells you what to do if that substance touches someone's eyes or skin or if it is swallowed. Different poisonings require different types of first aid. The operator will tell you what to do until help arrives.

Poison Control

LIVE IT OUT!

Write your area poison control phone number here. You can post it in your home or save it in your cellphone.

_____

Sports Injuries

Most sports-related injuries affect the muscular or skeletal system. Sometimes, muscles can be stretched to the point of tearing. A **strain** is a *pulled muscle or tendon resulting from a tear*. With rest, strained muscles repair themselves within a few days. A **sprain** is a *stretched or torn ligament*. The joint becomes stiff and swollen to protect the ligaments while they slowly heal. Sometimes, sprains require medical attention.

Sometimes, a sports accident causes injuries to the nervous system. Nervous system injuries are medical emergencies. Do not move someone who may have injured his neck or spine. Call 911 and wait for help to arrive. A **concussion** is a *brain injury in which the brain is shaken inside the skull*. Concussions can occur during falls or collisions, injuring the brain's soft tissue and causing nerve or blood vessel damage.

Some signs of a concussion are headaches, dizziness, confusion, vision problems, or feeling ill. Calling 911 is not always necessary for a concussion, but the person should be checked by a doctor as soon as possible. Someone who has a concussion needs to heal completely before returning to sports or other physical activities.

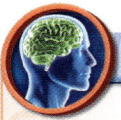

Comprehension Check 8.3

Short Answer: *Write the correct answer in the blank.*

1. What is first aid? _____

_____

2. Which type of burn goes down to the hypodermis? _____

3. What is a sudden loss of blood flow that causes blood pressure to drop?

_____

4. How should you perform first aid on a conscious choking victim? _____

_____

_____

5. When should CPR be performed? _____

_____

6. What is a poison? _____

_____

7. What is a concussion? _____

_____

Classify: *Circle the medical emergencies; cross through those that are not medical emergencies.*

choking	first-degree burn	severe bleeding	third-degree burn
coughing	muscle strain	scraped knee	unconsciousness

Think about It.

8. Why is it important to stay calm during a medical emergency? _____

_____

_____

8.4 Deciding to Say No!

God designed your physical body like an intricate machine. Similar to a manmade machine, how you care for your body determines how well it functions. This care includes choosing what substances go into your body.

A **drug** is a *chemical substance that causes changes in your body, mind, or behavior*. Medicines prescribed by doctors and sold in pharmacies are legal drugs. Other drugs are illegal to buy, sell, or use because they harm the body. When used properly, drugs can cure disease and relieve pain. **Drug misuse**, or *substance misuse*, is *using a drug in an improper way or for an improper purpose*. Taking more of a medicine than you should is using that medicine in an improper way. Taking a drug for a nonmedical purpose, such as to improve athletic performance, is using that drug for an improper purpose.

Harmful drugs interfere with the body systems, causing both immediate and long-term effects. They can harm the mind and decrease brain function; many affect the brain permanently. They may harm the body over time or may be deadly the first time they are misused. *Saying No: to drug misuse is an important part of being a healthy person.*

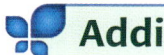 **Addiction**

Many commonly misused drugs can cause **addiction**, a *continual, controlling behavior that changes the way the brain functions*. You have learned that the *limbic system* in your brain acts as an emotional reward system. Normally, special hormones make you feel good when you do something that is healthy. An addictive drug breaks this system by causing neurons in the brain to make new connections. Because of these new connections, the limbic system tells the brain that it needs the drug to survive. When a person takes the drug, he feels good for a little while, but then he feels worse than before. He returns to that drug or to another drug to feel better again. This destructive cycle happens over and over in an addiction.

Changes in brain function make it difficult for someone with an addiction to stop on his own. If he stops taking the drug, he will go through withdrawal. **Withdrawal** is a *painful and sometimes deadly sickness that occurs when an addictive drug is no longer taken.* Professional help and support are often needed to stop an addictive behavior.

Addictive drugs do not damage only the body. They also harm the spirit, a person's invisible, personal part. These drugs cause spiritual suffering and bondage. They ruin relationships with loved ones. They hurt communities by harming families and bringing crime. Illegal drugs also have legal consequences, such as imprisonment, and can lead to other crimes. The power of God can give freedom from the spiritual bondage of addiction.

Whosoever committeth sin is the servant of sin. . . . If the Son therefore shall make you free, ye shall be free indeed. **John 8:34, 36**

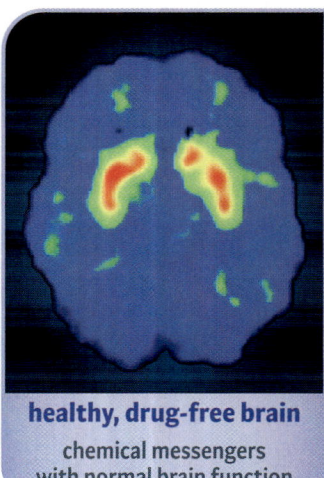

healthy, drug-free brain
chemical messengers
with normal brain function

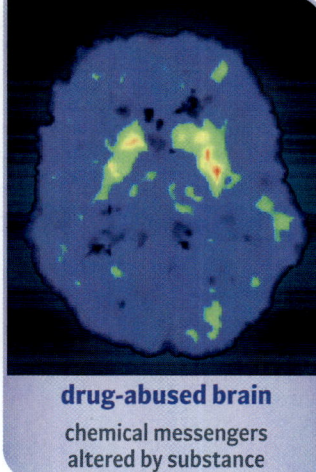

drug-abused brain
chemical messengers
altered by substance

Commonly Misused Drugs

Alcohol

One of the most widely misused drugs is alcohol. Alcohol creates a dreamy, floating feeling that many people use to escape their problems. Alcohol slows the brain's function and can influence a person to do things he would usually consider wrong. Because alcohol can greatly harm a young person's developing body, many countries prohibit children and teenagers from drinking alcohol.

Although it is legal for adults to drink alcohol, overconsumption can also cause great harm to their bodies. Alcohol is absorbed rapidly from the stomach and small intestine. It is then carried directly to the liver, where it is broken down into a poisonous chemical that destroys liver cells. Any alcohol that leaves the liver is carried by the blood to every part of the body. The poisonous chemicals can then damage the brain, heart, and other important organs.

Alcohol affects blood circulation by causing blood vessels to expand. When a person drinks alcohol, the heart pumps less blood with each contraction, causing the pulse to become very rapid and increasing the heart's workload. Continued heavy drinking eventually weakens the heart and increases blood pressure, causing greater risk of heart disease or heart attack.

Nicotine

Tobacco products contain a drug called **nicotine**, which is highly addictive and harms the body. Nicotine affects the nervous system, causing headaches, irritability, and weakened senses of taste and smell. It also increases the heart rate and makes the arteries become narrower. This makes the heart work harder and increases blood pressure. *A person who uses tobacco products has a greater risk of heart disease and heart attack than a nonsmoker.*

Smoked tobacco products, such as cigarettes, damage the lungs and cause lung cancer. The smoke contains tar, which coats the lungs and prevents them from functioning properly. *Secondhand smoke* is taken into the body when someone near you is smoking; it can harm your body just as much as firsthand smoke can.

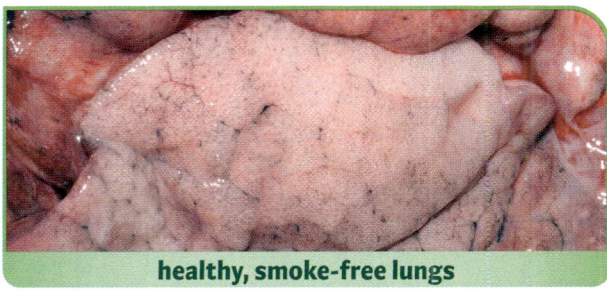
healthy, smoke-free lungs

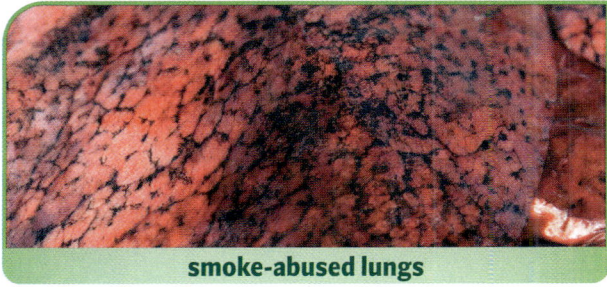
smoke-abused lungs

Smokeless tobacco products can damage the mouth and nose. Using smokeless tobacco greatly increases the risk of cavities; gum disease; and cancer of the mouth, throat, larynx, and esophagus.

Since tobacco products poison the respiratory and circulatory systems, *smoking affects a person's ability in physical activities.* Those who injure their lungs and heart with tobacco will experience decreased athletic performance.

Nicotine is found in *electronic cigarettes,* also called *e-cigarettes* or *vapes.* These contain liquid nicotine, which is heated into a vapor and inhaled. Vaping was originally marketed as safer than cigarettes, but *vaped nicotine is just as addictive and harmful as smoked nicotine.* Some research suggests that vaping is dangerous in other ways.

Other Misused Drugs

Marijuana [măr′ə·wä′nə] *is a commonly misused drug made from the leaves and blossoms of the hemp, or cannabis* [kăn′ə·bĭs]*, plant.* It contains many chemicals that affect the body. Some of them have medical uses, but others can cause serious health problems.

Some people use **inhalants**, *chemicals that are breathed in through the nose or mouth as a vapor.* Many inhalants are deadly poisons that can kill on the first use. Repeated use of inhalants can cause brain damage or organ failure.

Over-the-counter, or OTC, **drugs**, are *medicines that can be purchased without a prescription.* Many cough syrups and common pain medicines, such as ibuprofen, are OTC drugs. OTC drugs are generally safe when used correctly but harmful if misused. Read the label carefully and follow the directions to properly use any OTC drug.

How to Say No!

There are many reasons that people misuse drugs, but a major reason is *peer pressure.* If those around you misuse drugs, you may be tempted to fit in by misusing drugs yourself. People who do not have a support system are often drawn to drugs. A strong support system is made of family and friends who encourage you to do right and help you in difficult situations. Some people are tempted to use drugs to avoid dealing with stressful challenges. Media can also influence people to use harmful substances. Advertisements, social media, television shows, and music can all show drug misuse as if it were harmless.

You have every reason not to use drugs or alcohol. You were created in God's image and for His glory. If you trust in Jesus, your body is God's temple, or dwelling place. You are set apart to serve Him and to serve others for Him. Addictions will hinder that service. Care for your health in a way that brings honor to God. Decide now to avoid misusing drugs.

In your own strength, you cannot resist the temptation to sin. You need God's help to say no to sin. You also need a support system of those who encourage you to live a godly life. Talk to parents or other trusted adults about the peer pressure you feel and the temptations you face. Choose friends who want to live for Jesus and support each other in their decisions to say no.

Watch and pray, that ye enter not into temptation: the spirit indeed is willing, but the flesh is weak. **Matthew 26:41**

Saying no to drugs is not a skill that you develop immediately. It is like a muscle that you train. Your flesh, or humanness, is weak. Daily ask God for the strength to resist temptation.

- Learn to recognize when you need to say no. When offered a substance that you don't recognize, ask what it is and where it came from. Do not accept anything that might be harmful to your body.

- Say no and walk away. Do not stay near a temptation. The Bible tells us to flee sin, or to run in the opposite direction.

- Pray. Call out to God when you are tempted in any way. Ask Him to help you.

- If you still feel tempted, tell a trusted adult that you are struggling.

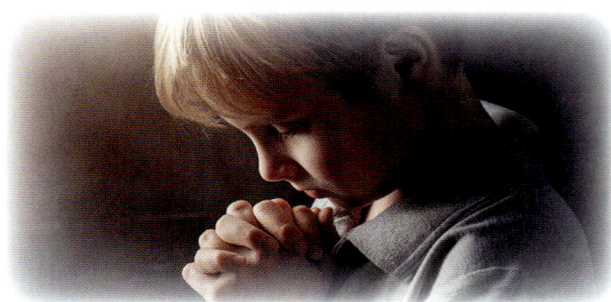

Build on TRUTH

Read each of the verses below. Explain how you can use each verse to say no to drugs.

1. Proverbs 11:14 _____

_____

_____

2. Proverbs 13:20 _____

_____

3. 1 Corinthians 10:13 _____

_____

_____

4. 1 Peter 5:8 _____

_____

_____

5. James 4:7 _____

_____

_____

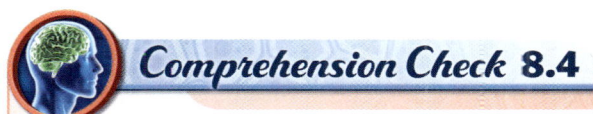

Matching: *Write the letter of the correct answer in the blank.*

_____ 1. one of the most widely misused drugs

_____ 2. drug found in tobacco products

_____ 3. drug made from the leaves and blossoms of the cannabis plant

_____ 4. chemical that is breathed in through the nose or mouth as a vapor

_____ 5. medicine that can be purchased without a prescription

A. alcohol

B. inhalant

C. marijuana

D. nicotine

E. OTC drug

F. prescription drug

Short Answer: *Write the correct answer in the blank.*

6. What is a drug? _____

_____

7. What is using a drug in an improper way or for an improper purpose?

_____

8. What is a continual, controlling behavior that changes the way the brain functions? _____

9. What sickness occurs when an addictive drug is no longer taken?

_____

Think about It.

10. What are two reasons that people misuse drugs? _____

_____

_____

LEARN WHEN
TO SAY NO.

SAY NO AND
WALK AWAY.

PRAY.

1 Staying Safe (8.1)

A. True/False: *If the statement is true, write* true *in the blank. If the statement is false, replace the underlined word(s) with a word or phrase that will make the statement true. Do not write* false *in any blank.*

_____ 1. The freezing of body tissue is called <u>dehydration</u>.

_____ 2. Minerals that help regulate the body's water balance are <u>electrolytes</u>.

_____ 3. A condition in which the body cannot control its internal temperature is <u>dehydration</u>.

_____ 4. The harmful rays from the sun are called <u>infrared</u> rays.

_____ 5. Each bedroom in your house should have a working <u>smoke detector</u> nearby.

_____ 6. If your clothes catch on fire, you should <u>run</u>, drop, and roll.

B. Short Answer: *Write the correct answer in the blank.*

1. You decide to join a football team. What should you do before you start playing?

_____

_____

_____

2. Why is it important to apply sunscreen? _____

_____

_____

3. What are two reasons that drowning accidents occur? _____

_____

_____

4. Why should you put out a campfire before leaving the area? _____

_____

_____

2 Being Aware, Alert, and Careful (8.2)

A. Short Answer: *Write the correct answer in the blank.*

1. What should you do if someone tries to force you to leave with him? _____

_____

2. What is a gang? _____

_____

3. What are two types of information that it is not safe to give out while using the
internet? _____

B. List: *Write the steps that you should take if you find yourself in a dangerous or violent
situation. Explain what you should do in each step.*

1. _____

_____

2. _____

_____

3. _____

_____

C. Fill in the Blank: *Write the correct word in the blank.*

1. A bully taunts someone else or makes him feel unsafe to gain _____
over the person.

2. If you see someone being bullied, stand up for the person and be an
_____ bystander.

3. Using electronic devices to send, post, or share harmful or embarrassing content
is _____.

D. Think!

1. What are characteristics that you can use to identify a safe adult when you are in a
store? _____

_____

2. What are boundaries? _____

_____

Why are boundaries important? _____

_____

3 First Aid (8.3)

A. Multiple Choice: *Write the letter of the correct answer in the blank.*

_____ 1. In order, what are the three general steps for dealing with a medical emergency?
  a. Call—Care—Check
  b. Check—Call—Care
  c. Check—Call—Consent
  d. Consent—Call—Check

_____ 2. Which type of burn damages only the epidermis?
  a. first-degree burn
  b. second-degree burn
  c. third-degree burn
  d. fourth-degree burn

_____ 3. What condition occurs when a sudden loss of blood flow causes blood pressure to drop?
  a. choking
  b. concussion
  c. shock
  d. strain

_____ 4. What first-aid procedure should be performed when someone's heart stops beating?
  a. abdominal thrusts
  b. back blows
  c. CPR
  d. direct pressure

B. Short Answer: *Write the correct answer in the blank.*

1. What is emergency care given to an injured person until professional medical help arrives? _____

2. What is a medical emergency? _____
_____

3. If someone is conscious, what must you do before beginning care? _____
_____

4. What should you do if someone swallows poison? _____
_____

5. What is the difference between a strain and a sprain? _____
_____

C. Think!

What is the difference between a medical emergency and a minor injury?

_____
_____
_____

4 **Deciding to Say No! (8.4)**

A. Crossword Puzzle: *Fill in the answers to complete the crossword puzzle.*

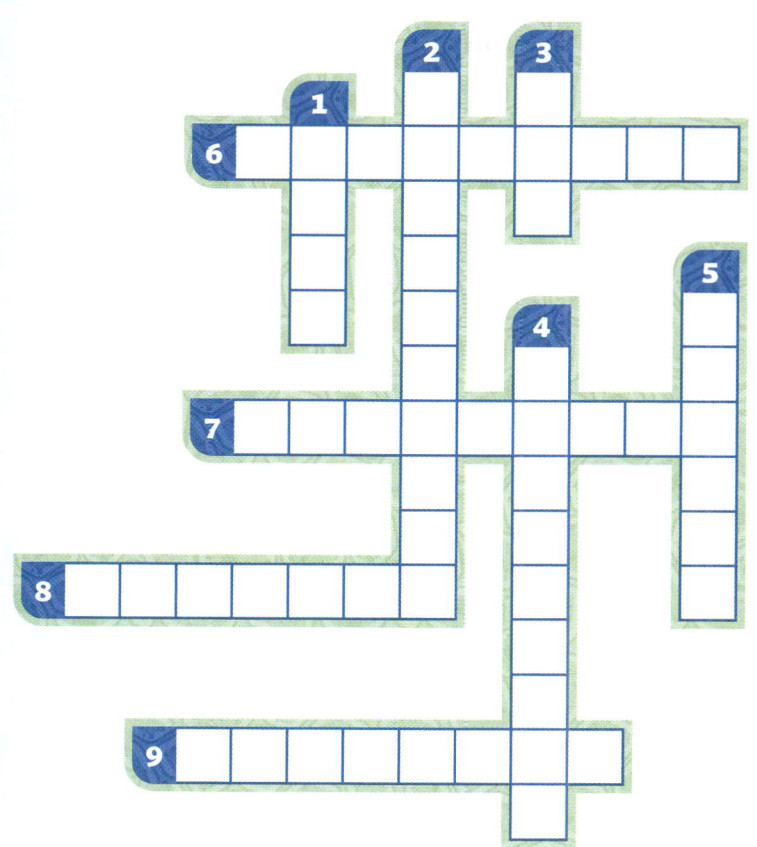

Down

1. chemical substance that causes changes in your body, mind, or behavior

2. sickness that occurs when an addictive drug is no longer taken

3. medicine that can be purchased without a prescription

4. drug made from the leaves and blossoms of the cannabis plant

5. using a drug in an improper way or for an improper purpose

Across

6. continual, controlling behavior that changes the way the brain functions

7. chemicals that are breathed in through the nose or mouth as a vapor

8. one of the most widely abused drugs

9. drug found in tobacco products

B. Think!

1. Why is it difficult to quit an addictive drug? _____

_____

2. Why is vaping not a safe alternative to smoking? _____

_____

_____

3. What are two things that you can do to avoid drug misuse and addiction?

_____

_____

_____

Pursuing a Healthy Spirit

9.1 Spiritual Wellness

You are a unique person both in your body and in your spirit, the invisible, eternal part of you that can learn to love and know God. A healthy spirit is one that is also growing socially, mentally, and emotionally.

> *I beseech* [plead] *you therefore, brethren, by the mercies of God, that ye present your bodies a living sacrifice, holy, acceptable unto God, which is your reasonable service. And be not conformed to this world: but be ye transformed by the renewing of your mind, that ye may prove what is that good, and acceptable, and perfect, will of God.* **Romans 12:1–2**

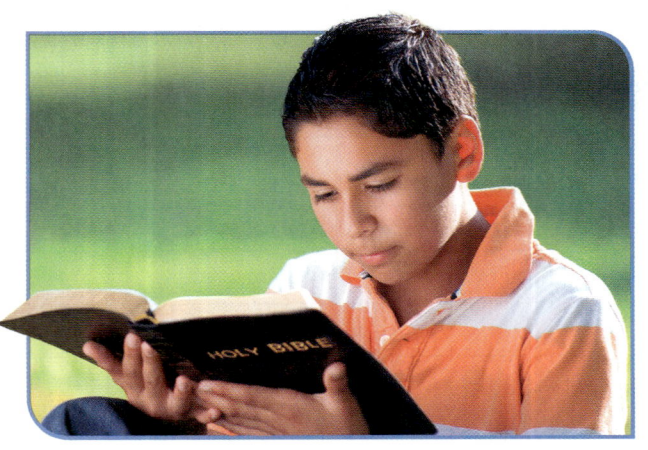

Spiritual Birth

Genesis 3 records how Satan, God's enemy, tempted Adam and Eve to disobey God. Because of Adam's sin, every person born into the world is a sinner—physically alive, but spiritually dead (Rom. 5:12–14). Sin separates us from God, but our sin does not ruin God's perfect love. In punishing Adam and Eve for their sin, He also promised a Savior Who would come and defeat Satan, the enemy of God (Gen. 3:15). Throughout the Old Testament, the prophets continued to tell of the coming Savior.

Thousands of years after Adam and Eve, Jesus Christ, the Son of God, came to Earth as a baby. He lived a perfect life on Earth. He died on the cross, taking the eternal punishment for every person's sin. After Jesus died, His body was buried in a tomb, but on the third day, He rose from the dead! *Jesus conquered sin, death, and Satan! God's promise had been fulfilled.*

God calls every person to receive the forgiveness of sins and salvation that Jesus paid for on the cross. When someone trusts Jesus to save him, he receives God's gift of eternal life and has fellowship with God. He is made spiritually alive and becomes part of God's family forever. When he dies, he will be with God for all eternity.

> For God so loved the world, that He gave His only begotten Son, that whosoever believeth in Him should not perish, but have everlasting life. For God sent not His Son into the world to condemn the world; but that the world through Him might be saved. **John 3:16–17**

Spiritual Growth

You need spiritual food to grow and stay healthy in your spiritual relationship with God. The Bible, God's Word, provides this spiritual food. *Set aside some time each day to read God's Word and talk to Him in prayer.* The Bible teaches you Who God is, what He has done, and what He will continue to do. It tells you how much He loves you, how to live for Him, and how to remain spiritually healthy.

> I am the bread of life: he that cometh to Me shall never hunger; and he that believeth on Me shall never thirst. **John 6:35**

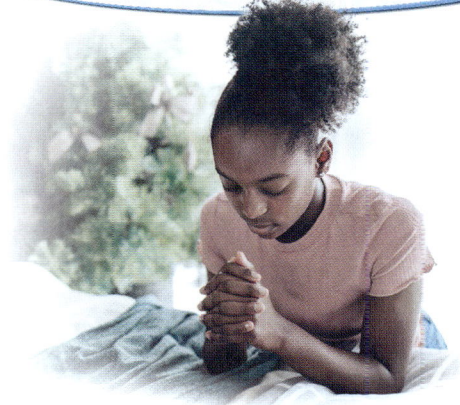

Applying God's Word

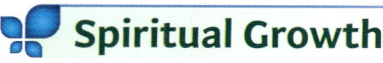

Read Romans 12:1–8 and apply the verses by answering these questions:

- How can I be a living sacrifice to God?
- Are there areas in which I shape myself to the world instead of to God's will?
- Do I think proudly of myself?
- How can I serve the body of Christ?

Spiritual Cleansing

When you believe in Jesus, you become a Christian, part of God's family. Unfortunately, there are times when we sin instead of obeying God's Word. Sin may make us feel guilty and fear that God does not love us anymore. Always remember, *God will always love you, even when you sin.* Your sin may cause you to avoid spending time with Him. But there is a remedy. *Confessing your sin to God restores your fellowship with Him, which removes your guilty feelings.* God has given us the following promise in the Bible: "If we confess our sins, He is faithful and just to forgive us our sins, and to cleanse us from all unrighteousness" (1 John 1:9).

Sin can also affect your health. Bitterness, anger, jealousy, and self-pity can upset how your body systems work, causing you to feel ill. God has provided three gifts to resist the temptation to sin—the Holy Spirit Who dwells in you; God's Word, the Bible; and prayer to talk directly to God. When you memorize and study God's Word, the Holy Spirit will bring those verses to your mind and help you make the choices that will please God.

What do you do when you keep committing the same sins? The apostle Paul had the same struggle that we do. In Romans 7:15, he admits, "For that which I do I allow not: for what I would, that do I not; but what I hate, that do I." In anguish, he cries out, "O wretched man that I am! who shall deliver me from the body of this death?" Paul then turns to Jesus: "I thank God through Jesus Christ our Lord" (Rom. 7:24–25). Paul knew God's promise of the forgiveness of sins and trusted that God's forgiveness, not his own works, saved him and made him righteous before God.

Character Development

God's plan for all of His children includes growing in Christian character. Growing in character is learning to think and act in a way that honors God. Jesus is our greatest example of Christian character, but many other individuals in Scripture also demonstrate the character traits of courage, trustworthiness, and godly leadership.

Sometimes, acting how God desires you to will require courage. You show courage by trusting God and doing what is right even when it is difficult or unpopular. Daniel 3 records how Shadrach, Meshach, and Abed-nego had to make a choice: worship Nebuchadnezzar's idol or be thrown into the fiery furnace. They revealed their godly courage by refusing to bow to the idol, no matter the consequence. They had faith in God to take care of them, whether in life or in death. You can also trust God's promises and show the same courage that they did.

We have all been let down by someone who failed to fulfill a promise. Unlike us, God is trustworthy; He always keeps His word (Num. 23:19). Trustworthiness is an important part of Christian character; you should be dependable and "let your yea be yea; and your nay, nay" (James 5:12). When you fail, ask God to help you be a person others can depend upon.

In Luke 22:24–27, Jesus taught His apostles how a godly leader should act. He is not to exercise harsh rule and command over others. Instead, he should view his leadership as a service to God and others. He should be willing to take on the humblest tasks of service, as Jesus did when He washed the apostles' feet.

Christian leadership begins with an attitude of service, but it also requires developing competence, or skilled ability, to organize people and manage tasks. These skills can be taught, but developing competence requires practice. Seek mentors in your home, church, school, and community who can teach you these leadership skills. Find opportunities like clubs, organizations, and committees that will let you develop competence in these skills. But as you practice these skills, always remember to follow Jesus' attitude of humble service.

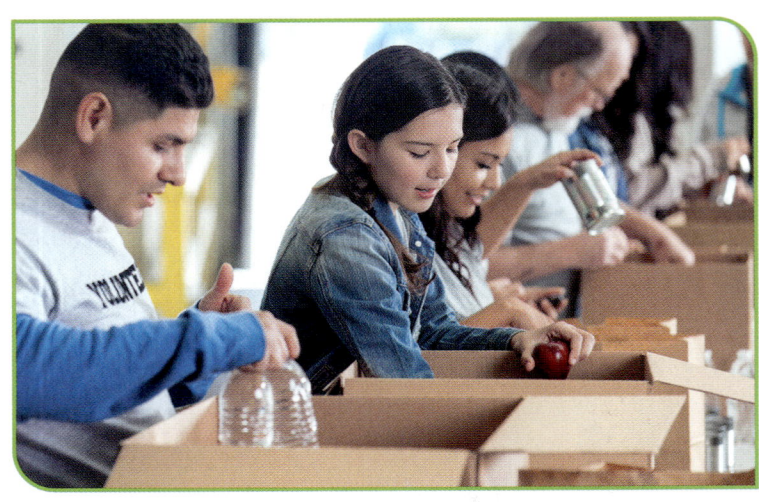

Spiritual Peace

God has promised to give peace to all who put their faith and trust in Him. God designed your body to be able not only to move but also to rest and recharge. There are times each day or night that we lie down and sleep, ending all physical activity. We may just rest, enjoying the quiet time. Do you remember a time when you could not relax and rest? Christians are privileged to give problems that affect their sleep over to God.

> *Be careful* [anxious] *for nothing; but in every thing by prayer and supplication with thanksgiving let your requests be made known unto God. And the peace of God, which passeth all understanding, shall keep your hearts and minds through Christ Jesus.* **Philippians 4:6–7**

Spiritual Development

Once a person is saved, he needs to deepen and strengthen his relationship with God. When the Holy Spirit enters a Christian's life, He gives the person a new spiritual nature. The Holy Spirit guides Christians and helps them joyfully obey and serve God. However, there is a continual battle between the old, sinful nature and the new nature. The Holy Spirit gives the strength to resist and choose what pleases God. He also causes the new nature to bear spiritual fruit. Submitting to the Holy Spirit's control of our attitudes and choices gives us peace and contentment as we serve God and others.

It is important for us to reflect God's love to others. When they see God's love in our lives, they may want to know how they can trust Jesus too. Telling others about Jesus is a special way that you can serve God. It is helpful to know a few verses that you can use to help others learn to trust in Jesus.

- We have all sinned, or done wrong things.

  For all have sinned, and come short of the glory of God. Romans 3:23

- The wrong we have done must be punished.

  For the wages of sin is death; but the gift of God is eternal life through Jesus Christ our Lord. Romans 6:23

- Jesus took all our sin and punishment on Himself when He died on the cross.

  But God commendeth His love toward us, in that, while we were yet sinners, Christ died for us. Romans 5:8

- If we believe in Jesus and receive His gift of forgiveness, He will save us and bring us into the family of God.

  That if thou shalt confess with thy mouth the Lord Jesus, and shalt believe in thine heart that God hath raised Him from the dead, thou shalt be saved. Romans 10:9

Prayer is an important part of spiritual development. We communicate with God through prayer. Our relationship with Him is strengthened by talking to Him every day. You can pray at any time and any place. A prayer can be as simple as expressing thanks for a new day or confessing an unkind word or action. You can whisper a prayer as you walk into class or think of a friend who is sick. You can speak a prayer silently in your heart when you are sad, nervous, or afraid

Prayer Journal

LIVE IT OUT!

Although you can talk to God at any time and anywhere, you may find that keeping a prayer journal helps your prayer time stay focused on God. You can use the word *PRAY* as a model for a simple prayer journal.

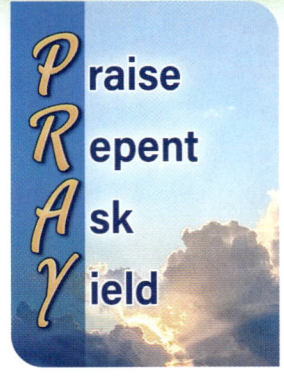

Praise—Praise God for Who He is and thank Him for what He has done.

> *Enter into His gates with thanksgiving, and into His courts with praise: be thankful unto Him, and bless His name.* Psalm 100:4

Repent—If you know of unconfessed sins in your life, name them and ask for forgiveness. Also ask God to forgive your secret faults, those sins that you are not aware of.

> *I acknowledged my sin unto thee, and mine iniquity have I not hid. I said, I will confess my transgressions unto the LORD; and Thou forgavest the iniquity of my sin.* Psalm 32:5
>
> *Who can understand his errors? cleanse Thou me from secret faults.* Psalm 19:12

Ask—Share your needs and the needs of others with God. Be thankful that He will answer in the best way.

> *Be careful for nothing; but in every thing by prayer and supplication with thanksgiving let your requests be made known unto God.* Philippians 4:6

Yield—Yield, or submit, to God by accepting His plan for your life. Trust that God's answer to your prayer is exactly what you need.

> *Thy kingdom come. Thy will be done in earth, as it is in heaven.* Matthew 6:10

Practice using the *PRAY* model to journal a prayer to God.

Praise: God, I praise You for being _____

_____.

Thank You for _____

_____.

Repent: I confess that _____

_____.

Thank You for forgiving me for _____

_____.

Ask: Please _____

_____.

Yield: I trust that _____

_____. Amen.

192   *Enjoying Good Health*

Social Wellness

As you get older and grow physically, you also grow socially. Jesus should be the model for our behavior when interacting with others. We should treat other people as Jesus did, showing care and compassion but giving loving rebuke when needed. As we grow spiritually, the Holy Spirit will make us more like Jesus in our social behavior.

> *A man that hath friends must show himself friendly.* **Proverbs 18:24**

Friendship

Making New Friends

Making new friends comes naturally to some people but is awkward for others. If you change schools or move to a new town, making friends can be challenging. Smiling is a good way to show others friendliness. Learning and using the names of new people will help you remember their names. If you are not sure how to respond in a new situation with new people, remember the Golden Rule—"*Do unto others as you would have them do unto you.*" Treat other people how you want to be treated.

> *And as ye would that men should do to you, do ye also to them likewise.* **Luke 6:31**

Being a Good Friend

> *Charity suffereth long, and is kind; charity envieth not; charity vaunteth not itself, is not puffed up, doth not behave itself unseemly, seeketh not her own, is not easily provoked, thinketh no evil.* **1 Corinthians 13:4–5**

Godly love is important for being a good friend. We should love others the same way Jesus loves us. Love is patient and kind with others, even when they are unkind. It is not jealous. It is humble instead of proud. Love is polite and puts others first. Love forgives wrongs done to us instead of becoming bitter.

Loving others is more than just saying that you love them. You demonstrate your love by the way you treat others. You love them for who they are, not for their toys, skills, or clothes. You pay attention by listening and trying to understand your friend's feelings. Be happy when he is happy. When he is sad, you may not understand why, but you can always listen. The Bible says it this way: "Rejoice with them that do rejoice, and weep with them that weep" (Rom. 12:15). Be faithful in good times and in bad times.

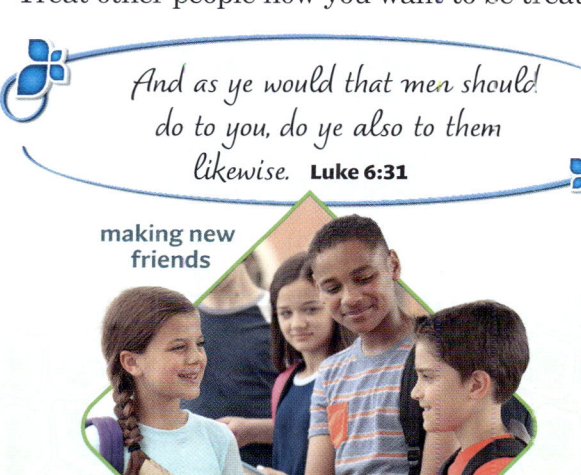
making new friends

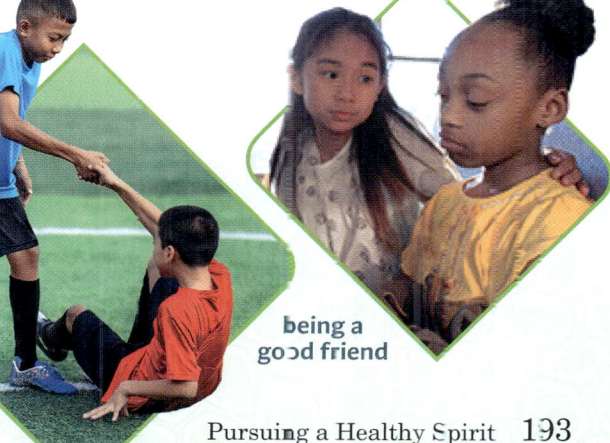
being a good friend

Being Considerate

Always be kind and courteous in your communication. Be a good listener; avoid interrupting people or causing a disturbance. Try to understand other peoples' views and opinions; even if you disagree, you can still treat people with respect because they are created in God's image. Be aware of your tone when you speak; even if your words are respectful, your tone may seem disrespectful. Avoid gossip, since you risk hurting someone by spreading information that may not be true.

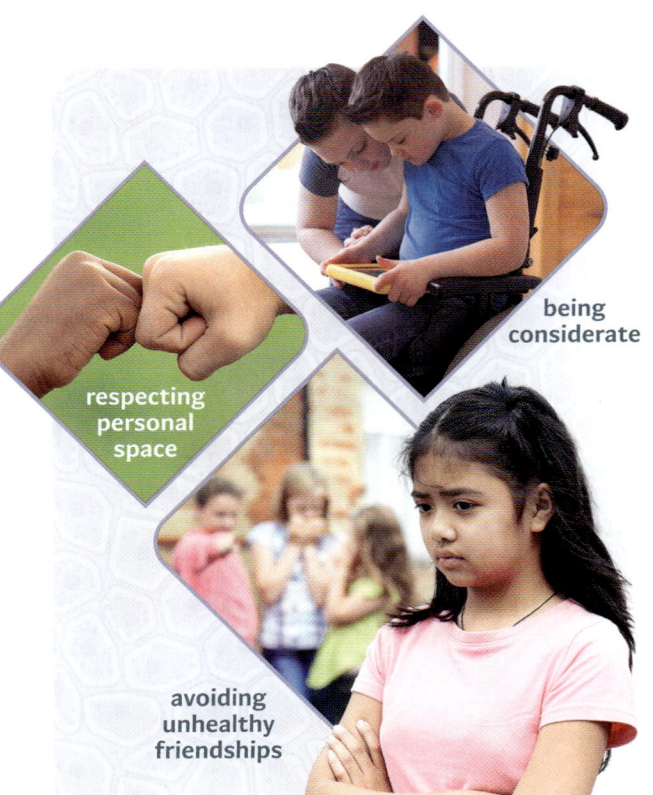

respecting personal space

being considerate

avoiding unhealthy friendships

Respecting Personal Space

Personal space is the area around a person that he considers his own. This space is different for each person, based on his preferences. Someone's personal space also depends on his relationship with another person; it represents how comfortable he is being close to the other person.

Respecting someone's personal space means that you do not get so close that you make him feel uncomfortable. It also means not touching him without his consent. For example, if someone does not want to give you a handshake or a high-five, show respect by not trying to make him give you one.

Respecting someone's personal space helps him feel comfortable and relaxed while interacting with you. It also lets him communicate with you freely. Consider how you feel about your own personal space. How may others' feelings differ? What can you do to respect personal space in your everyday life?

Avoiding Unhealthy Friendships

The people you spend the most time with have the most influence in your life. Therefore, *it is important to choose your closest friends wisely.* Friends should be kind to each other in both their words and actions. Friends should not be mean-spirited or cruel by making fun of others.

Do you know the difference between teasing and taunting? *Teasing is a silly way that people who care about each other interact to make each other laugh.* Both people usually participate, and it is never meant to hurt, embarrass, or control someone. *Taunting comes from just one person and is meant to hurt, embarrass, or control someone.* Teasing is usually fun and harmless, but you must take care that it does not become taunting by hurting or embarrassing others. Always be careful how you speak to your friends.

Do not be pressured to join a certain group to feel included, accepted, or popular. Negative peer pressure is not a quality of true friendship. If you feel excluded or ignored by a group, remind yourself that you are loved and accepted by God. Ask Him to give you true friends who accept you as you are. Remember, a good friend encourages you to do right and to be yourself. Your group of friends should be an open circle with plenty of room to receive others.

Peer pressure can happen at any age but especially during adolescence. Sometimes it is hard to say no to peer pressure. Do you practice standing up for the right even when it is hard? In Daniel 1:8, we read that "Daniel purposed in his heart that he would not defile himself." Stand up for what is right in God's eyes, even when doing so is hard. Ask God for help. Learn ways to assertively reject negative peer pressure.

LIVE IT OUT!

Refusing Peer Pressure

In each situation, explain how you can appropriately respond to peer pressure.

Your friend constantly says mean or embarrassing things about you. When you tell her to stop, she says, "I'm just teasing."

_____

_____

_____

_____

_____

Your best friend is pressuring you to watch a movie that you know your parents would not allow.

_____

_____

_____

_____

_____

A boy you just met has invited you to be part of his popular friend group. He insists that you must end your relationship with your best friend because your friend is not "cool" enough. _____

_____

_____

_____

_____

Communication

To grow and be healthy, your relationships with family members and friends must be developed and nurtured. An important part of building healthy relationships is communicating effectively. For the relationship to grow, you must understand each other and try to meet each other's needs.

To communicate is to share information. People communicate verbally and nonverbally. Verbal communication uses words, such as talking face to face, speaking on the phone, writing emails, and sending text messages. Nonverbal communication is communication without words; it includes facial expressions, eye contact, hand gestures, and body language. With practice, you can confidently communicate both verbally and nonverbally.

When you speak with someone, communicate effectively by looking into his eyes and using a respectful tone of voice. Speak clearly and use correct grammar. It is important to say things kindly. When the other person is speaking, do not interrupt; instead, think carefully about what he is saying and how you will respond. Be patient, and listen with empathy.

Your communication should be assertive but not aggressive. Assertive communication is speaking with confidence while still being respectful of the other person and what he has to say. Aggressive communication makes the other person feel as if he is being attacked. Be sure that your nonverbal communication also shows respect and empathy toward the person to whom you are speaking. A smile or thumbs-up may be just the encouragement your friend needs.

Which one of these situations demonstrates being assertive but not aggressive?

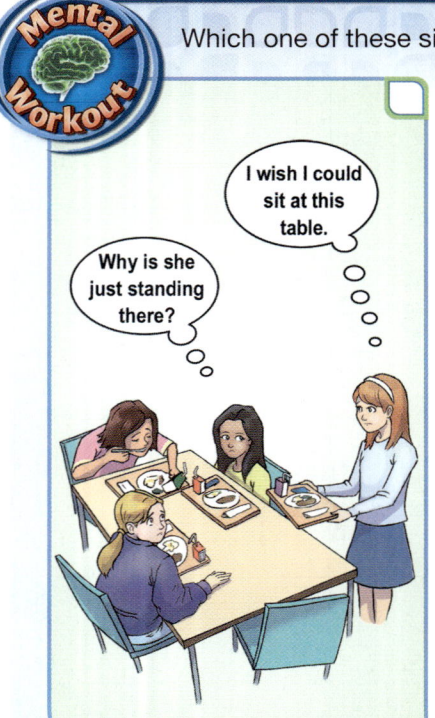

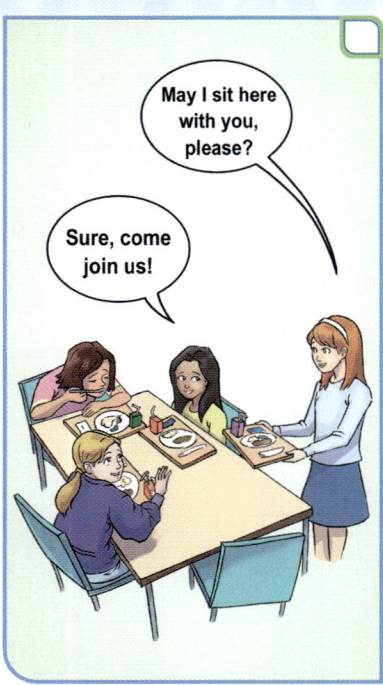

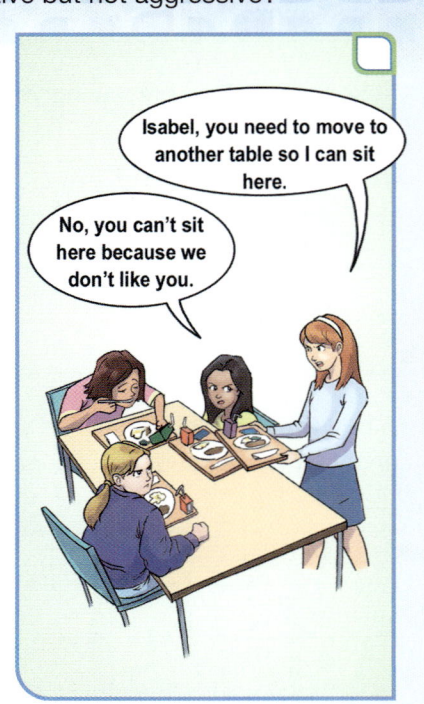

Communicating Online

It can be especially difficult to show empathy and respect in online communications. Remember that you are not talking to a machine or a screen; you are talking to an actual person. *Before you send a message, reread it to be sure that you were not unintentionally aggressive or disrespectful.* Words that are friendly teasing when spoken could seem mean or hurtful when typed out. Emoji can be useful for nonverbal communication, but beware that the other person may interpret them differently than you do.

Also consider whether you should post anything at all. Is what you are saying kind and helpful? If you would not say it in person, do not post it online. Avoid posting messages, photos, or videos that could embarrass you or another person; once something is on the internet, it is almost impossible to remove. A message to a specific person is better sent privately than posted publicly. Be careful even in private messages; you cannot control what the recipient does with what you send. Also follow the rules for online safety that you have learned.

Conflict Resolution

Every relationship will have disagreements and conflicts. Conflict may be caused by a simple misunderstanding or difference of opinion. Conflict may also be caused by sinful pride and selfishness. *Good communication can resolve many conflicts.*

No matter the cause, decide to resolve the conflict in a way that honors God. You have an opportunity to grow in maturity and build a stronger relationship with the person.

> *Wherefore, my beloved brethren, let every man be swift to hear, slow to speak, slow to wrath: for the wrath of man worketh not the righteousness of God* **James 1:19–20**

You may have a disagreement even with your family members or your closest friends. Remember that the person you are in conflict with is not your enemy. *Confront, or address, the problem rather than the person; work to solve the problem together.*

Before discussing the conflict, determine what problem needs solving and how to express the problem respectfully. After expressing the problem, let the other person share his view. Listen with empathy and try to understand his point of view. If you need to apologize, say exactly what you did without making excuses; then ask for forgiveness. If the other person apologizes, be quick to forgive.

> *Only by pride cometh contention: but with the well advised is wisdom* **Proverbs 13:10**

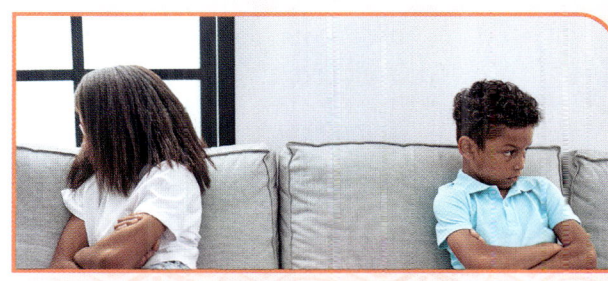

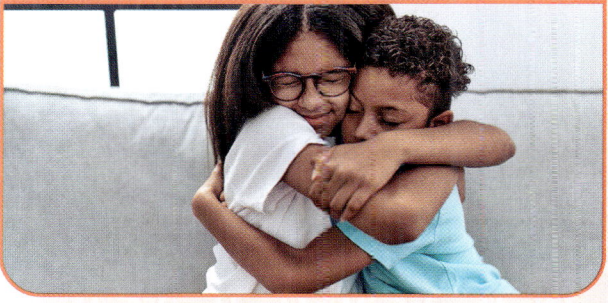

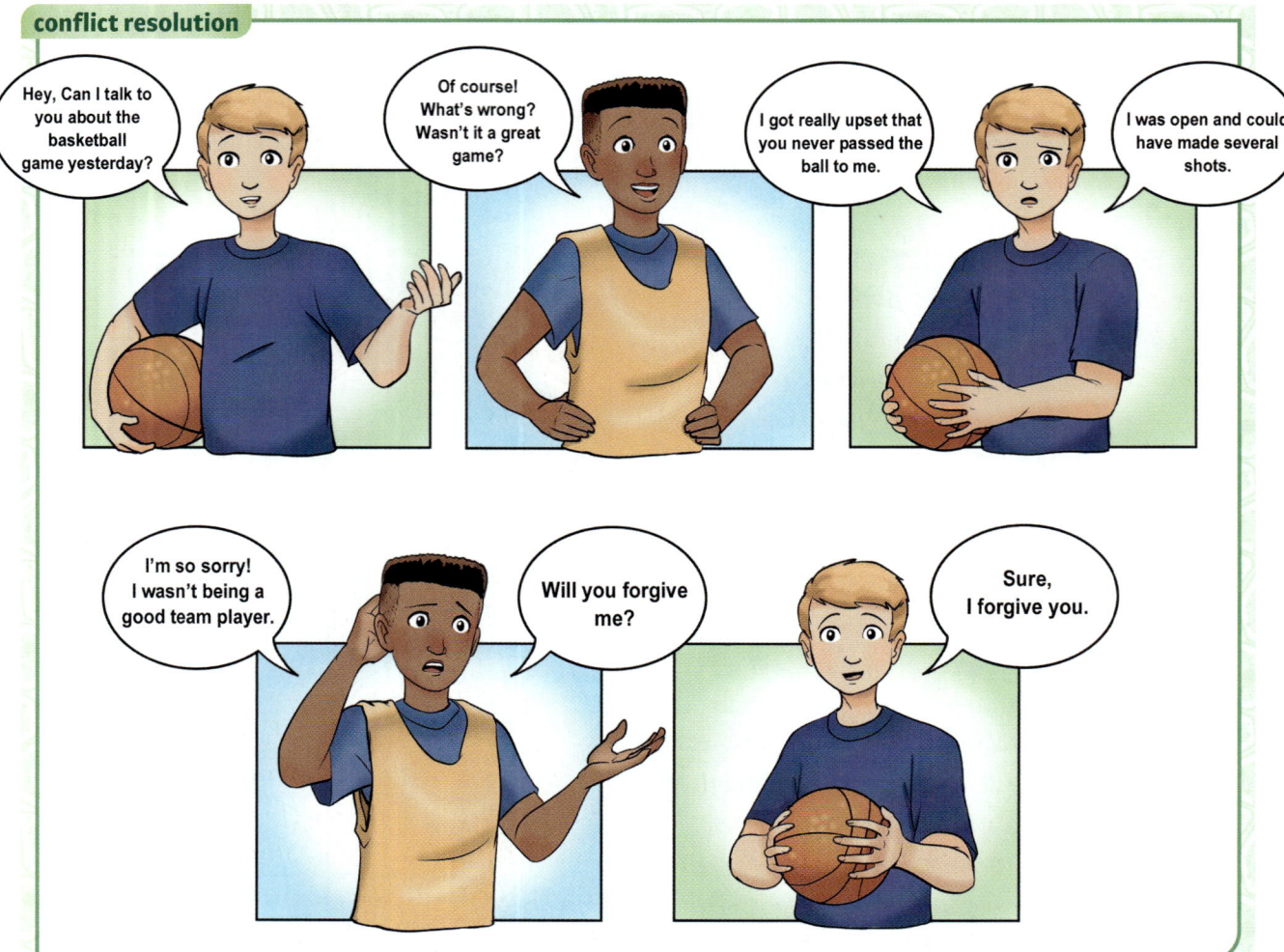

![Mental Workout logo] Think about the way you communicate with other people. Read the following questions and circle **Yes** or **No**. Decide which areas of communication you need to improve.

1. When someone is speaking to me, do I always listen intently?   **Yes   No**

2. When someone is speaking to me, do I look at their eyes?   **Yes   No**

3. Do I wait until the other person is done speaking before I start talking?   **Yes   No**

4. Do I share private information about others that can damage their reputations?   **Yes   No**

5. Do I use proper vocabulary to communicate accurately?   **Yes   No**

6. Do I often talk for a long time without actually getting to the point?   **Yes   No**

7. Do I speak clearly and audibly so that I can be understood?   **Yes   No**

8. Do I speak assertively without being aggressive?   **Yes   No**

> *Keep thy heart with all diligence; for out of it are the issues of life.* **Proverbs 4:23**

As you grow spiritually and socially, you will learn how to develop in your inner health—mentally, in your thoughts, and emotionally, in your feelings. Your thoughts and feelings are developed in your spirit, your inner self. Your thoughts influence your feelings, and your feelings are displayed publicly by your actions.

Healthy Thoughts

You are responsible for what you think about. The Bible tells us to take our thoughts captive so that they are obedient to Christ. In Genesis 4, God spoke to Cain because Cain was angry at and jealous of his brother, Abel. Cain disregarded God's warning and did not change his thinking. Allowing his anger and jealousy to control him, he murdered Abel. With God's help, we can control what we think about so that our thoughts lead us to do what is right in His sight.

> *Casting down imaginations, and every high thing that exalteth itself against the knowledge of God, and bringing into captivity every thought to the obedience of Christ.* **2 Corinthians 10:5**

Biblical thinking leads to right behavior. Your thoughts need to be on right things (Phil. 4:8). When you become a Christian, the Holy Spirit renews your mind and helps you use self-control in your thinking (Rom. 12:2). Thinking biblically from a right heart comes from your new nature as a child of God.

When your thoughts become overwhelming, take them to Jesus. It is easy to feel sorry for yourself when bad things happen. However, you should encourage yourself in the Lord, as David did in times of trouble (1 Sam. 30:6). Don't get trapped in overwhelming feelings; avoid dwelling on negative or unhelpful thoughts. Instead, turn your thoughts over to God. Reject thoughts that do not agree with God's truth and righteousness. Ask yourself how He can help you in your difficult situation. Reading and obeying God's Word will help your inner spiritual nature to grow and help you replace negative thoughts with positive ones.

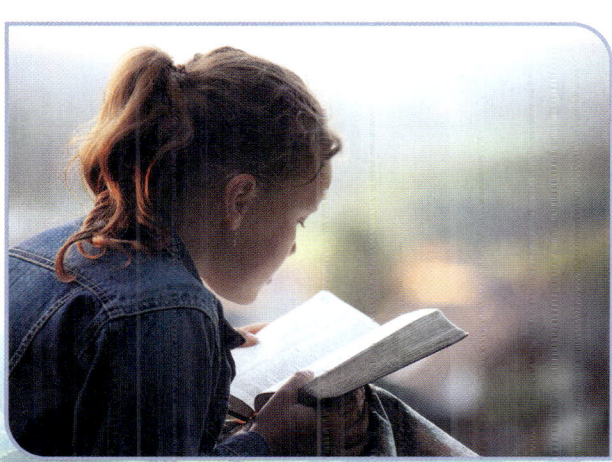

Self-Image

Each person has a mental picture of himself called his *self-image*. *Your self-image is the way you think about yourself and your value to yourself and others.* Throughout your life, you will face situations that develop your self-image. Your experiences and interactions with family, friends, and other people help form your opinion of yourself. Your self-image will affect your health behaviors and influence how you react in challenging situations.

Developing a correct self-image will help you live a life that brings glory to God. *The foundation of your self-image should be knowing that God created you—your body, mind, and soul—in His own image.* Because of sin, that image is damaged, and we all deserve God's eternal punishment. But God loves and cares about us so much that Jesus died to pay for our sins. *For the Christian, a correct self-image is a balance between what he was—an enemy of God, dead in sins—and what he is—a beloved child of God, saved by grace.*

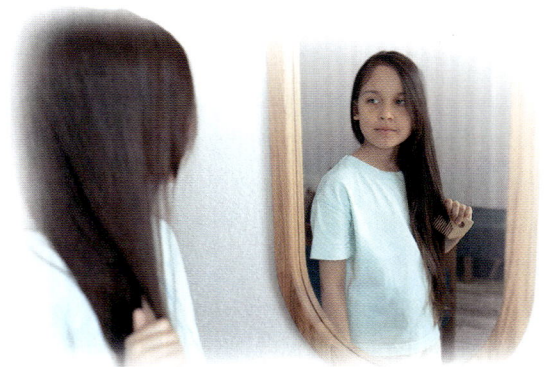

> But God, Who is rich in mercy, for His great love wherewith He loved us, even when we were dead in sins, hath quickened us together with Christ, (by grace ye are saved;) and hath raised us up together, and made us sit together in heavenly places in Christ Jesus. **Ephesians 2:4–6**

Think. Feel. Act.

	Self-Centered		God-Centered
Think	I am alone. No one loves me. I never get what I want. I can't do it.	**Think**	God is with me. God loves me. God cares for me. God will help me.
Feel	fear, discontentment, bitterness	**Feel**	confidence, gratitude, joy
Act	distrusting God, being unkind to others, disobeying parents, giving up, etc.	**Act**	trusting God, sharing with others, obeying parents, doing my best in school, etc.

When I think...	God says...	When I feel...	God says...
I'm all alone.	I am with you. *Deuteronomy 31:6*	fearful	I will protect you. *Psalm 27:1*
No one loves me.	I love you. *1 John 3:1*	discontented	I will provide for your needs. *Philippians 4:19*
I can't do it.	I will help you. *Psalm 32:8*	overwhelmed	I am your hope. *Psalm 42:11*
I'm not good enough.	I created you. *Genesis 1:27*	tired	I will give you rest. *Matthew 11:28–30*

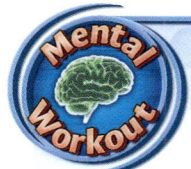

Can you identify right thinking? Circle right thoughts: cross out wrong thoughts.

1. No one can tell me what to do or not to do.

2. I am thankful for my brother because he helps me with arithmetic.

3. God knows my future, and I can trust Him to take care of me.

4. I will never understand how to solve proportions.

5. Everyone on the baseball team thinks I should quit.

6. I like helping my sister learn to ice skate.

7. God's Word helps me to think good thoughts.

8. My teacher doesn't like me.

9. I can trust God to help me when I am sad.

Spirit-Controlled Emotions

God created you with a full range of emotions, or feelings, including happiness, sadness, excitement, fear, and anger. It is normal to experience several emotions during a typical day. Some are enjoyable, while others can be difficult to deal with. Our emotions influence the way we act. We need to remember that God has given us everything we need in His Word to learn how to glorify Him, even with our emotions.

Every person has felt anger, sadness, worry, and fear. God has a purpose for these negative emotions, but carrying them for a long time is not healthy for your body or spirit. God knows your thoughts; ask Him to help you interpret your feelings based on the truth of His Word. Share your emotions with a parent or trusted adult. He can pray with you and give the comfort you need from the Bible.

Overcoming Anger

Be ye angry, and sin not: let not the sun go down upon your wrath: neither give place to the devil. **Ephesians 4:26–27**

Anger is a normal human emotion, but it becomes sinful when you react by hurting others or holding on to bitterness. To control the emotion of anger, walk away from the situation and ask for God's help. The Holy Spirit will help a Christian overcome anger. Talk to a parent or trusted adult about the situation that made you angry; ask for help to resolve the situation in a way that honors God.

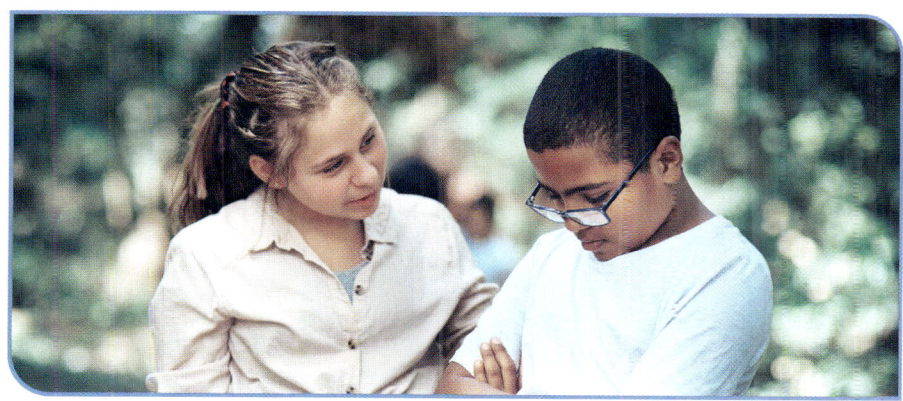

Conquering Fear

Fear is a powerful emotion. Knowing how to handle our fears can help us overcome them. We need to remind ourselves that God is always with us. King David wrote, "I sought the LORD, and He heard me, and delivered me from all my fears" (Ps. 34:4). As Christians, David's God is also our God; we can trust Him to take care of us in our fears.

Dealing with Jealousy

Our human nature tempts us to compare ourselves with others. When we compare our physical appearance, our belongings, our home, and our abilities to those of others, we can become dissatisfied with what God has given us. Instead of being content and thankful for God meeting our needs, we let dissatisfaction lead to the sin of jealousy, or coveting.

> *Thou shalt not covet thy neighbor's house, thou shalt not covet thy neighbor's wife, nor his manservant, nor his maidservant, nor his ox, nor his ass, nor any thing that is thy neighbor's.* **Exodus 20:17**

If you become jealous of another person, ask God to remind you of the many ways He has cared for you. Jealousy is a sin that comes from a lack of trust in God's goodness; repenting is the first step in dealing with it. Learn to be patient and accept the tasks you are given, rather than wishing for something that you think is more important. Trust God for strength and seek His will.

When You Feel Sad

We all feel disappointed at times. We feel sad when we do poorly at a task or quarrel with a close friend. You may feel that you have disappointed those around you. This sadness should not last very long. Be patient with yourself and give yourself time to feel better. Also get enough exercise, water, healthy food, and rest, so that your nervous system is able to help you respond to your emotions.

When you feel confusing emotions, take your thoughts and feelings to God. Ask Him to help you replace wrong thoughts with true thoughts about God and yourself. Talk to a parent or a trusted adult who can help you process your negative feelings. He can pray with you, listen, and give you godly advice to overcome your sad feelings.

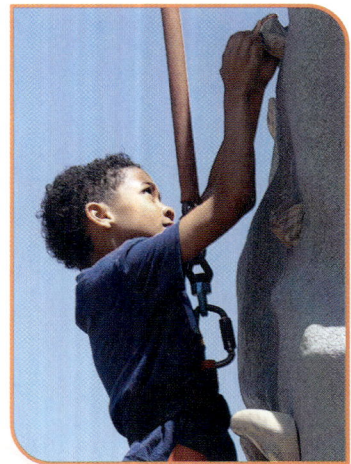

conquering fear

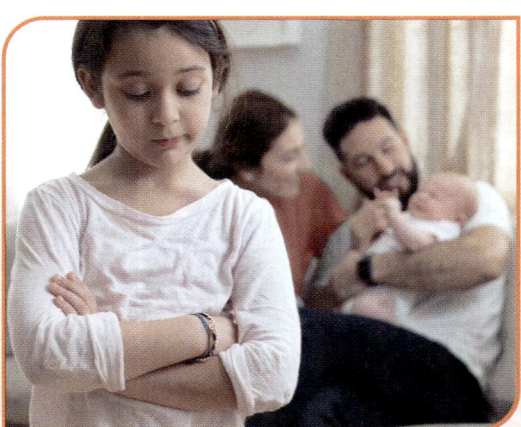

dealing with jealousy

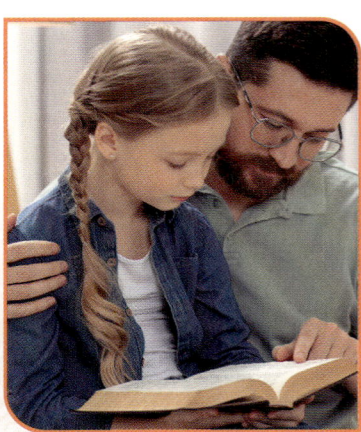

overcoming sadness

If you continue to feel sadness for a long time even after you have done all these things, speak up and ask for help. This is especially important if your sadness has no obvious cause, if it makes ordinary living difficult, or if you have thoughts of hurting yourself. Your parents may decide to seek biblical counseling or medical advice.

The LORD is nigh unto them that are of a broken heart. **Psalm 34:18**

Grieving a Personal Loss

Grief is the normal emotional response that happens after a personal loss. The loss could be the death of a family member or friend. Grief can also accompany the loss of a special pet or moving away from a good friend. When you lose someone you love, the hurt is very deep. God is with you in times of sorrow and knows the deep hurts of your heart; take your thoughts and feelings to Him, because He cares for you. Allow yourself the time you need to grieve. Tell someone you trust whenever you are feeling difficult emotions.

How can you comfort a friend who is grieving a loss? You may not know all the right words to say, but just being with him is one way that you can comfort him. Tell him that you are sorry for his loss. Pray for him faithfully and keep being his friend.

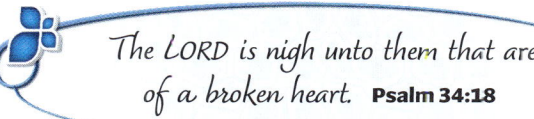

Identifying Emotions

Look up and read each verse. Decide what emotion is being described by the verse; write the reference in the correct box.

Proverbs 19:11	John 14:27	Hebrews 13:5
Proverbs 24:19	Romans 8:25	Revelation 21:4
Isaiah 41:10	Philippians 4:4	
Matthew 11:28	1 Thessalonians 5:18	

Positive Emotions		Negative Emotions	
contentment		anger	
hope		fear	
joy		jealousy	
peace		sadness	
thankfulness		tiredness	

Coping with Emotions

Think about ways that you can handle the weight of heavy emotions.

1. Getting fresh air is good for your mind and spirit. What are some outdoor activities that help you feel better? _____

_____

_____

2. Physical activity releases hormones in the body that help your mind and spirit to feel better. Write about a time when exercising helped you feel better. _____

_____

_____

3. Finding a creative outlet can help you take your mind off difficult emotions. What are some creative hobbies that you enjoy? _____

_____

_____

4. Peaceful, soothing music helps your brain to overcome stress and process emotion. Write about a time when music helped you to overcome difficult emotions. _____

_____

_____

_____

_____

God's Special Plan

God created you with a unique plan for a relationship with Him. Your physical, spiritual, social, mental, and emotional well-being are all parts of His special plan for you. Sometimes, we might wish that God had created us differently than He did, but that does not change His plan.

God designed a special place for each person to grow and learn. Do you know what that place is? It's your home! Your home is filled with your family—the special people that God created for you to grow and learn with.

When God created the first man, Adam, and the first woman, Eve, He uniquely designed Adam to be male and Eve to be female

(Gen. 1:27). Did you know that God also designed marriage? Genesis 2:24 tells us that His special plan is for a man to leave his father and mother to be joined to his wife so that they can form a new family and home. Perhaps you've seen wedding pictures of your parents in that special time in their lives. *A husband and wife have a special relationship designed only for them.* They share a closeness with each other that is not to be shared with anyone else. That closeness is a picture of the close relationship that God desires to have with each person who puts his faith in God for salvation. Because of this picture, God designed marriage to last for a lifetime.

Have you ever felt like your parents talked about things that they didn't share with you? That is likely true! There are many adult conversations your parents share that are not appropriate for you to know or be concerned about yet. As you get older, your parents may share more things with you that will help you be prepared for decisions you will make as you reach adulthood.

Just as God created Adam and Eve to be distinctly male and female, *He created you to be a boy or a girl according to His good plan for your life.* God's design for you as a boy or a girl is often referred to as your sex. As you grow older, you may find that your friendship with someone of the opposite sex starts to become special to you. It is important to remember that a special friendship is not the same thing as being married. You can discuss these feelings with your parents or a trusted adult; they will be able to help you learn things that will be important as you continue maturing. They can also help you set boundaries to protect your physical, emotional, and spiritual safety.

Conclusion

In *Enjoying Good Health*, you have learned that you are a masterpiece of God's creation. He made you with an intricate design. You have many parts—your heart, your lungs, your brain, your stomach, your kidneys, your white blood cells, your muscles and bones, and many more. As different as they are from each other, all of these parts work together as one unified whole—you. God also gave you a spirit that lets you think and feel emotions; most importantly, it lets you know and learn to love Him.

You have also learned that your body and spirit need care to work correctly and be healthy. You have learned about behaviors that help your health and others that harm your health. You know that habits you develop now will last as you grow into your teenage and adult years. Will you be a good steward of the body and spirit God has given you? Will you use what you know by making goals and planning to meet them? Will you seek to show love to others by helping them also live healthy lives? *Knowing how to be healthy is not enough. Only by *doing* can you continue to enjoy good health.

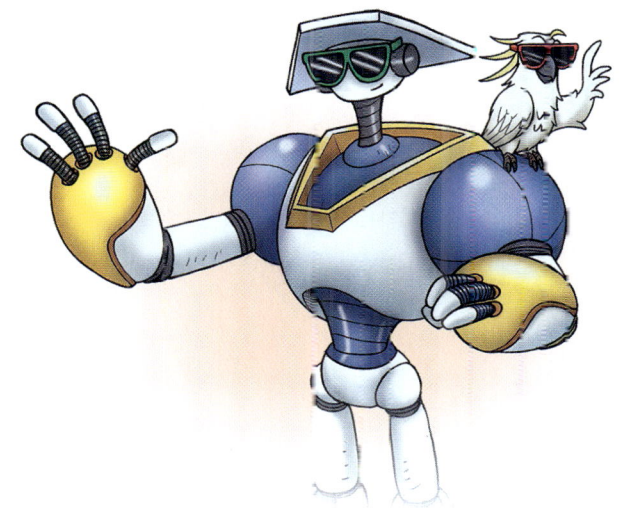

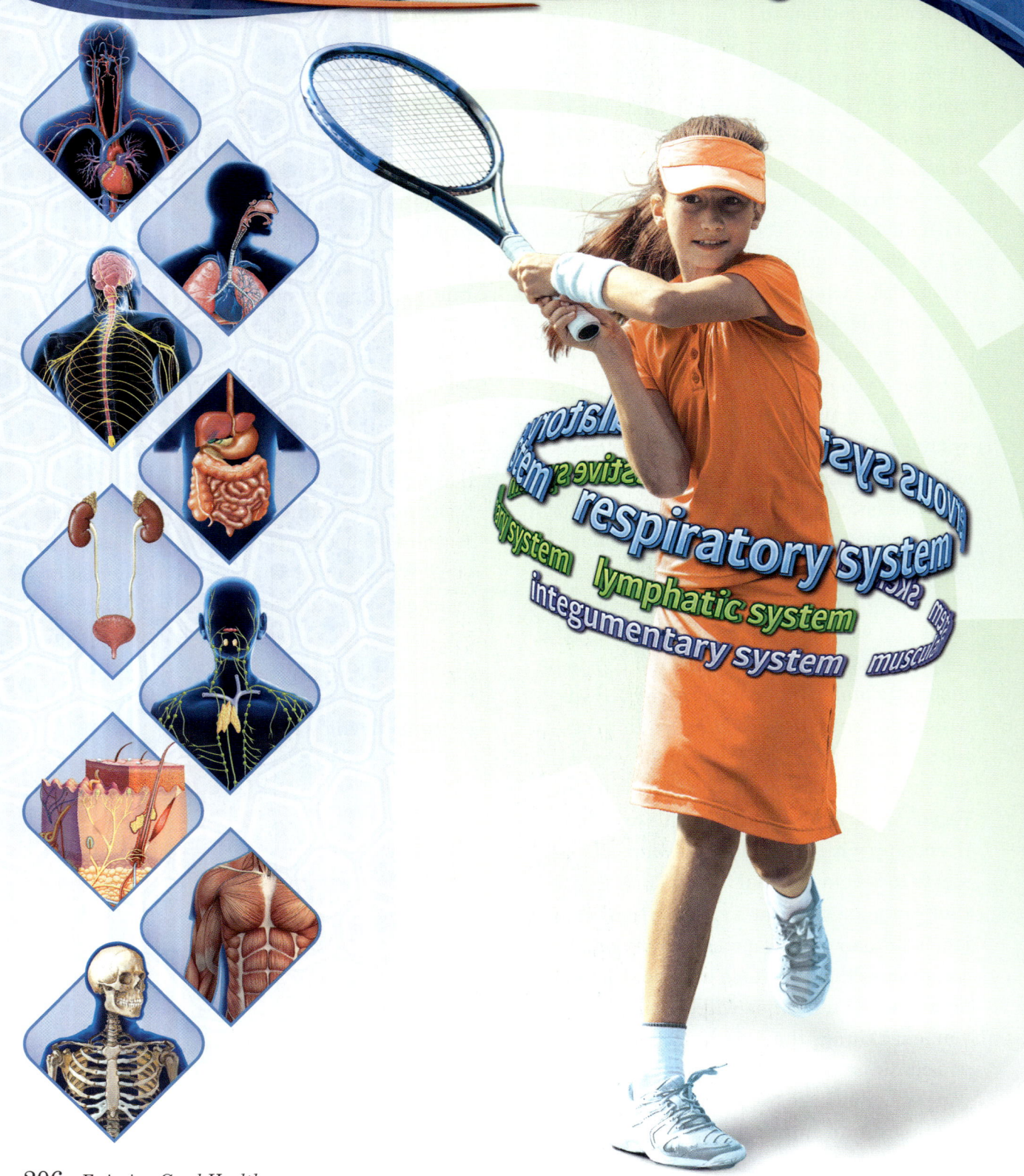

respiratory system

lymphatic system

integumentary system

Circulatory System

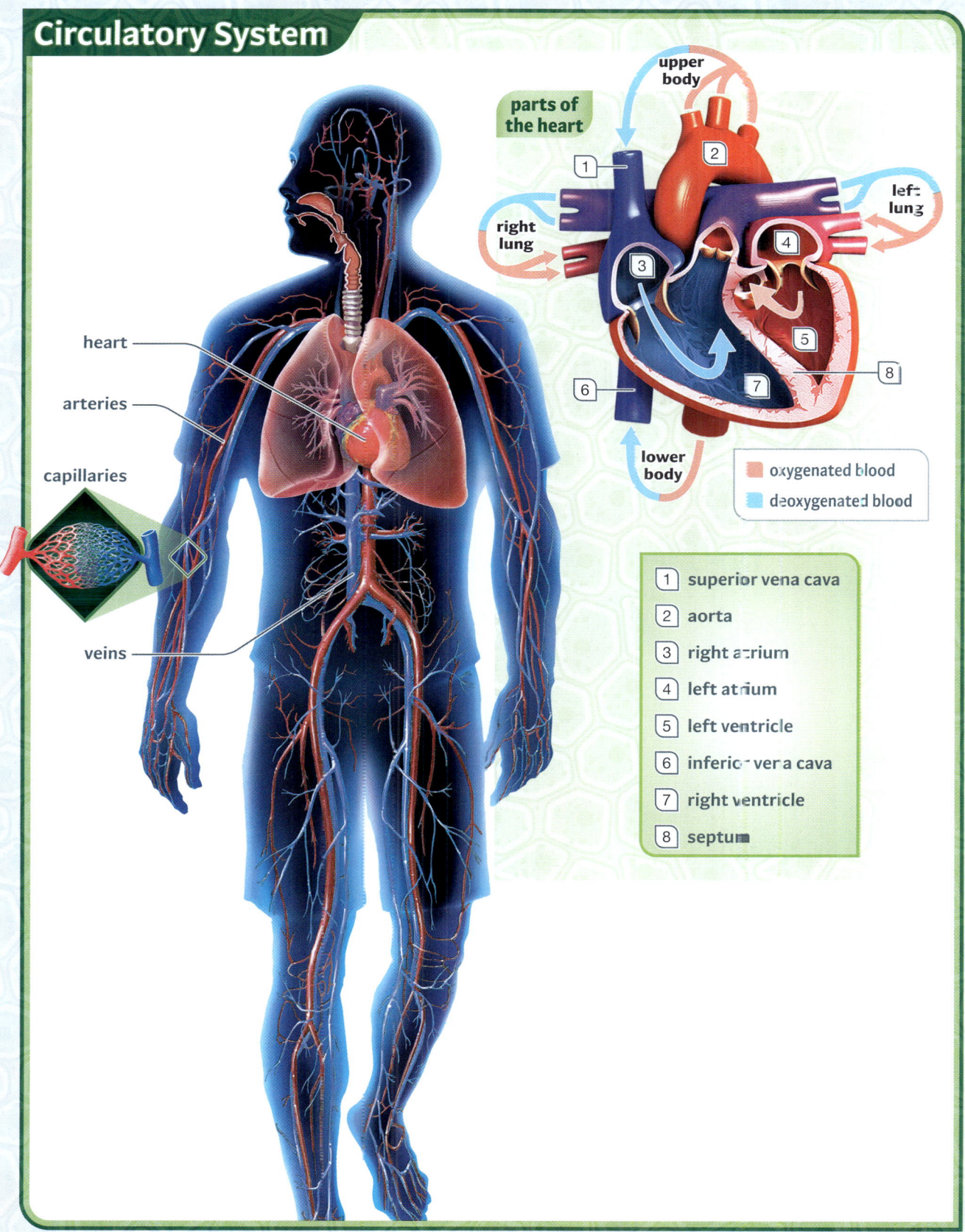

parts of the heart

upper body

right lung

left lung

lower body

heart

arteries

capillaries

veins

- oxygenated blood
- deoxygenated blood

1. superior vena cava
2. aorta
3. right atrium
4. left atrium
5. left ventricle
6. inferior vena cava
7. right ventricle
8. septum

Circulatory System

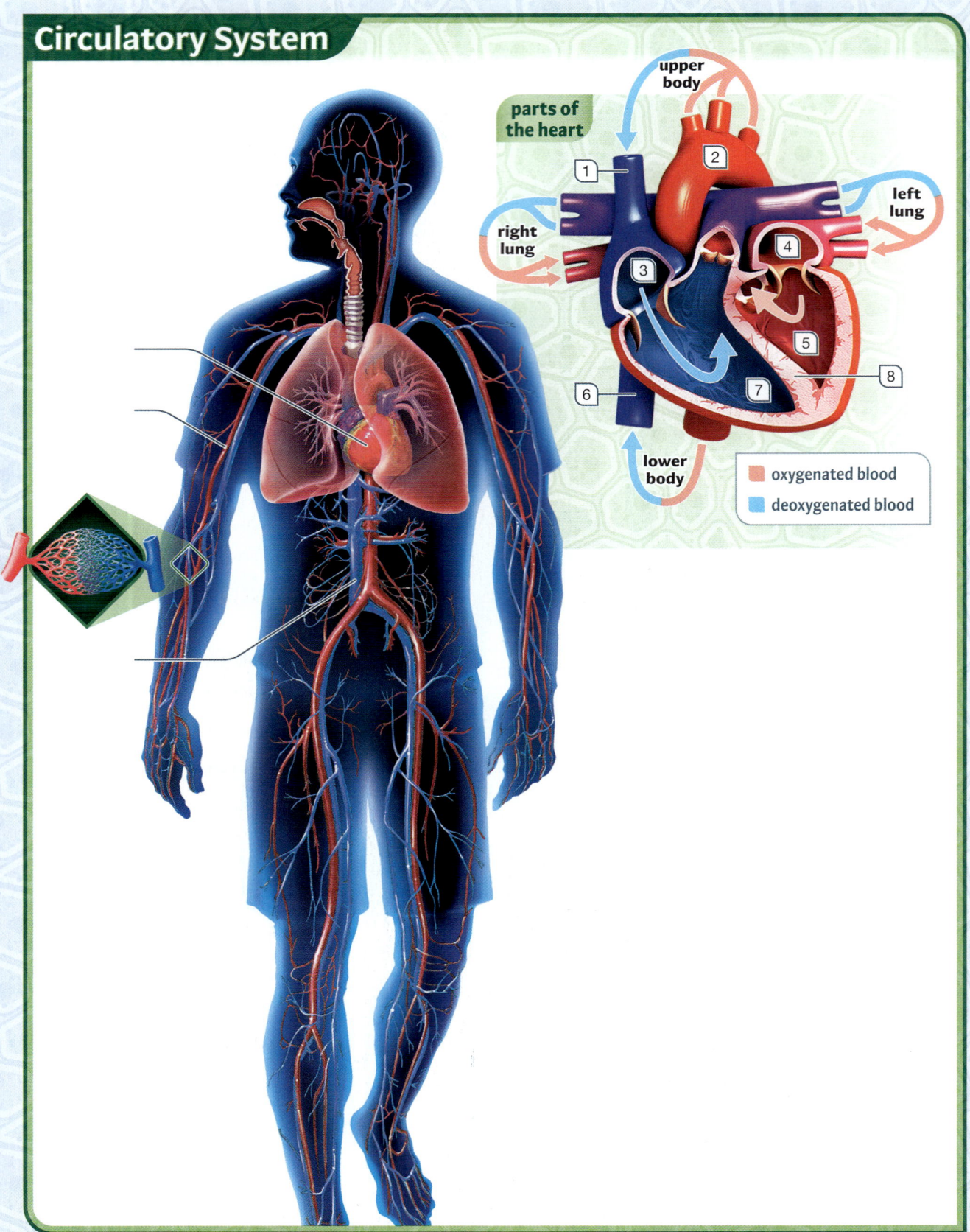

parts of the heart

upper body

left lung

right lung

lower body

1

2

3

4

5

6

7

8

oxygenated blood

deoxygenated blood

Respiratory System

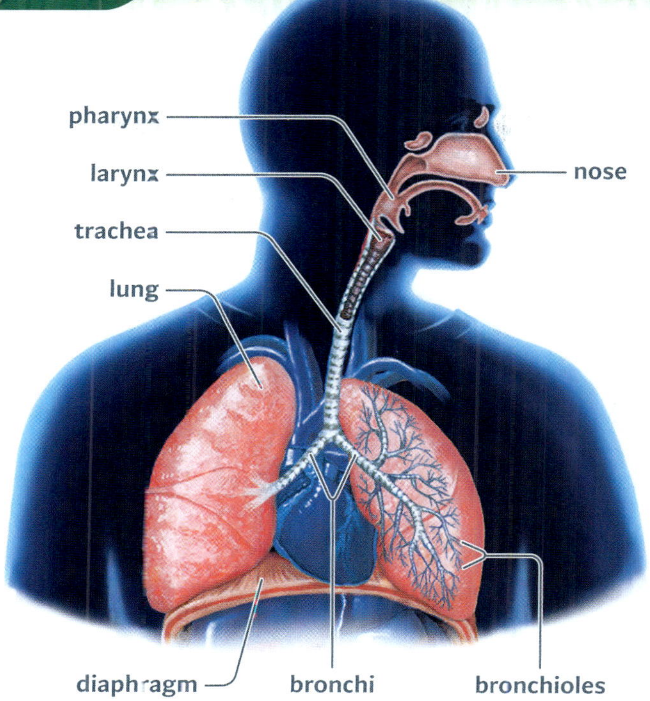

pharynx

larynx

trachea

lung

nose

diaphragm — bronchi — bronchioles

Nervous System

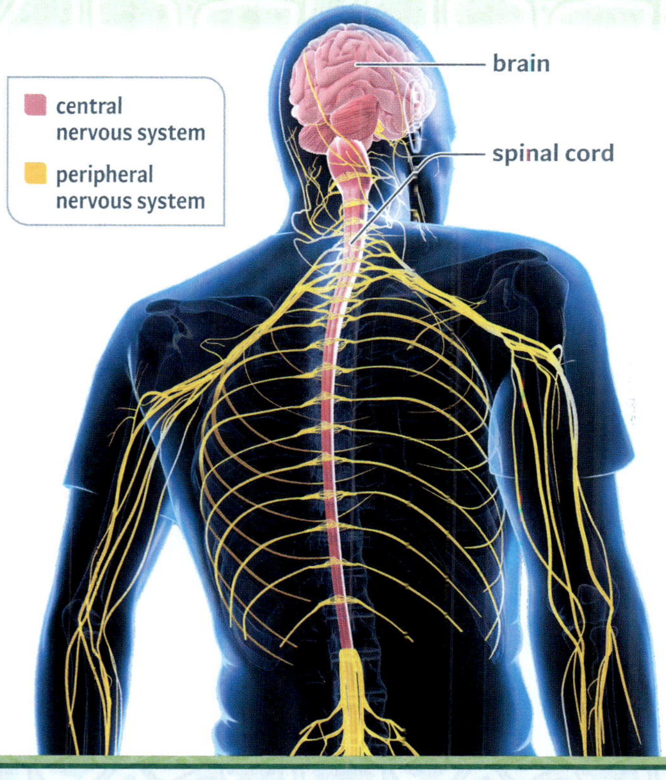

brain

spinal cord

central nervous system

peripheral nervous system

main parts of the brain

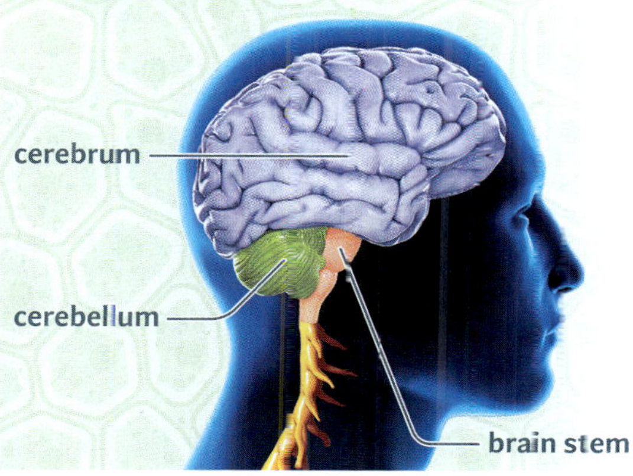

cerebrum

cerebellum

brain stem

Respiratory System

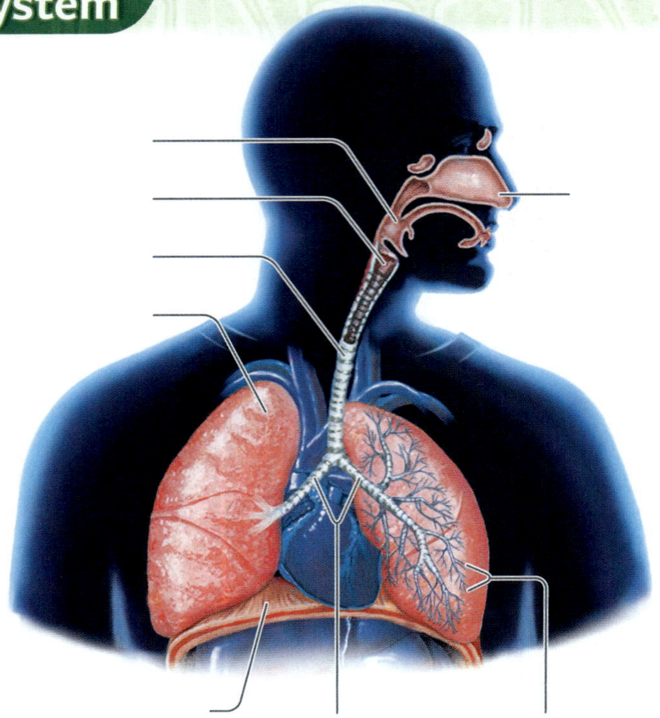

Nervous System

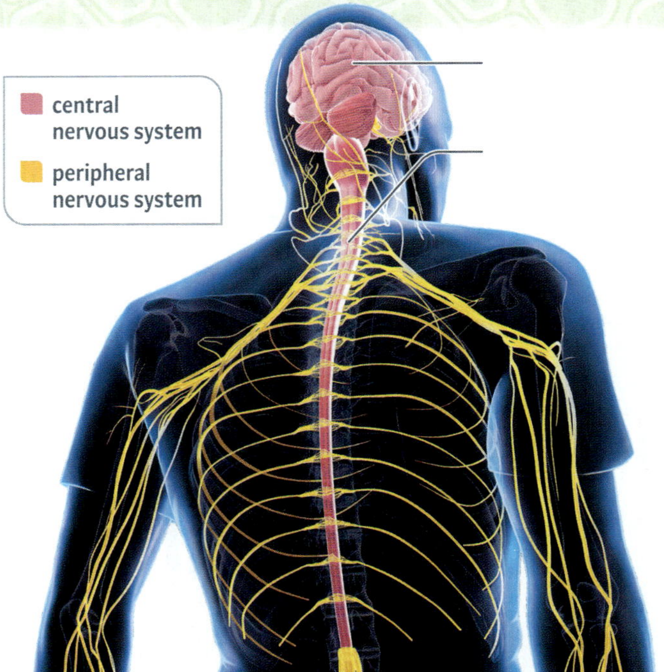

central
nervous system

peripheral
nervous system

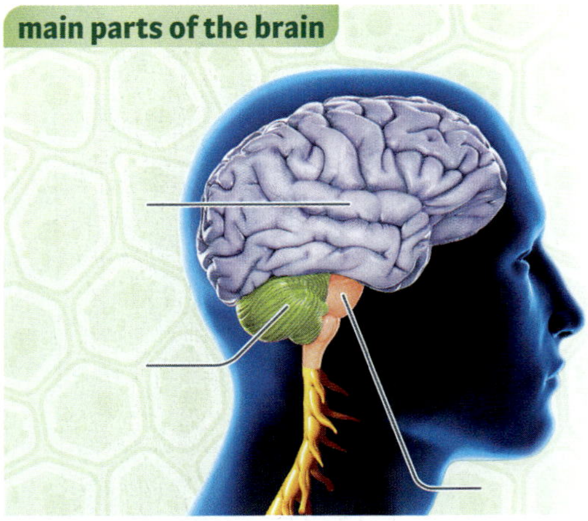

main parts of the brain

Digestive System

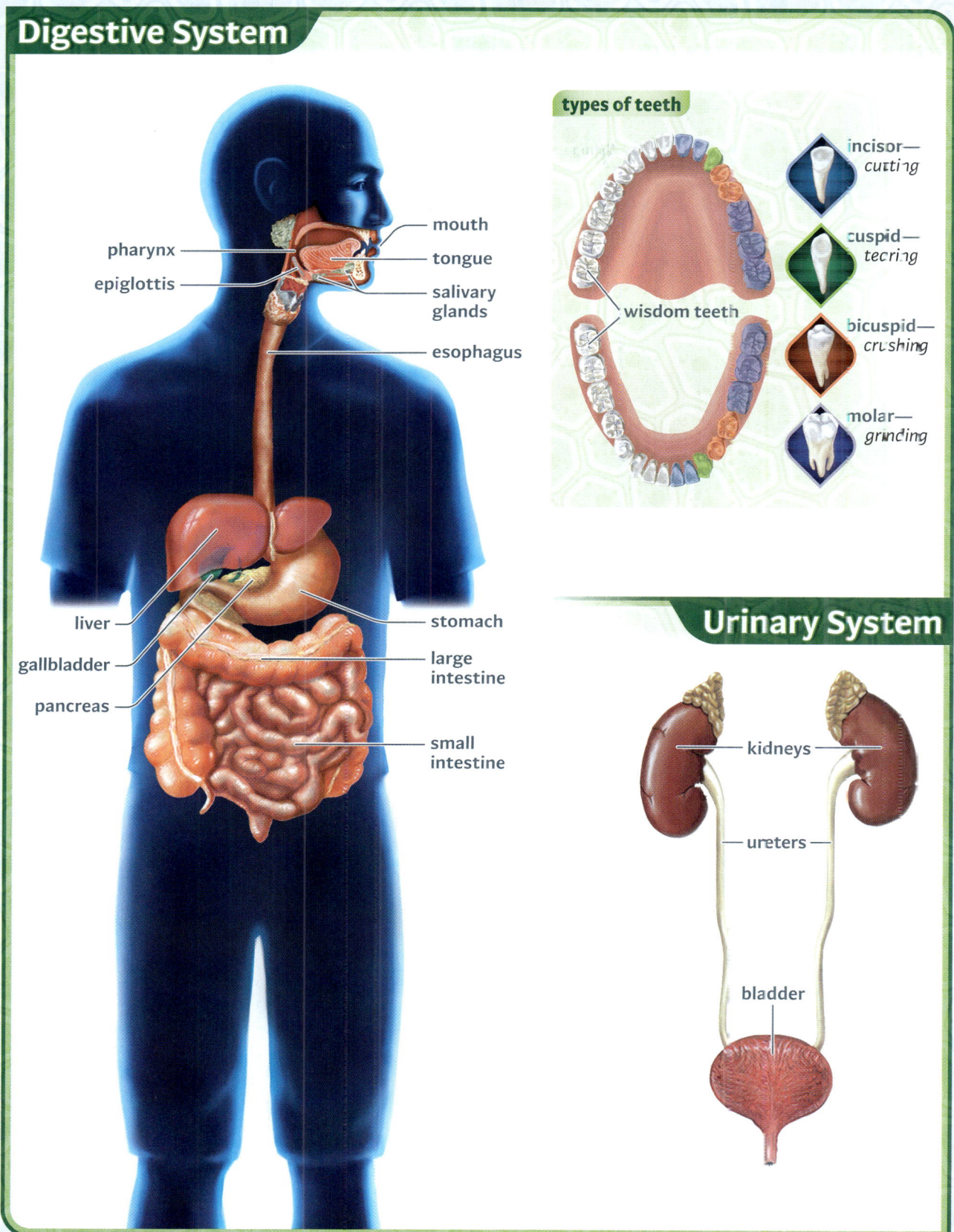

pharynx

epiglottis

mouth

tongue

salivary glands

esophagus

liver

gallbladder

pancreas

stomach

large intestine

small intestine

types of teeth

wisdom teeth

incisor—*cutting*

cuspid—*tearing*

bicuspid—*crushing*

molar—*grinding*

Urinary System

kidneys

ureters

bladder

Digestive System

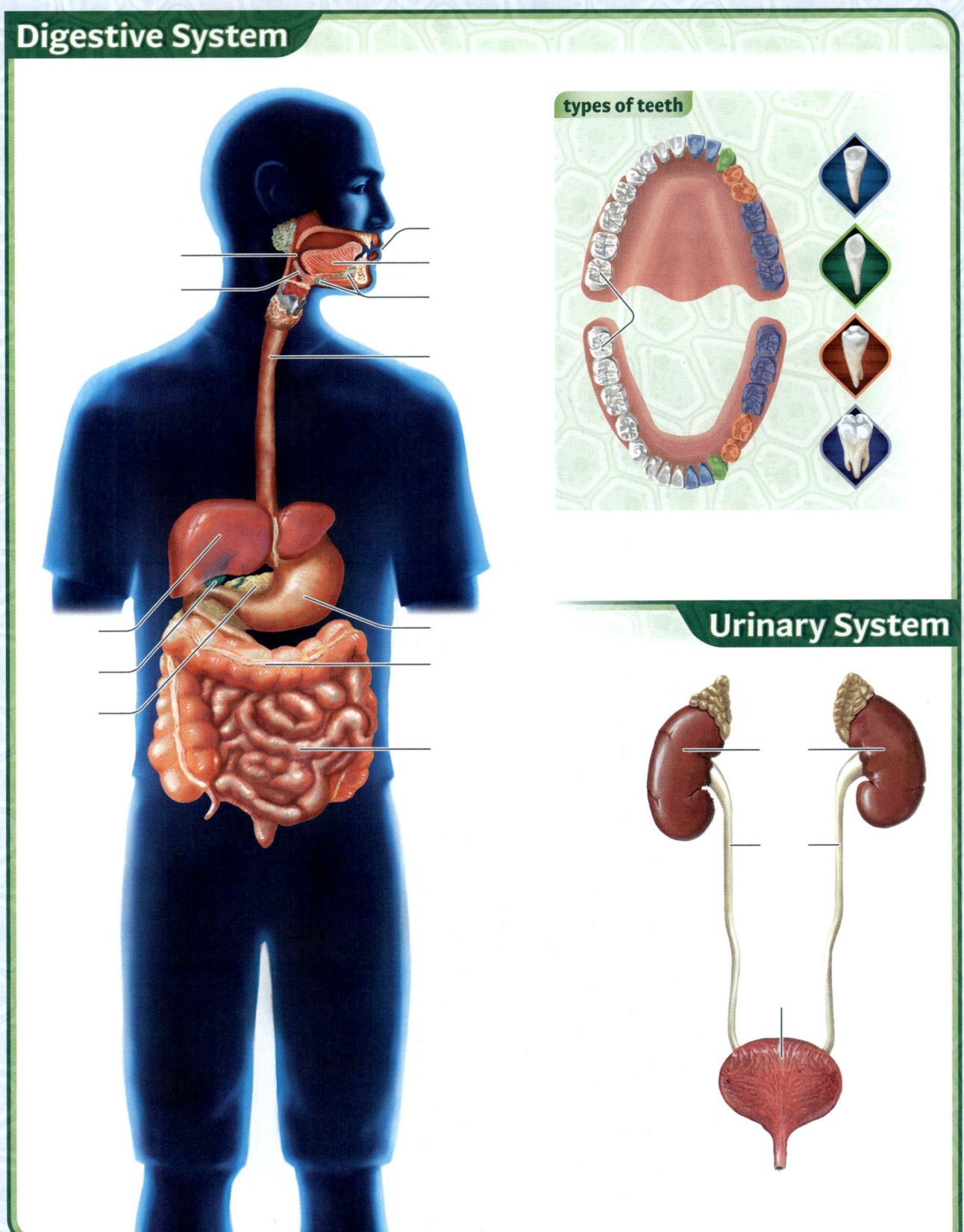

types of teeth

Urinary System

Lymphatic System

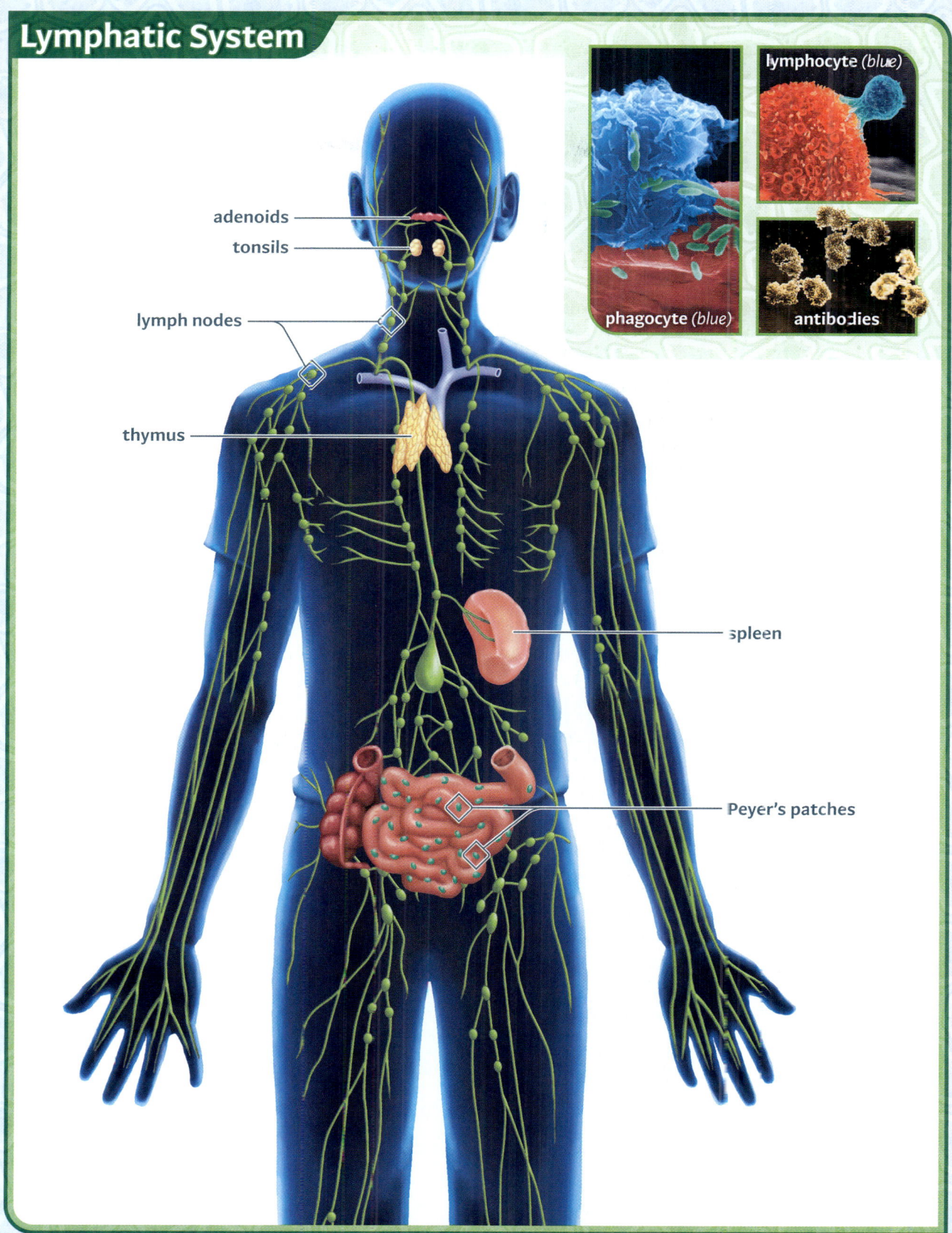

adenoids

tonsils

lymph nodes

thymus

lymphocyte *(blue)*

phagocyte *(blue)*

antibodies

spleen

Peyer's patches

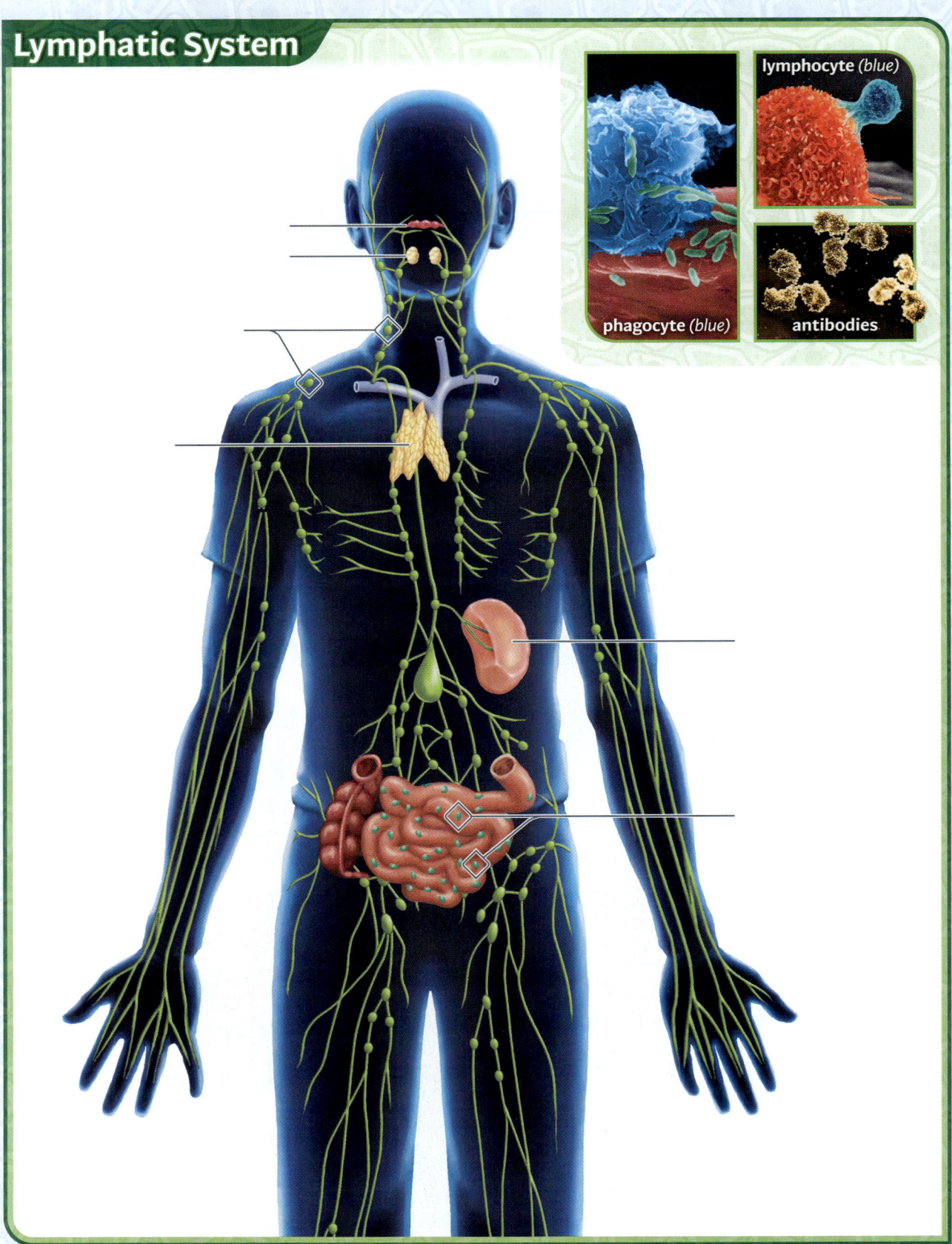

lymphocyte (*blue*)

phagocyte (*blue*)

antibodies

Integumentary System

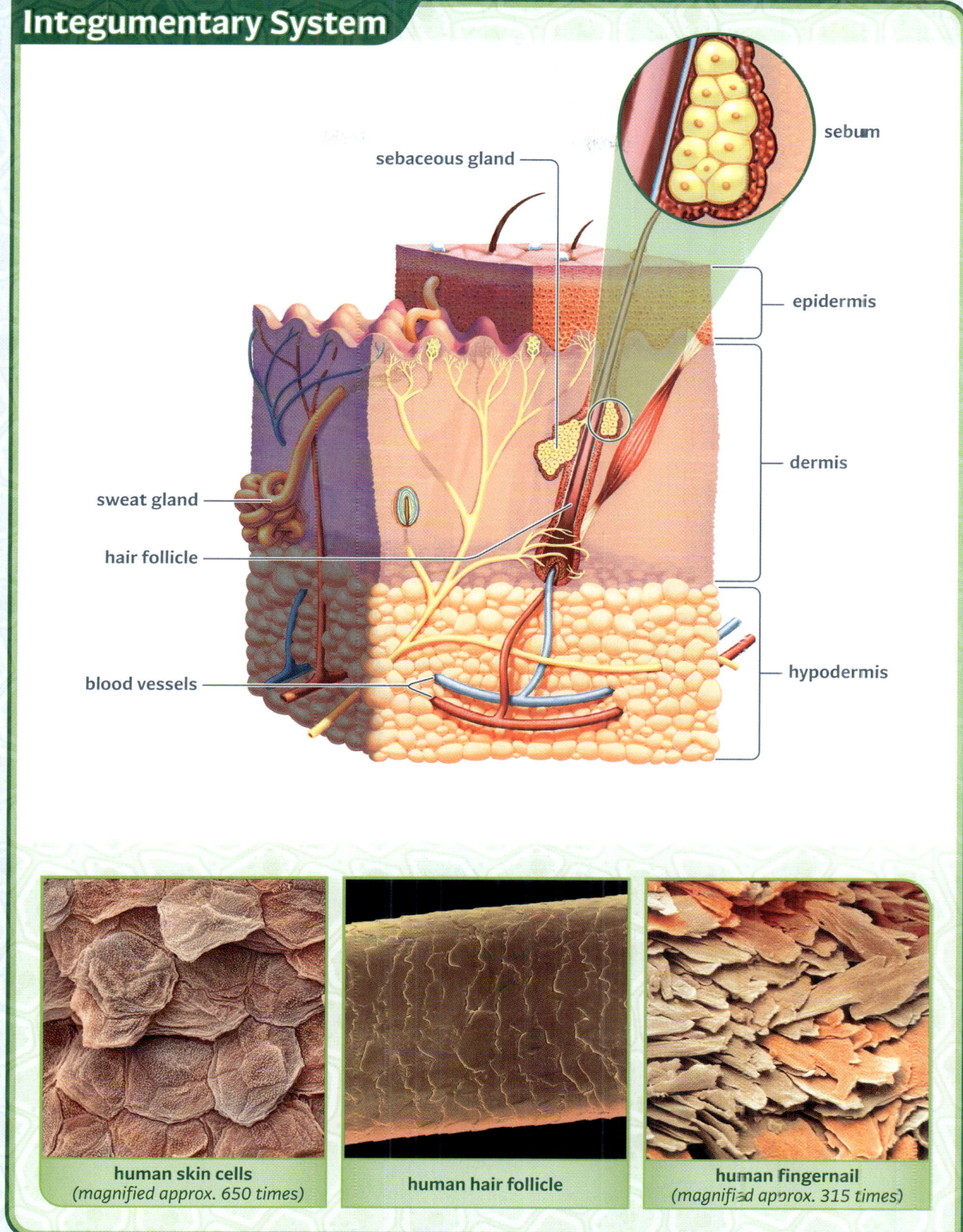

sebum

epidermis

dermis

hypodermis

sebaceous gland

sweat gland

hair follicle

blood vessels

human skin cells
(magnified approx. 650 times)

human hair follicle

human fingernail
(magnified approx. 315 times)

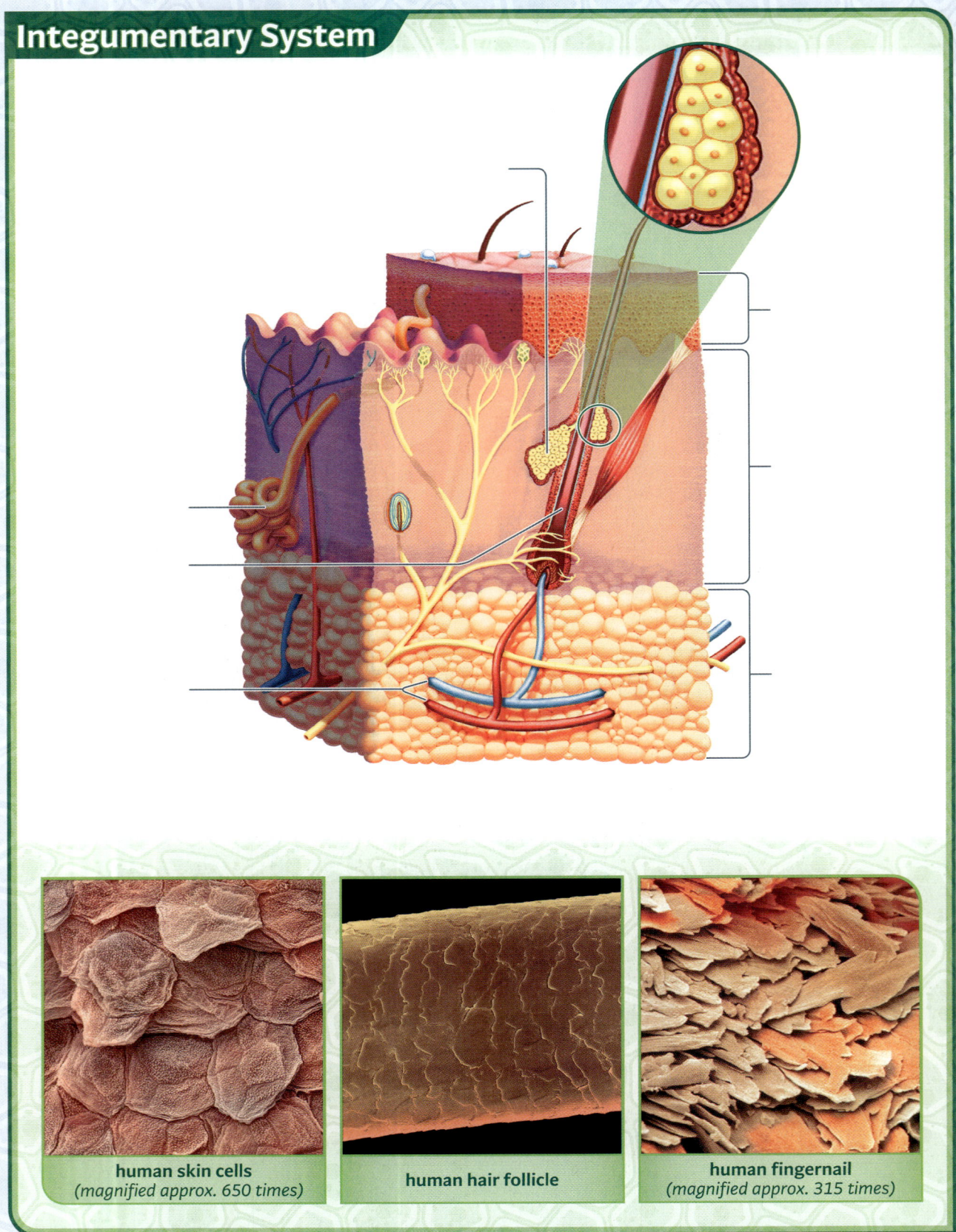

human skin cells
(magnified approx. 650 times)

human hair follicle

human fingernail
(magnified approx. 315 times)

Muscular System

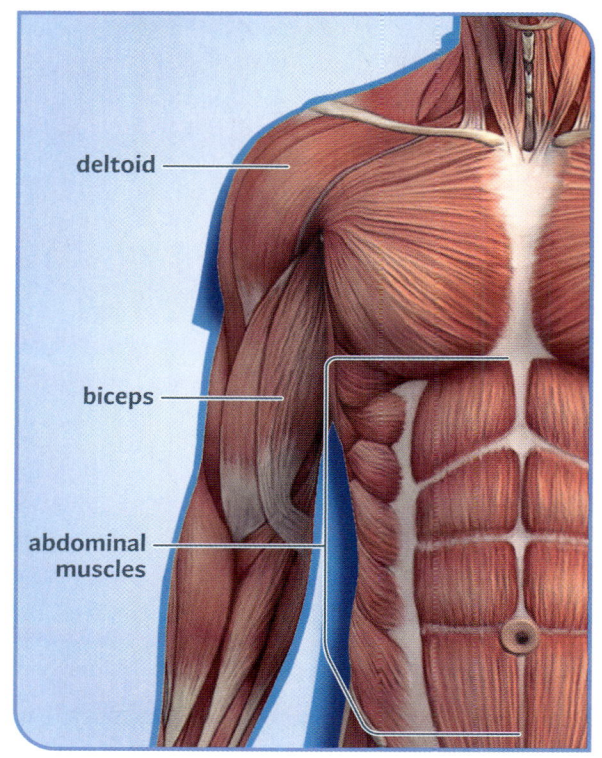

deltoid

biceps

abdominal muscles

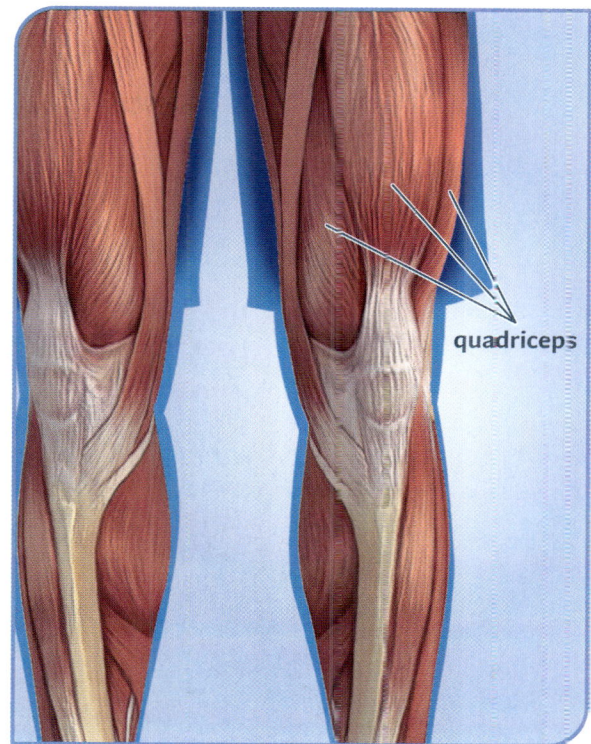

quadriceps

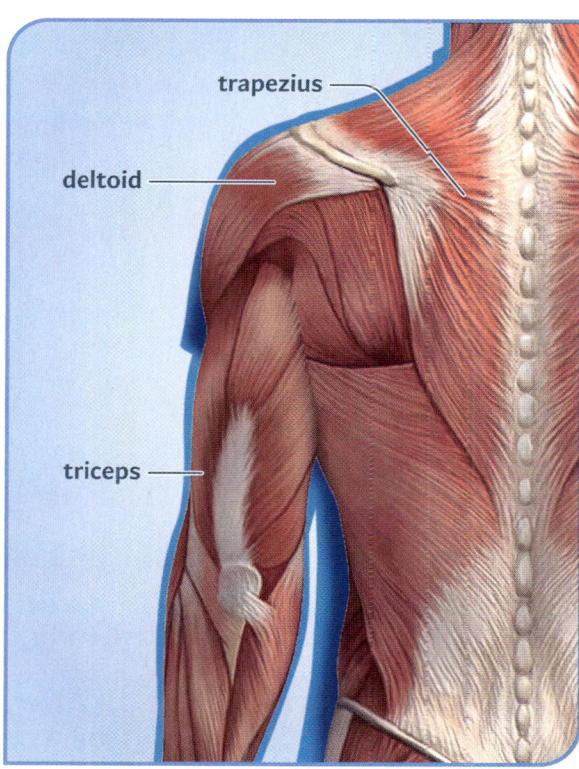

trapezius

deltoid

triceps

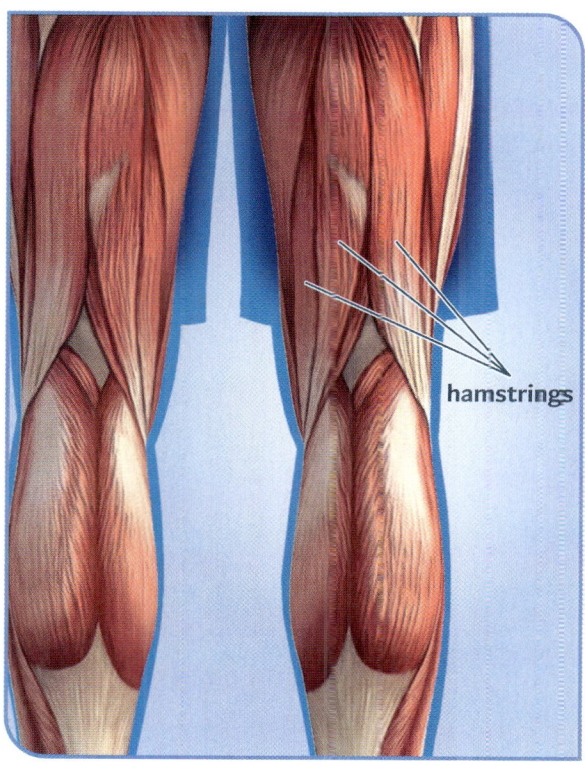

hamstrings

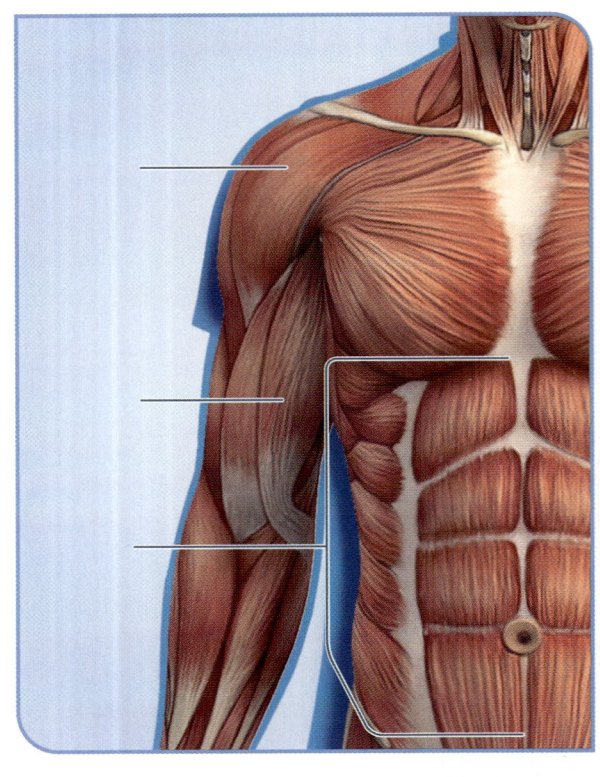
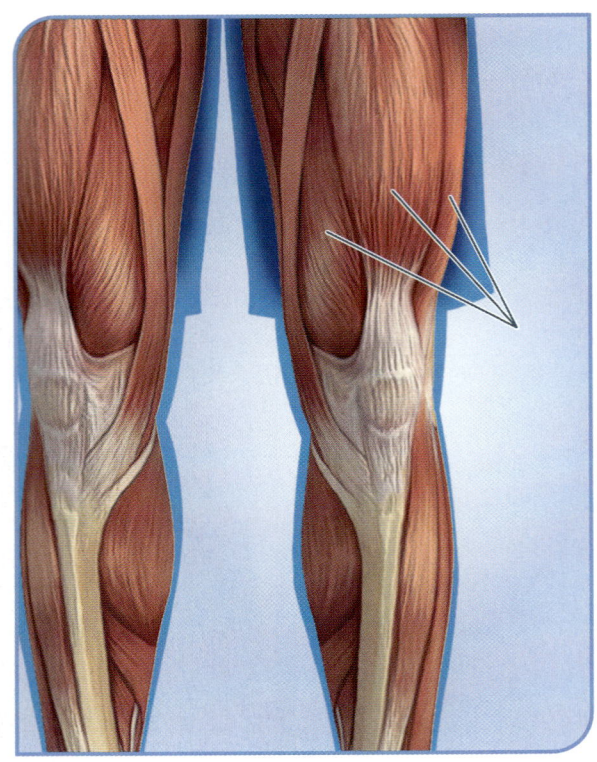
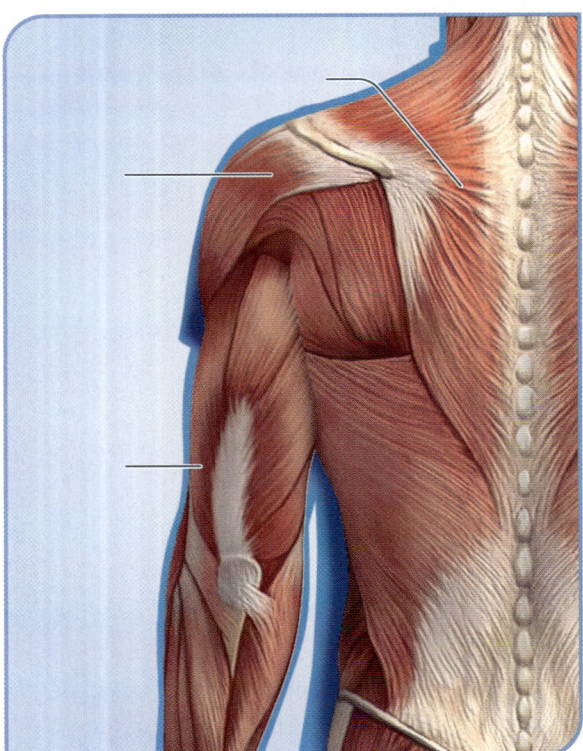
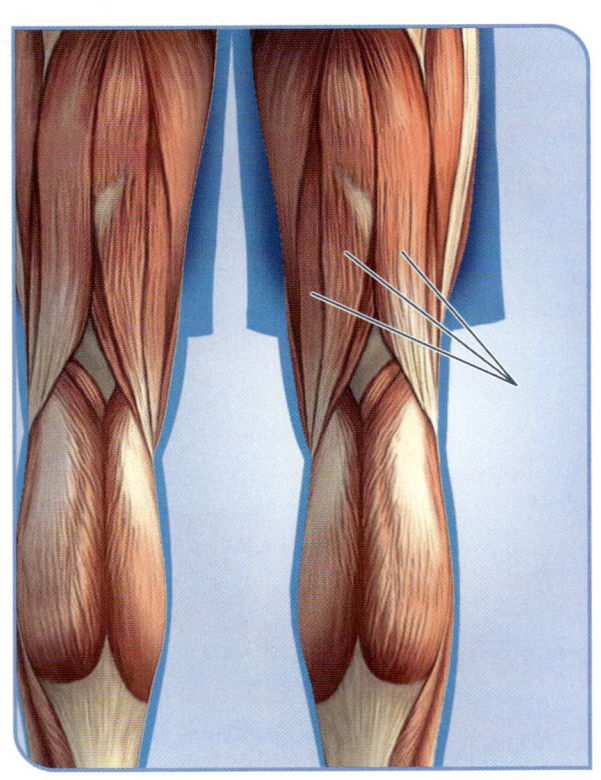

Skeletal System

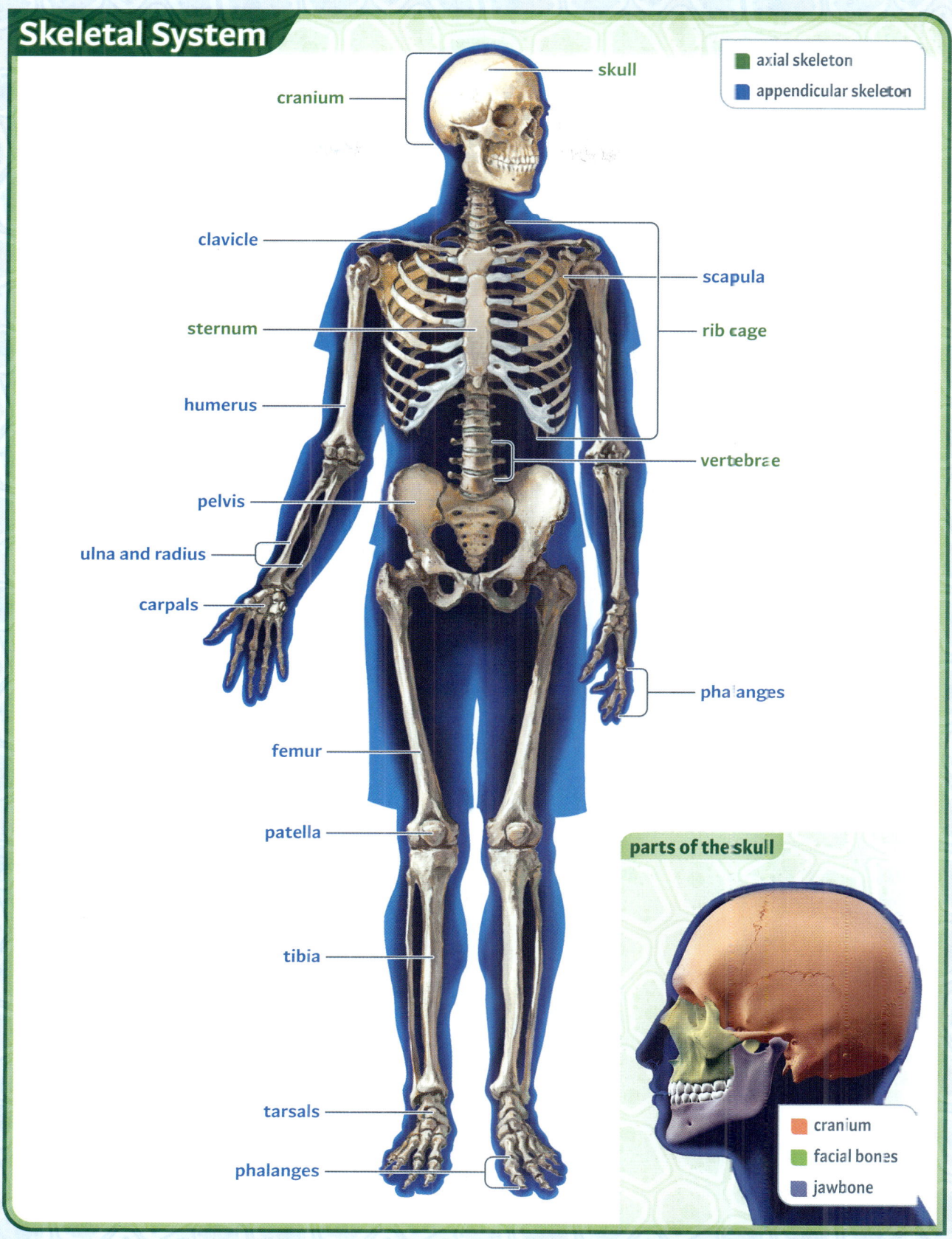

axial skeleton
appendicular skeleton

skull

cranium

clavicle

scapula

sternum

rib cage

humerus

vertebrae

pelvis

ulna and radius

carpals

phalanges

femur

patella

parts of the skull

tibia

tarsals

phalanges

cranium
facial bones
jawbone

Skeletal System

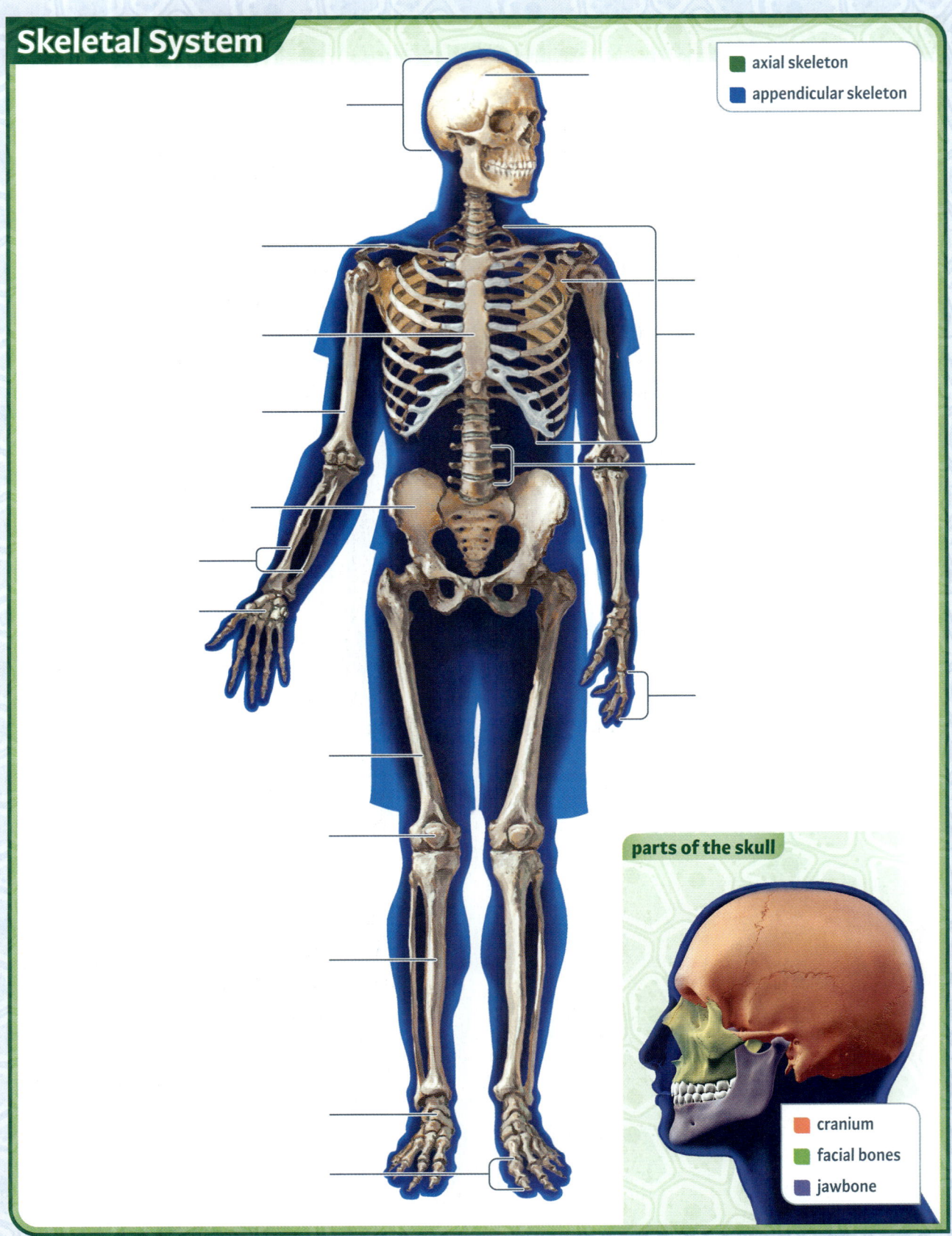

parts of the skull

■ cranium
■ facial bones
■ jawbone

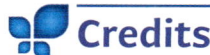

Credits

Photo credits are listed in the order images appear on each page from top to bottom, left to right. Materials provided by the publisher (Abeka) are credited only to clarify location of other images.

Cover: front–FGorgun/iStock via Getty Images, Ian Hooton/Science Photo Library via Getty Images, CasarsaGuru/E+ via Getty Images, Sebastian Kaulitzki/Science Photo Library via Getty Images, newphotoservice/iStock via Getty Images, Ibrahim Akcengiz/iStock via Getty Images; back–Henrik5000/iStock via Getty Images, Hank Grebe/ Stocktrek Images/Science Source, eranicle/iStock via Getty Images; images and design elements used throughout–Natallia Yatskova/iStock via Getty Images, eb75/DigitalVision Vectors via Getty Images, creator76/iStock via Getty Images, ekapanova/iStock via Getty Images, serkorkin/iStock via Getty Images, Image by starline on Freepik, comotion_design/E+ via Getty Images, janulla/iStock via Getty Images, nathaphat/iStock via Getty Images, cnythzl/DigitalVision Vectors via Getty Images, logonest/ Shutterstock.com, artvea/DigitalVision Vectors via Getty Images, artvea/ DigitalVision Vectors via Getty Images, Trifonenko/iStock via Getty Images, Baretsky/iStock via Getty Images, Raman_Shapavalau/iStock via Getty Images, Karolina Madej/iStock via Getty Images, simon2579/DigitalVision Vectors via Getty Images, samarets1984/iStock via Getty Images, bubaone/ DigitalVision Vectors via Getty Images, Bigmouse108/iStock via Getty Images, Mai Vu/iStock via Getty Images, DragonImages/iStock via Getty Images; i–Sebastian Kaulitzki/Science Photo Library via Getty Images; ii–Image by Jomkwan on Freepik; iv–gradyreese/iStock via Getty Images; 2–Image by Freepik (notebook, hands, girl), Image by daniel-007 on Freepik (pen), LSOphoto/iStock via Getty Images, D. Lentz/E+ via Getty Images; 3–AscentXmedia/iStock via Getty Images; 5–simonkr/iStock via Getty Images; 6–Image by Freepik, Image by johnniedavid12412 on Freepik, Image by benzoix on Freepik, Bevan Goldswain/E+ via Getty Images, sturti/ E+ via Getty Images, AndrewSoundarajan/iStock via Getty Images; 8–Jose Luis Pelaez Inc/DigitalVision via Getty Images, Image by Jomkwan on Freepik, Steven McDowell/Science Photo Library via Getty Images, nobeastsofierce/Science Source; 9–someone25/iStock via Getty Images; 10–SciePro/Science Photo Library via Getty Images, Kateryna Kon/Science Source, Innerspace Imaging/Science Source, Sebastian Kaulitzki/ Shutterstock.com; 11–sturti/E+ via Getty Images, Akarawut Lohacharoenvanich/iStock via Getty Images; 13–tassel78/iStock via Getty Images, David Mack/Science Source; 14–PhonlamaiPhoto/iStock via Getty Images, Artur Plawgo/iStock via Getty Images, Kateryna Kon/Science Photo Library via Getty Images, Abeka/Dan Phyllaier, BSIP/Science Source(2), Abeka, 7activestudio - stock.adobe.com; 15–ruizluquepaz/iStock via Getty Images, gorodenkoff/iStock via Getty Images; 16–undefined undefined/ iStock via Getty Images; 17–Image by zacon_studio on Freepik, Image by repinanatoly on Freepik, www.airnow.gov, Image by Macmontree on Freepik, 18–PhotoInc/iStock via Getty Images; 20–Image by Freepik, DWalker44/E+ via Getty Images; 21–Alex Potemkin/E+ via Getty Images, Image by hemul3059 on Freepik; 25–PhotoSG - stock.adobe.com, Ian Hooton/Science Photo Library via Getty Images, Dr_Microbe - stock.adobe .com; 26–monkeybusinessimages/iStock via Getty Images; 27–Traceydee Photography/Moment via Getty Images, Bill Cheyrou/Alamy Stock Photo, Axel Kock - stock.adobe.com; 29–BSIP/Science Source, 7activestudio - stock .adobe.com; 32–Science Photo Library - PASIEKA/Brand X Pictures via Getty Images, Asia-Pacific Images Studio/E+ via Getty Images iLexx/iStock via Getty Images, hudiemm/iStock via Getty Images; 33–SciePro/iStock via Getty Images; 34–Peakstock - stock.adobe.com, Science Photo Library/ Alamy Stock Photo, NIH/Science Source, Ferno Da Cunha/Science Source; 38–pixologicstudio/iStock via Getty Images, Sebastian Kaulitzki - stock .adobe.com; 38, 42–pixologicstudio/Science Photo Library via Getty Images; 39–pepifoto/iStock via Getty Images, Image by yaseen22100 on Freepik, Universal Images Group North America LLC/Alamy Stock Photo, Liudmila Chernetska/iStock via Getty Images, Image by dzlab on Freepik, Image by Freepik, _human/iStock via Getty Images, Image by alexextrememail on Freepik; 40, 42, 57–Sebastian Kaulitzki - stock.adobe.com, 40, 57, 209-210–Sebastian Kaulitzki/Science Photo Library via Getty Images; 41–Olha Rohulya/iStock via Getty Images; 42–Hank Grebe/iStock via Getty Images, Sebastian Kaulitzki/Science Photo Library via Getty Images(5), SciePro/iStock via Getty Images, Adam Smigielski/E+ via Getty Images; 44–pixologicstudio/iStock via Getty Images, Evan Oto/Science Source; 47–FGorgun/iStock via Getty Images, Image by chandlervid85 on Freepik, Diy13/iStock via Getty Images, PeopleImages/iStock via Getty Images, Liudmila Chernetska/iStock via Getty Images; 49–vm/E+ via Getty Images; 51–Six_Characters/iStock via Getty Images, Ekkasit Jokthong/iStock via Getty Images, FG Trade/iStock via Getty Images, Juanmonino/iStock via Getty Images, PrathanChorruangsak/iStock via Getty Images;

53–ediebloom/iStock via Getty Images, indigolotos/iStock via Getty Images, Mukhina1/iStock via Getty Images, peakstock/iStock via Getty Images; 54–Image by xb100 on Freepik, skynesher/E+ via Getty Images; 55–Image by EyeEm on Freepik, Image by fabrikasimf on Freepik, Elena Bioryisheva-Abramova/iStock via Getty Images, ka i9/E+ via Getty Images; 59–Sissoupitch/iStock via Getty Images; 62–Ekaterina79/iStock via Getty Images, kali9/E+ via Getty Images, Yir Yang/E+ via Getty Images, karandaev/iStock via Getty Images, Image by user6694312 on Freepik; 63–Image by Freepik (bread), Image by anja ikulathunga on Freepik (honey), Image by azerbaijan_stockers on Freepik (pasta), Image by splitov27 on Freepik (bananas), Image by stockking on Freepik (potatoes), Image by voyager_human on Freepik (seeds); 64–DNY59/E+ via Getty Images, Bohdan Bevz/iStock via Getty Images; 65–Image by user6170755 on Freepik (sirloin, pork chops), Image by gofurxp2 on Freepik (chicken), Image by kues1 on Freepik (black background), Image by timolina on Freepik (salmon), Image by Freepik (eggs), Image by komthong wongsangiam on Freepik (red beans), Image by Pineapple_Studio on Freepik (almonds), Image by artyomstock89 on Freepik (olive oil), Image by Freepik (butter), Image by KamranAydinov on Freepik french fries), Image by Freepik (honey bun), Image by azerbaijan_stockers on Freepik (sunflower seeds), Image by Racool_studio on Freepik (coconut), Image by user6170755 on Freepik (fish), Image by tania.kitura on Freepik (plate); 66–Image by artyomstock89 on Freepik (olive oil), Image by da-ga on Freepik (butter), Image by idea route on Freepik (hamburger), Image by Turbo Render on Freepik (French fries), Image by user6170755 on Freepik (chicken), Image by fernatiroman on Freepik (hot dogs), Image by timolina on Freepik (coconut), Image by AI Artwork on Freepik (pastry), Image by topntp26 on Freepik (cookies), Image by chandlervid85 on Freepik (olive oil), Image by atlascompany on Freepik (salmon), Image by AndreyStar on Freepik (sunflower seeds), Image by opasstudio on Freepik (mackerel); 67–pipat wongsawang/Moment via Getty Images, olegkalina/iStock via Getty Images; 69–Image by user20119892 on Freepik, Image by EyeEm on Freepik; 70–Image by Freepik (food group, bread), Image by arso74 on Freepik (egg), Image by azerbaijan_stockers on Freepik (oranges), Image by timolina on Freepik (salmon), Image by kues1 on Freepik (black baground), Image by dmitr1ch on Freepik (sunflower seeds), Image by user14908974 on Freepik (spinach), fcafotodigital/iStock via Getty Images (pills); 71–Image by Freepik (food group), Image by atlascompany on Freepik (salmon), Image by toonsangaroon on Freepik (carrots), Image by zacon_studio on Freepik (spinach), Image by korarkar on Freepik (yellow bell pepper), Image by da-ga on Freepik (butter), Image by vasyl24 on Freepik (broken egg), Image by Freepik (milk, grapefruit), Image by yulia mikhaylova on Freepik (bread), angorius - stock.adobe.com (liver); Image by user6170755 on Freepik (chicken), Image by agartish on Freepik (oats), Image by Nhay Gallery on Freepik (eggs), Image by holiday.photc.top on Freepik (almonds) Image by jonganu on Freepik (orange), Image by 8photo on Freepik (lemon), Image by niksads on Freepik (lime), Image by maryloco22 on Freepik (red bell pepper), Image by azerbaijan_stockers on Freepik (green bell pepper), Image by julia-buz on Freepik (pineapple), Image by repinanatoly on Freepik (broccoli), Image by wadeeda on Freepik (cauliflower), Image by t_limura on Freepik (strawberries), Image by frendcornerkim on Freepik (papaya), Image by kossovskiy on Freepik (cheese), Image by chestorm66 on Freepik (sardines), Image by Johndon on Freepik (yogurt), Image by asier_ relampagoestudio on Freepik (tuna), Image by holiday.photo.top on Freepik (almonds), Image by sommail on Freepik (mango), Image by user13662878 on Freepik (peanuts), Image by Shipors Creative on Freepik (avocado), Image by AndreyStar on Freepik (sunflower seeds), Image by Esin Deniz on Freepik (hazelnuts), Image by mikeos on Freepik (blueberries), Image by Macmontree on Freepik (kale); 72–Image by zacon_studio on Freepik (carrots), Image by jcomp on Freepik (milk), Image by sweethomeandroom88 on Freepik (oysters), Image by stockking on Freepik (cheese), JohnnyMad/ iStock via Getty Images (iodized salt), Image by romandbree on Freepik (granola), Image by timolina on Freepik (steak), Image by artemshon Freepik (salt), Image by user31792867 on Freepik (orange); 73–Image by zacon_studio on Freepik (carrots), Image by chestorm66 on Freepik (sardines), Image by Racool_studio on Freepik (broccoli), Image by holiday. photo.top on Freepik (almonds), Image by kcssovskiy on Freepik (cheese), Image by zacon_studio on Freepik (spinach) Image by Freepik (milk), Image by mikeos on Freepik (figs), Image by JSakorn on Freepik (red beans) Image by Johndon on Freepik (yogurt), Image by user25234940 on Freepik (soybeans), Image by yuliamikhaylova on Freepik (bread), Image by

Glossary

Location in Terms box indicated by bold page number.

A

abdominal muscles: muscles that cover the abdomen; help balance and posture (pp. **140**, 142)

absorption: process by which digested nutrients are taken into the bloodstream (p. **99**)

abuse: situation in which someone deliberately ignores another person's boundaries for the purpose of causing harm (pp. **169**, 170)

acne: skin condition in which clogged pores cause blemishes, or pimples (pp. **132**, 135)

added sugar: sugar that is not naturally present in a food but has been added in its preparation (pp. **77**, 80)

addiction: continual, controlling behavior that changes the way the brain functions (p. **179**)

adenoids: a group of lymph nodes at the back of the nose (pp. **123**, 124)

adolescence: transitional time of growth and development between childhood and adulthood (p. **132**)

aerobic endurance: ability of the body to do strenuous work over long periods of time (pp. **23**, 25)

aerobic exercise: exercise that causes muscles to use more oxygen; endurance exercise (pp. **140**, 143)

alimentary canal: long, muscular tube through which food travels in the digestive system; includes the mouth, esophagus, stomach, small intestine, and large intestine (p. **94**)

allergen: protein or other substance that causes an allergic reaction (pp. **77**, 80)

alveoli: the tiny air sacs in the lungs; thin walls allow the exchange of gases between the air and blood (alveolus, *sing.*) (pp. **18**, 19)

anaerobic exercise: exercise in which muscles do not use more oxygen; requires strength, speed, and agility rather than endurance (pp. **140**, 143)

anaphylaxis: most severe allergic reaction; affects the whole body by causing difficulty breathing, a drop in blood pressure, and swelling of various body parts (pp. **77**, 80)

anatomy: study of the structure and parts of the body (p. **2**)

antibodies: Y-shaped molecules made by lymphocytes to help protect the body from disease and infection (pp. **118**, 120)

aorta: the body's largest artery; receives blood from the left ventricle of the heart; branches into arteries that carry blood to the rest of the body (pp. **23**, 24)

appendicular skeleton: division of the skeleton that includes the shoulders, hips, arms, and legs (p. **149**)

artery: blood vessel that takes blood away from the heart (pp. **12**, 15)

atherosclerosis: buildup of fatty deposits in an artery (pp. **23**, 25)

atrium: upper chamber of the heart (atria, *plural*) (pp. **23**, 24)

auditory canal: tube of the outer ear through which sound waves travel (pp. **49**, 52)

auditory nerve: nerve that carries messages of hearing from the cochlea to the brain (pp. **49**, 52)

axial skeleton: division of the skeleton that includes the head, spine, and ribs (p. **149**)

axon: long, straight part of a neuron that extends from the cell body (pp. **32**, 35)

bacterium: single-celled microorganism that does not have a cell nucleus (bacteria, *plural*) (pp. **112**, 113)

balanced diet: diet containing all the nutrients necessary to keep you healthy (p. **83**)

B-complex vitamins: eight vitamins that help to digest food and use it for energy (p. **70**)

biceps: upper-arm muscle that bends the arm (pp. **140**, 141)

bile: a greenish digestive juice produced by the liver; performs emulsification of fats (pp. **99**, 101)

bladder: expandable pouch that stores urine (pp. **104**, 106)

blood: liquid tissue that carries substances throughout the body; main parts are plasma, red blood cells, white blood cells, and platelets (p. **12**)

blood pressure: the pressure of blood against the artery walls (pp. **23**, 25)

blood vessels: tubes that carry blood throughout the body; arteries, capillaries, and veins (pp. **12**, 15)

bone marrow: soft tissue in the open spaces of a bone (p. **149**)

boundaries: rules or guidelines for appropriate behavior from yourself and others (pp. **169**, 170)

brain: main organ of the nervous system; controls the body (p. **38**)

brain stem: controls involuntary functions of the body; "turns off" and "turns on" cerebrum for sleeping and waking (pp. **38**, 40)

bronchi: the air tubes that allow air to enter the lungs (bronchus, *sing.*) (p. **18**)

bronchioles: the smallest air tubes in the lungs (pp. **18**, 19)

bullying: trying to gain control over someone by taunting him or by making him feel unsafe (pp. **169**, 171)

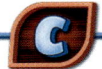

caffeine: drug that is naturally found in the leaves or fruits of some plants; forces the kidneys to give up more water, increasing the amount of urine produced and the amount of water lost by the body (pp. **104**, 106)

calcium: the most common mineral found in the body (p. 72)

calorie: measure of the amount of energy stored in food (p. **77**)

cancer: disease caused by the uncontrolled growth of body cells (pp. **112**, 116)

capillary: the smallest type of blood vessel; links arteries and veins (pp. **12**, 15)

carbohydrates: group of macronutrients that includes sugars and starches; the body's main source of energy (pp. **62**, 63)

cardiac arrest: serious medical emergency in which a person's heart stops beating (pp. **174**, 177)

cardiopulmonary resuscitation (CPR): life-saving procedure that can be used when the heart stops beating (pp. **174**, 177)

carotene: chemical found in green or deep-yellow fruits and vegetables (p. 70)

carpals: bones of the wrist (pp. **152**, 154)

cell: smallest unit of any living thing (pp. **8**, 9)

cell body: central part of a neuron containing the nucleus and organelles (pp. **32**, 35)

central nervous system (CNS): major part of the nervous system consisting of the brain and spinal cord (pp. **32**, 33)

cerebellum: part of the brain that controls balance and coordination of voluntary muscles (pp. **38**, 39)

cerebrum: largest part of the brain; controls the process of thinking and reasoning; receives and interprets information from sense organs (pp. **38**, 39)

cilia: hair-like projections that keep pathogens from getting into the lungs (cilium, *sing.*) (pp. **118**, 119)

circulation: the continuous flow of blood within the body (pp. **12**, 14)

circulatory system: body system that circulates blood throughout the body; main parts are blood, heart, and blood vessels (p. **12**)

clavicle: collarbone; attaches to the top of the sternum (pp. **152**, 153)

cochlea: part of the ear that detects sound waves and sends them as messages to the brain (pp. **49**, 52)

communicable disease: disease that can be spread from person to person (pp. **112**, 113)

complex carbohydrates: large molecules made of many connected sugar molecules; also called starches (pp. **62**, 63)

concussion: brain injury in which the brain is shaken inside the skull (pp. **174**, 177)

cornea: transparent front portion of the eye; lets light into the eye (pp. **49**, 50)

cranial nerve: nerve that branches directly from the brain (pp. **44**, 46)

cranium: part of the skull that covers the brain (pp. **152**, 153)

cross-contamination: transfer of harmful microorganisms from one object to another (pp. **83**, 88)

cyberbullying: use of electronic devices to bully by sending, posting, or sharing harmful or embarrassing content (pp. **169**, 172)

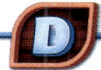

dehydration: loss of water from body tissues (pp. **162**, 164)

deltoid: muscle that forms the curve of the shoulder and lifts the arm (pp. **140**, 141)

dendrite: short, branching part of a neuron that extends from the cell body (pp. **32**, 35)

dental caries: disease caused by bacteria inside the mouth; also called cavities (pp. **132**, 136)

dentin: hard, bone-like tissue that gives a tooth its shape (pp. **132**, 136)

dermis: inner layer of skin beneath the epidermis (pp. **132**, 134)

diabetes mellitus: disease that causes extra sugar to collect in the blood (pp. **112**, 116)

diaphragm: main muscle of breathing; moves down to inhale and up to exhale (pp. **18**, 19)

digestion: the process of breaking down food into a form that the body can use (p. **94**)

digestive system: body system that performs digestion (p. **94**)

disease: any condition that causes the body to work in an incorrect way (p. **112**)

drug: a chemical substance that causes changes in your body, mind, or behavior (p. **179**)

drug misuse (substance misuse): using a drug in an improper way or for an improper purpose (p. **179**)

eardrum: thin piece of tissue that separates the outer ear from the middle ear (pp. **49**, 52)

electrolytes: minerals that help regulate the body's water balance (pp. **162**, 163)

enamel: protective outer covering of a tooth's crown; hardest substance in the body (pp. **132**, 136)

enzyme: any of the special chemicals that perform chemical reactions within the body (pp. **94**, 96)

epidermis: outer layer of skin (pp. **132**, 134)

esophagus: muscular tube that carries food from the pharynx to the stomach (pp. **94**, 96)

excretion: removal of unneeded substances from the body (pp. **104**, 105)

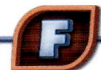

fats: nutrients that help the body to store energy, make cell parts, and use certain vitamins (pp. **62**, 65)

fat-soluble vitamins: vitamins that can be stored in your body; vitamins A, D, E, and K (p. **69**)

femur: long bone in the upper leg (pp. **152**, 154)

fiber: carbohydrates that the body cannot break down and absorb (pp. **62**, 64)

first aid: emergency care or treatment given to a person who is injured or suddenly becomes ill until professional medical help arrives (p. **174**)

food allergy: situation in which the immune system overreacts to a food protein that has entered the bloodstream (pp. **77**, 80)

frostbite: the freezing of body tissue (pp. **162**, 163)

gang: group of people who use violence or crime to gain power and who identify themselves with a group name or symbol (pp. **169**, 172)

grains: the seeds and fruits of certain types of grass plants (pp. **83**, 85)

---

hair follicle: small tube in the dermis that makes hair (pp. **132**, 134)

hamstrings: group of muscles in the back of the upper leg; bend the knee (pp. **140**, 142)

health: complete well-being of a person; includes the material body and immaterial spirit (pp. **2**, 3)

heart: main organ of the circulatory system; powerful muscle that circulates blood throughout the body (pp. **12**, 14)

heat exhaustion: condition in which heat and dehydration limit the body's ability to control its internal temperature (pp. **162**, 164)

hemoglobin: special protein that red blood cells use to carry oxygen; contains the mineral iron (pp. **12**, 13)

histamine: chemical messenger that triggers inflammation (pp. **118**, 120)

hormone: chemical messenger that regulates how the body works (pp. **132**, 133)

humerus: long bone in the upper arm (pp. **152**, 153)

hydration: replacing water that has been lost from the body (p. **104**)

hydrogenated oil: unsaturated vegetable oil that has had hydrogen atoms added to make the oil more solid (pp. **62**, 66)

hygiene: cleanliness habits that prevent disease and promote health (pp. **132**, 134)

hypodermis: layer of fat cells below the dermis; deepest layer of the integumentary system (pp. **132**, 134)

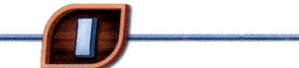

immune system: the body system that defends against pathogens (p. **118**)

immunity: the body's ability to resist and protect itself against infectious diseases (p. **118**)

inflammation: increased blood flow caused by histamine; makes the tissue become red, swollen, and tender (pp. **118**, 120)

inhalants: chemicals that are breathed in through the nose or mouth as a vapor (pp. **179**, 181)

inner ear: division of the ear that contains the cochlea and semicircular canals (pp. **49**, 52)

insulin: hormone, or chemical messenger, made in the pancreas; helps the body remove excess sugar from the blood (pp. **99**, 102)

integumentary system: the body system that covers and protects the body; includes the skin, hair, and nails (pp. **132**, 134)

involuntary muscles: muscles that work automatically without your thinking about them (p. **140**)

iodine: helps the thyroid gland to do its job; helps in proper bone and brain development during pregnancy and infancy (p. 73)

iris: ring of muscles that surrounds the pupil and controls its size; colored part of the eye (pp. **49**, 50)

iron: helps the body make hemoglobin (p. 73)

joint: place where two or more bones join (pp. **149**, 151)

kidneys: bean-shaped organs that filter the blood (pp. **104**, 105)

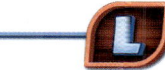

lactic acid: waste product formed during strenuous exercise (pp. **140**, 144)

large intestine: the last organ of the alimentary canal; prepares undigested food to be removed from the body as waste (pp. **99**, 100)

larynx: voice box (p. **18**)

lens: focuses light that enters the eye by refracting it; changes shape to focus on objects at different distances (pp. **49**, 50)

ligament: strong, elastic band of fibrous tissue that connects bones and stabilizes joints (pp. **149**, 151)

limbic system: part of the brain that helps you coordinate emotions, alerts you of physical needs, and is important for forming memories; includes an emotional reward system (pp. **38**, 40)

liver: the largest organ inside the body; recycles red blood cells to produce bile salts, stores and processes nutrients, and filters blood (pp. **99**, 101)

long bone: bone that is longer than it is wide and has enlarged ends (p. **149**)

lungs: main organs of the respiratory system; absorb oxygen from the air into the blood and release carbon dioxide from the blood into the air (p. **18**)

lung capacity: the amount of air that the lungs can hold (pp. **23**, 25)

lymph: tissue fluid that has been forced into lymph vessels (p. **123**)

lymph capillaries: the smallest vessels of the lymphatic system (p. **123**)

lymph nodes: large bunches of lymphatic tissue located throughout the body (pp. **123**, 124)

lymph vessel: a transportation vessel for lymph (p. **123**)

lymphatic system: part of the immune system that collects tissue fluid and cleans the body of pathogens (p. **123**)

lymphocytes: white blood cells that recognize and attack invading pathogens, produce antibodies, and can become memory cells (pp. **118**, 120)

lysozyme: special enzyme found in tears that can kill bacteria (pp. **118**, 119)

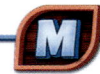

macronutrients: nutrients that the body needs in relatively large amounts; can be used by the body as sources of energy (p. **62**)

magnesium: affects how the nervous system works and regulates muscle contractions (p. 72)

marijuana: drug made from the leaves and blossoms of the hemp, or cannabis, plant (pp. **179**, 181)

medical emergency: any illness or injury requiring immediate care (p. **174**)

metabolism: the process by which the body produces and uses energy from food (p. **77**)

micronutrients: nutrients that are needed by the body in small amounts; help protect body systems and help them work properly (p. **69**)

microorganism: microscopic organism; also called microbe (pp. **112**, 113)

middle ear: division of the ear that is a cavity inside the skull; contains three tiny bones: the hammer, the anvil, and the stirrup (pp. **49**, 52)

minerals: chemical elements that are needed as micronutrients (pp. **69**, 72)

motor nerve fiber: nerve fiber that controls some part of the body by delivering messages from the central nervous system; carries a single message to an individual cell or group of cells (pp. **44**, 45)

mucus: thick, sticky fluid that traps pathogens; produced by mucous membranes (pp. **118**, 119)

muscle tone: the steady contraction of muscles against each other (pp. **140**, 143)

muscular system: body system that provides movement (p. **140**)

MyPlate: tool, prepared by the U.S. Department of Agriculture, that helps you choose a variety of foods to obtain the nutrients that your body needs each day; divides foods into fruits, vegetables, protein, grains, and dairy (p. **83**)

nerve: organ made of bundles of nerve fibers; transmits messages between the central nervous system and one or more specific regions of the body (p. **44**)

nervous system: body system that coordinates and controls all activities of the body; brain, spinal cord, and nerves (p. **32**)

neurology: medical study of the nervous system (pp. **32**, 33)

neuron: nerve cell; cell that transmits messages within the body (pp. **32**, 35)

nicotine: drug found in tobacco products (pp. **179**, 180)

noncommunicable disease: disease that cannot be spread from person to person (pp. **112**, 113)

nonperishable food: food that does not require refrigeration or freezing; includes fresh fruits and vegetables, most foods in unopened cans and bottles, baked goods, and most types of dried foods (pp. **83**, 88)

nutrients: substances in food that the body uses to grow, have energy, and stay healthy (p. **62**)

Nutrition Facts label: tool that tells the most important nutritional information for every kind of packaged food (pp. **77**, 78)

obesity: the condition of having too much body fat (pp. **112**, 117)

optic nerve: cranial nerve that carries messages of sight to the cerebrum (pp. **49**, 51)

organ: structure made of several types of tissue to perform a definite function for a system (pp. **8**, 9)

outer ear: division of the ear that consists of the cup-shaped structure on the side of the head and of the auditory canal (pp. **49**, 52)

over-the-counter (OTC) drugs: medicines that can be purchased without a prescription (pp. **179**, 181)

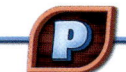

pancreas: digestive organ located between the stomach and small intestine; produces pancreatic juice and insulin (pp. **99**, 101)

patella: kneecap (pp. **152**, 154)

pathogen: microorganism that can cause disease; a germ (pp. **112**, 113)

pelvis: hipbone (pp. **152**, 154)

percent Daily Value (% Daily Value or %DV): how much one serving of a food contributes to a nutrient's total daily amount (pp. **77**, 79)

peripheral nervous system (PNS): major part of the nervous system consisting of nerves and of sense organs (pp. **32**, 33)

perishable food: food that can spoil easily and must be refrigerated or frozen; includes most foods containing meat, eggs, or dairy products (pp. **83**, 88)

Peyer's patches: groups of lymph nodes in the walls of the small intestine (pp. **123**, 124)

phagocytes: white blood cells that find, surround, and destroy pathogens (pp. **118**, 119)

phalanges: finger, thumb, and toe bones (pp. **152**, 154)

pharynx: throat (p. **18**)

phosphorus: helps give rigidity, or hardness, to the bones and teeth (p. 72)

physical fitness: body's ability to function at its best during daily physical activities without tiring easily (p. **140**)

plaque: film of harmful bacteria that forms on teeth (pp. **132**, 136)

plasma: straw-colored liquid part of the blood; makes up over 50% of blood (pp. **12**, 13)

platelets: part of blood that covers open wounds and enables blood to clot (pp. **12**, 14)

poison: substance that causes harm, illness, or death when it is consumed or absorbed into the body (pp. **174**, 177)

potassium: helps regulate the movement of muscles, including the heart, and helps deliver nerve messages (p. 72)

protein: macronutrients that provide material for body growth and repair (pp. **62**, 65)

puberty: process of physical changes during adolescence (p. **132**)

pulp: soft tissue within the dentin that contains nerves and blood vessels (pp. **132**, 136)

pulse: the expanding of the arteries after each heartbeat; used to measure heart rate (pp. **23**, 25)

pupil: round hole that lets light into the eye (pp. **49**, 50)

quadriceps: group of muscles in the front of the upper leg; straighten the knee (pp. **140**, 142)

Recommended Dietary Allowance (RDA): the typical daily amount of a nutrient that a healthy individual needs, considering age and other factors (pp. **77**, 78)

red blood cells: blood cells that absorb oxygen in the lungs and carry it throughout the body (pp. **12**, 13)

reflex: quick, automatic action that the body does in response to something else (pp. **38**, 42)

respiration: the process of inhaling (breathing in) and exhaling (breathing out) air (pp. **18**, 19)

respiratory system: body system that brings oxygen into the body and exchanges it with carbon dioxide (p. **18**)

retina: layer of nerve cells in the back of the eye; contains rod cells and cone cells (pp. **49**, 51)

rib cage: bones that protect the heart and lungs (pp. **152**, 153)

ruptured eardrum: injury of a torn eardrum (pp. **49**, 53)

saliva: digestive juice in the mouth (pp. **94**, 96)

salivary glands: digestive glands in the mouth that produce saliva (pp. **94**, 96)

saturated fats: fats that are usually solid at room temperature (pp. **62**, 66)

scapula: shoulder blade (pp. **152**, 153)

sclera: white of the eye (pp. **49**, 50)

sebum: oily substance produced by sebaceous glands (pp. **132**, 135)

semicircular canals: three inner-ear structures that detect movements of the head; send information that the brain uses to help keep balance (pp. **49**, 52)

sense receptor: special cell or group of cells that detects a sensation and sends a message on a sensory nerve fiber (pp. **44**, 45)

sensory nerve fiber: nerve fiber that carries signals from the body to the central nervous system (pp. **44**, 45)

septum: wall of muscle that separates the right side of the heart from the left side (pp. **23**, 24)

serving size: the portion of a food that an adult will usually eat in one sitting (pp. **77**, 78)

shock: sudden loss of blood flow that causes blood pressure to drop (pp. **174**, 176)

simple carbohydrates: sugars; have molecules that are small and relatively simple (pp. **62**, 63)

skeletal system: framework of bones that support and protect the body (p. **149**)

skull: group of bones that protect the brain, ears, and eyes (pp. **152**, 153)

small intestine: twenty-foot-long tube of muscle and other tissues that is coiled up just below the stomach; digests most food and absorbs most nutrients (p. **99**)

sodium: helps regulate water balance in the body (p. 72)

SPF: sun protection factor; tells the amount of UV rays being filtered (pp. **162**, 164)

spinal cord: bundle of nerve cells attached to the base of the brain stem; carries messages between the brain and the rest of the body (pp. **38**, 42)

spinal nerve: nerve that branches from the spinal cord and travels to the muscles and organs (pp. **44**, 46)

spleen: largest organ of the lymphatic system; cleanses the blood (pp. **123**, 124)

spongy bone: lightweight, porous tissue that reduces a bone's weight (p. **149**)

sprain: stretched or torn ligament (pp. **174**, 177)

sternum: breastbone (pp. **152**, 153)

stewardship: managing what belongs to someone else as a caretaker (pp. **2**, 3)

stomach: digestive organ that is a small elastic bag made of bands of muscles; breaks down and stores food (pp. **94**, 97)

strain: pulled muscle or tendon resulting from a tear (pp. **174**, 177)

stress: the way that the body responds to unfamiliar or difficult circumstances (pp. **44**, 46)

system: group of organs working together to do a specific job for the body (pp. **8**, 10)

tarsals: bones of the ankle (pp. **152**, 154)

tendon: cord of white fibers that connects muscle to bone (pp. **140**, 141)

thymus: lymphatic organ that prepares lymphocytes to fight pathogens (pp. **123**, 125)

tibia: main bone of the lower leg; shinbone (pp. **152**, 154)

tissue: group of cells working together to perform a single function for the body (pp. **8**, 9)

tissue fluid: fluid that surrounds cells, keeps cells clean and balanced with liquid (p **123**)

tonsils: a group of lymph nodes at the back of the throat (pp. **123**, 124)

trace elements: minerals that the body needs extremely tiny amounts of (pp. **69**, 73)

trachea: windpipe (p. **18**)

trapezius: back muscle that moves the shoulder and turns the head (pp. **140**, 141)

triceps: upper-arm muscle that straightens the arm (pp. **140**, 141)

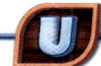

ulna and radius: bones of the forearm (pp. **152**, 153)

ultraviolet radiation (UV rays): invisible rays beyond the violet end of the light spectrum (pp. **162**, 164)

unsaturated fats: fats that are liquid at room temperature; found in oils (pp. **62**, 63)

urinary system: body system that removes liquid waste products and regulates the amount of water in the body; part of the excretory system (pp. **104**, 105)

vector: animal that can carry a pathogen and transmit it to humans (pp. **112**, 114)

vegan: type of diet in which a person does not eat meat or animal products (pp. **83**, 85)

vein: blood vessel that returns blood to the heart (pp. **12**, 15)

vena cava: large vein that brings blood from the body to the right atrium of the heart (venae cavae, *plural*) (pp. **23**, 24)

ventricle: lower chamber of the heart (pp. **23**, 24)

vertebrae: small bones that make up the vertebral column, or backbone; protect the spinal cord (vertebra, *sing.*) (pp. **152**, 153)

villi: hair-like projections in the small intestine through which food is absorbed (villus, *sing.*) (pp. **99**, 100)

virus: pathogen much smaller than a bacterium; reproduces by using a host cell of the body (pp. **112**, 114)

vitamin A: helps keep the eyes and skin healthy; helps fight infections and maintain bone growth (p. 70)

vitamin C: helps the body to resist and fight infection (p. 70)

vitamin D: helps build strong bones and teeth (p. 70)

vitamin E: protects cells from damage and helps the body use nutrients from food (p. 70)

vitamin K: stops bleeding by helping the blood to clot (p. 71)

vitamins: micronutrients manufactured by living things in their body cells; support the body systems' normal function and development (p. **69**)

voluntary muscles: skeletal muscles that can be moved when you want them to move (pp. **140**, 141)

water-soluble vitamins: vitamins that are easily eliminated from the body and must be eaten every day; vitamin C and the B-complex vitamins (p. **69**)

white blood cells: blood cells that defend the body by fighting disease and infection (pp. **12**, 13)

withdrawal: painful and sometimes deadly sickness that occurs when an addictive drug is no longer taken (pp. **179**, 180)

zinc: mineral needed for normal growth, wound healing, and immune-system function (p. 73)